CARDIAC RESYNCHRONIZATION THERAPY IN HEART FAILURE

WILLIAM T. ABRAHAM, MD, FACP, FACC, FAHA

Professor of Medicine, Physiology and Cell Biology
Director, Division of Cardiovascular Medicine
Deputy Director, Davis Heart and Lung Research Institute
The Ohio State University
Columbus, Ohio

RAGAVENDRA R. BALIGA, MD, MBA, FRCP, FACC

Editor in Chief
Heart Failure Clinics of North America
Assistant Division Director
Division of Cardiovascular Medicine
Professor of Internal Medicine
The Ohio State University
Columbus, Ohio

 Wolters Kluwer | Lippincott Williams & Wilkins
Health

Philadelphia · Baltimore · New York · London
Buenos Aires · Hong Kong · Sydney · Tokyo

Acquisitions Editor: Frances R. DeStefano
Product Manager: Leanne McMillan
Production Manager: Bridgett Dougherty
Senior Manufacturing Manager: Benjamin Rivera
Marketing Manager: Kimberly Schonberger
Design Coordinator: Teresa Mallon
Production Service: Spearhead Global, Inc.

530 Walnut Street
Philadelphia, PA 19106 USA

LWW.com

Printed in China

Library of Congress Cataloging-in-Publication Data

Cardiac resynchronization therapy in heart failure / editors, William T. Abraham, Ragavendra R. Baliga.
     p. ; cm.
   Includes bibliographical references.
   ISBN-13: 978-0-7817-9844-0
   ISBN-10: 0-7817-9844-2
1. Heart failure—Treatment. 2. Cardiac pacing. I. Abraham, William T. II. Baliga, R. R.
   [DNLM: 1. Heart Failure—therapy. 2. Cardiac Pacing, Artificial—methods. WG 370 C2677 2010]
   RC685.C53C38 2010
   616.1±29—dc22

                                                                           2009032206

To purchase additional copies of this book, call our customer service department at (800) 638-3030 or fax orders to (301) 223-2320. International customers should call (301) 223-2300.

Visit Lippincott Williams & Wilkins on the Internet: at LWW.com. Lippincott Williams & Wilkins customer service representatives are available from 8:30 am to 6 pm, EST.

                                                              10 9 8 7 6 5 4 3 2 1

CONTRIBUTORS

Theodore P. Abraham, MD
Associate Professor of Medicine
Division of Cardiology
John Hopkins University
Baltimore, Maryland

Philip B. Adamson, MD, FACC
Adjunct Associate Professor
University of Oklahoma Health Sciences Center
Director, The Heart Failure Institute
Oklahoma Heart Hospital
Oklahoma City, Oklahoma

Jeroen J. Bax, MD, PhD
Professor, Department of Cardiology
Leiden University Medical Center
Leiden, The Netherlands

Khalid Chakir, MS, PhD
Post-doctoral Fellow
Medicine/Cardiology
Johns Hopkins University
Baltimore, Maryland

Victor G. Davila-Roman, MD, FALL, FASE
Professor of Medicine, Radiology and Anesthesiology
Cardiovascular Division
Washington University School of Medicine
Staff cardiologist, Barnes-Jewish Hospital
St. Louis, Missouri

Veronica Lea J. Dimaano, MD
Senior Research Fellow
Division of Cardiology
John Hopkins University School of Medicine
Baltimore, Maryland

Michael R. Donnally, MD
Fellow, Division of Cardiovascular Medicine
The Ohio State University
Columbus, Ohio

Anne M. Dubin, MD
Associate Professor Pediatrics
Stanford University
Pediatric Arrhythmia Service
Lucile Packard Children's Hospital
Palo Alto, California

Lisa de las Fuentes, MD
Assistant Professor of Medicine
Cardiovascular Division
Washington University School of Medicine
Staff Cardiologist
Barnes-Jewish Hospital
St. Louis, Missouri

Mikhael F. El-Chami, MD
Assistant Professor of Medicine
Cardiology/Electrophysiology Division
Emory University School of Medicine
Atlanta, Georgia

David S. Feldman, MD, PhD, FACC, FAHA
Medical Director of Heart Failure, VAD and Cardiac
    Transplant Programs
The Minneapolis Heart Institute
Abbott-Northwestern Hospital
Minneapolis, Minnesota

Ayesha K. Hasan, MD, FACC
Assistant Professor, Internal Medicine
The Ohio State University
Medical Director, Cardiac Transplant Program
The Ohio State University Medical Center
Columbus, Ohio

Nathaniel M. Hawkins, MB ChB
Specialist Registrar
Department of Cardiology
Liverpool Heart and Chest Hospital
Liverpool, United Kingdom

Robert H. Helm, MD
Assistant Professor of Medicine
Cardiology Section
Boston University
Boston Medical Center
Boston, Massachusetts

Mark A. Hlatky, MD
Professor of Health Research and Policy
Professor of Cardiovascular Medicine
Stanford University School of Medicine
Stanford, California

Ping Jia, PhD
Consultant, CardioInsight Technologies Inc.
Cleveland, Ohio

David A. Kass, MD
Abraham and Virginia Weiss Professor of Cardiology
Professor of Medicine
Professor of Biomedical Engineering
Johns Hopkins University Medical Institutions
Baltimore, Maryland

Dhruv S. Kazi, MD, MSc
Fellow, Division of Cardiology
University of California
San Diego, California

Angel R. Leon, MD, FACC
The Linton and June Bishop Professor of Medicine
Department of Cardiology
Emory University School of Medicine
Chief, Department of Cardiology
Emory University Hospital Midtown
Atlanta, Georgia

William H. Maisel, MD, MPH
Assistant Professor of Medicine
Harvard Medical School
Director, Pacemaker and Defibrillator Service
Beth Israel Deaconess Medical Center
Boston, Massachusetts

John J.V. McMurray, MD
Professor of Medical Cardiology
BHF Cardiovascular Research Centre
University of Glasgow
Honorary Consultant Cardiologist
Western Infirmary
Glasgow, United Kingdom

Vincent M. Pestritto, MD
Fellow, Cardiovascular Medicine
Department of Internal Medicine
The Ohio State University College of Medicine/
    The Ohio State University Medical Center
Columbus, Ohio

Mark C. Petrie, MD
Consultant Cardiologist
West of Scotland Heart Centre
Golden Jubilee National Hospital
Glasgow, United Kingdom

Luis A. Pires, MD, FACC
Associate Professor of Medicine
Wayne State University School of Medicine
Director, Heart Rhythm Center
St. John Hospital and Medical Center
Detroit, Michigan

Hind W. Rahmouni, MD
Senior Research Investigator, Cardiology
University of Pennsylvania
Philadelphia, Pennsylvania

Subha V. Raman, MD, MSEE, FACC
Associate Professor
Department of Internal Medicine/Cardiovascular Medicine
The Ohio State University
Columbus, Ohio

Yoram Rudy, PhD
The Fred Saigh Distinguished Professor
Director of the Cardiac Bioelectricity and Arrhythmia Center
Washington University
St. Louis, Missouri

Eric S. Silver, MD
Assistant Professor, Pediatric Arrhythmia Service
Division of Pediatric Cardiology
Columbia University
New York, New York

Martin J. Schalij, MD, PhD
Professor, Department of Cardiology
Leiden University Medical Center
Leiden, The Netherlands

David D. Spragg, MD
Associate Professor, Division of Cardiology
Johns Hopkins University
Director, Cardiac Electrophysiology Laboratory
Johns Hopkins Bayview Medical Center
Baltimore, Maryland

Martin G. St. John Sutton, MD
Professor of Medicine, Cardiology Department
University of Pennsylvania
Director, Cardiovascular Imaging
Hospital of the University of Pennsylvania
Philadelphia, Pennsylvania

Laurens F. Tops, MD
Research Fellow
Department of Cardiology
Leiden University Medical Center
Leiden, The Netherlands

Emilio Vanoli, MD
Associate Professor, Cardiology
University of Pavia
Head, Cardiac Rehabilitation Unit
Policlinico di Monza
Monza, Italy

Niraj Varma, MA, DM, FRCP
Pacing and Electrophysiology Section
Heart and Vascular Institute
Cleveland Clinic
Cleveland, Ohio

Alan D. Waggoner, MHS
Research Associate Professor of Medicine
Cardiovascular Division
Washington University School of Medicine
St. Louis, Missouri

PREFACE

Cardiac Resynchronization Therapy for All HF Patients?

When the MIRACLE (Multicenter InSync Randomized Clinical Evaluation) study[1] reported benefits of cardiac resynchronization therapy, there was hesitation to adopt this new technology. The extent of the benefits was not entirely clear—the study showed improvements in 6-minute walk distance, New York Heart Association (NYHA) functional class ranking, and quality of life. These observations, however, provided impetus for the COMPANION (Comparison of Medical Therapy, Pacing and Defibrillation in Heart Failure)[2] and CARE HF (Cardiac Resynchronization—Heart Failure) trials,[3] which confirmed not only improvements in functional capacity but also survival benefits for cardiac resynchronization therapy with defibrillation and for cardiac resynchronization therapy alone. Based on these findings, the 2005 American College of Cardiology and American Heart Association guideline statement[4] recommended cardiac resynchronization therapy for chronic NYHA Class III and ambulatory Class IV heart failure patients with a reduced ejection fraction and ventricular dyssynchrony as a Class I indication with a level of evidence "A." Despite these unequivocal recommendations, there has been reluctance by some to use cardiac resynchronization therapy with a penetration of around 40% in the indicated heart failure population.[5] Thus, approximately 60% of eligible patients are currently denied or otherwise not receiving this evidence-based, guideline-recommended, life-sustaining therapy. The medical community simply must do better than this.

More recent data from the REVERSE (REsynchronization reVErses Remodeling in Systolic left vEntricular dysfunction)[6] and MADIT-CRT[7,8] trials demonstrate that the benefits of cardiac resynchronization therapy extend to NYHA Class I and Class II heart failure patients with ventricular dyssynchrony. Taken together, these trials should expand the clinical indication for cardiac resynchronization therapy to patients with asymptomatic or mildly symptomatic heart failure. The 2-year REVERSE study showed that cardiac resynchronization therapy significantly reduces the risk for heart failure hospitalization and improves ventricular structure and function in NYHA Class I and Class II patients. The MADIT-CRT (Multicenter Automatic Defibrillator Implantation Trial-CRT) trial evaluated the benefits of cardiac resynchronization therapy in mild to moderate heart failure (NYHA Class I and II) when compared to defibrillator alone. The Data Monitoring and Safety Board stopped the study, which enrolled 1,820 patients, because the use of cardiac resynchronization therapy with a defibrillator resulted in a statistically significant 29% reduction in the risk of death from any cause or heart failure hospitalizations, when compared to a defibrillator alone. Thus, the future looks bright for cardiac resynchronization

therapy as a standard treatment across all NYHA classes of heart failure, in patients with ventricular dyssynchrony.

Heart failure hospitalizations continue to have both clinical and economic impact (billions of dollars) in the management of heart failure. As new data continues to emerge, regarding the benefits of cardiac resynchronization therapy in reducing length of stay, avoiding re-hospitalizations, and saving lives, it is inevitable that cardiac resynchronization therapy will be appropriately used in most if not all heart failure patients. Keeping this in mind, we have put together a panel of experts who have provided a comprehensive and cutting-edge overview of cardiac resynchronization therapy. This book should be useful to the practicing family care physician, internist, cardiologist, and other healthcare professionals, who will continue to manage an increasing number of patients eligible for and subsequently treated with cardiac resynchronization therapy.

Ragavendra R. Baliga, MD
William T. Abraham, MD

REFERENCES

1. Abraham WT, Fisher WG, Smith AL, et al. Cardiac resynchronization in chronic heart failure. The New England journal of Medicine. 2002; 346(24):1845–1853.
2. Bristow MR, Saxon LA, Boehmer J, et al. Cardiac-resynchronization therapy with or without an implantable defibrillator in advanced chronic heart failure. *N. Engl J Med.* 2004;350(21):2140–2150.
3. Cleland JG, Daubert JC, Erdmann E, et al. The effect of cardiac resynchronization on morbidity and mortality in heart failure. *N. Engl J Med.* 2005;352(15):1539–1549.
4. Hunt SA, Abraham WT, Chin MH, et al. 2009 focused update incorporated into the ACC/AHA 2005 Guidelines for the Diagnosis and Management of Heart Failure in Adults: a report of the American College of Cardiology Foundation/American Heart Association Task Force on Practice Guidelines: developed in collaboration with the International Society for Heart and Lung Transplantation. *Circulation.* 2009;119(14):e391–479.
5. Piccini JP, Hernandez AF, Dai D, et al. Use of cardiac resynchronization therapy in patients hospitalized with heart failure. *Circulation.* 2008; 118(9):926–933.
6. Linde C, Abraham WT, Gold MR, et al. Randomized trial of cardiac resynchronization in mildly symptomatic heart failure patients and in asymptomatic patients with left ventricular dysfunction and previous heart failure symptoms. *J. Am. Coll Card.* 2008;52(23):1834–1843.
7. Moss AJ, Brown MW, Cannom DS, et al. Multicenter automatic defibrillator implantation trial-cardiac resynchronization therapy (MADIT-CRT): design and clinical protocol. *Ann Noninvasive Electrocardiol* 2005;10 (4 Suppl):34–43.
8. News Release: MADIT-CRT Trial Meets Primary Endpoint. June 23, 2009. Accessed on July 24, 2009 at http://bostonscientific.mediaroom.com/index. php?s=43&item=843.

ACKNOWLEDGMENTS

We dedicate this book to our heart failure patients, who have taught us first-hand about the benefits and limitations of cardiac resynchronization therapy, and to all the physician investigators, research coordinators, and patients who participated in clinical trials of cardiac resynchronization therapy, helping to establish it as a standard of care and saving countless lives.

In addition, we would like to acknowledge authors of the individual chapters for their dedication to the production of this book. And finally, we would also like to acknowledge our families for their love and support of our professional activities, including the editing of this book.

CONTENTS

Pathophysiology of Ventricular Dyssynchrony and Mechanisms of Cardiac Resynchronization Therapy

Robert H. Helm • David D. Spragg • Khalid Chakir • David A. Kass

HEART FAILURE AND RESYNCHRONIZATION THERAPY

Heart failure (HF) is a systemic disease, which typically begins with an initial cardiac insult resulting in acute ventricular dysfunction. To maintain pump function and systemic perfusion, a series of neurohormonal and adrenergic adaptations occur. Chronically, these changes lead to remodeling and maladaptation at the molecular and cellular levels resulting in sustained pump dysfunction.[1, 2] Neurohumoral stimulation occurs at both the systemic and local myocardial levels, and myocardial responses can be induced by hormone-receptor interactions, or mechanical stress.[3] Catecholamines acutely recruit myocardial reserve; however sustained stimulation results in abnormal calcium handling and worsened myocyte survival.[4] Intersitial fibrosis, vascular insufficiency, activation of fibroblasts and matrix remodeling protein (metalloproteinase), and other factors contribute to chronic maladaptive remodeling.[1] The result is impaired basal and reserve heart function manifested by blunted responses to neurohumoral stimulation (i.e., sympathetic stimulation), loading, and increases in heart rate. Many factors contribute to this behavior, including down-regulation of G-coupled receptor pathways, abnormal calcium cycling,[5,6] activation of multiple stress response signaling pathways,[7,8] energetics,[9] and sarcomere changes. Impaired Ca^{2+} cycling into and out of the sarcoplasmic reticulum blunts myocardial force generation and delays relaxation. Activation of stress kinases, phosphatases, and associated transcription factors alters contractile function, calcium handling, growth remodeling, and cell survival. Cardiac bio-energetics is rendered inefficient with depressed fatty acid utilization. Lastly, myofilament proteins are altered in the failure state, including the type of myosin, and post-translational modifications of regulatory and structural proteins such as titin.[1,10] These and other pathologic alterations all contribute to the HF phenotype.[1]

On top of this disease *landscape*, about one-third of patients develop electrical conduction delays resulting in marked discoordinate contraction.[11–12] Dyssynchrony reduces chamber function and efficiency in a normal heart, and its superimposition in HF worsens an already compromised state. Furthermore, dyssynchrony effects may not be simply additive; they may trigger more complex pathophysiology and a unique form of heart failure. Understanding how and what is achieved by CRT is increasingly important, as it has become standard therapy for groups of heart failure patients. In this chapter, we update current understanding of the mechanical, cellular, and molecular changes induced by dyssynchrony in the failing heart and how CRT affects them.

Mechanics of Dyssynchrony

His-Purkinje disease and intra myocardial conduction delay in the failing heart result in regionally delayed electrical excitation,[13] yielding early- and late-activated regions that contract out of phase with each other to generate dyssynchrony. Both left-bundle branch block (LBBB) and right ventricular (RV) pacing delay lateral wall stiffening and are the most common causes of left ventricular (LV) dyssynchrony. With both, septal activation occurs first, but as the lateral wall remains quiescent, forces from septal contraction do not raise LV pressure but are largely converted into prestretch of the lateral wall. This slows the rise of pressure (dP/dt) and increases lateral wall stress. When the free wall does contract, it generates systolic forces late, which are partly dissipated by restretching the already relaxing septal region, lowering net cardiac output. Delayed papillary muscle activation can contribute to mitral regurgitation, further reducing forward ejection. This common pattern of mechanical dyssynchrony is shown in Figure 1.1A. Tagged magnetic resonance imaging (MRI) was used to assess regional strain in a canine with mechanical dyssynchrony induced by radiofrequency ablation of the left bundle.[14] Strain is plotted as a function of LV region. In early systole (dashed line), the septum contracts (negative strain), whereas the lateral wall stretches (positive strain). In late systole (solid line), this pattern is reversed; as the lateral wall contracts, the septum stretches. Regional disparities in cardiac stiffening can be appreciated by portraying dyssynchrony as two time-varying elastance curves representing the early- and late-activated regions (Fig. 1.1B). The vertical distance between curves reflects disparities in wall stiffening that generate discoordinate motion. This is most marked in early

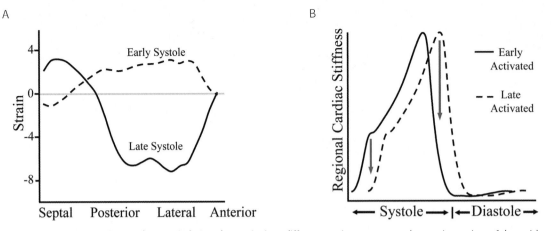

FIG. 1.1. **A**: Circumferential strain (relative shortening) at different regions across a short-axis section of the mid-LV in a dyssynchronous heart. Data for early (dashed) and late (solid) systole are shown, and reveal septal and lateral regions out of phase with each other. **B**: Model of dyssynchrony based on a time-delay of ventricular activation (stiffening). Plots of early-(solid) and late-(dashed) activated myocardial regions. Vertical distance between the curves indicates transfer of forces from one region to the other, and the arrows highlight two times—early contraction and late systole where this disparity is greatest and where discoordinate motion most manifests. (A, adapted from Byrne MJ, Helm, RH, Daya, S, et al. Diminished left ventricular dyssynchrony and impact of resynchronization in failing hearts with right versus left bundle branch block. *J Am Coll Cardiol.* 2007;50:1484–1490.)

systole (isovolumic contraction, lowering dP/dt_{max}), and late systole as one territory enters relaxation ahead of the other. The latter is when echoDoppler measures of dyssynchrony are typically observed.[15,16] The evolution and resolution of dyssynchrony highlight a critical time course and provide insight into how delayed contraction affects cardiac function throughout the cardiac cycle.

In contrast to LBBB and RV-paced associated dyssynchrony, right-bundle branch block (RBBB) results in delayed right-sided activation relative to LV free wall. The impact of RBBB on chamber synchrony and function is significantly less than with LBBB[14] largely due to the lack of symmetric heart geometry. Unlike the LV free wall, the septum is loaded not just by regional LV forces but also those from the RV. The size of the delay-activated region and its location are key factors that determine the net impact on global LV function and mechanical synchrony.

Dyssynchrony, Relaxation, and Loading

Cardiac dyssynchrony can delay ventricular relaxation. In an acute pacing study in dogs, Aoyagi et al.[17] demonstrated a significant correlation between left ventricular dyssynchrony (measured in early diastole) induced with ventricular pacing and prolongation in relaxation (increase in Tau, time constant of relaxation, Fig. 1.2A). Increased LV afterload can also induce relaxation delay and dyssynchrony. With acute aortic constriction in an otherwise normal canine, Yano et al.[18] showed an acute increase in Tau and onset of regionally delayed contraction (Fig 1.2B and Fig. 1.2C). Nearly 15 years later, attention is principally focused on cardiac dyssynchrony due to conduction delay (typically LBB pattern) but certainly

abnormal loading associated with heart failure can contribute to chamber dyssynchrony. Wang et al.[19] further substantiated these data by showing that vasodilators and diuretics could improve dyssynchrony (measured during the diastolic period) and relaxation in HF patients (Fig. 1.2D). These data are particularly important because dyssynchrony due to abnormal loading is far less likely to be amenable to electrical resynchronization.[20]

Effect of Dyssynchrony on Pump Function and Efficiency

One critical consequence of LV dyssynchrony is reduced pump function, which can be demonstrated by pressure-volume loops.[21] Figure 1.3A shows example relations, and with dyssynchrony induced by RV pacing, the end-systolic pressure-volume relationship (ESPVR) shifts rightward, indicating a fall in net function. Both stroke volume (loop width) and stroke work (loop area) also decline without a fall in end-diastolic volume. Furthermore, end-systolic wall stress is increased as the end-systolic volume rises. Rate of pressure development (dP/dt_{max}) declines by ~20%, stroke work by 10–15%, and relaxation (Tau) prolongs by ~10–15%.[22–23]

A second critical consequence of dyssynchrony is that LV efficiency is reduced. Work performed by one region of the heart is wasted by means of stretching the contralateral wall (intracavity energy sink). In a canine model of dyssynchrony induced with RV pacing, Prinzen et al.[24] assessed regional myocardial strain and work using tagged MRI. At baseline (right atrial pacing) regional work was fairly homogeneous; whereas with RV pacing a marked disparity in local work including a 125% increase in the lateral wall and a reciprocal

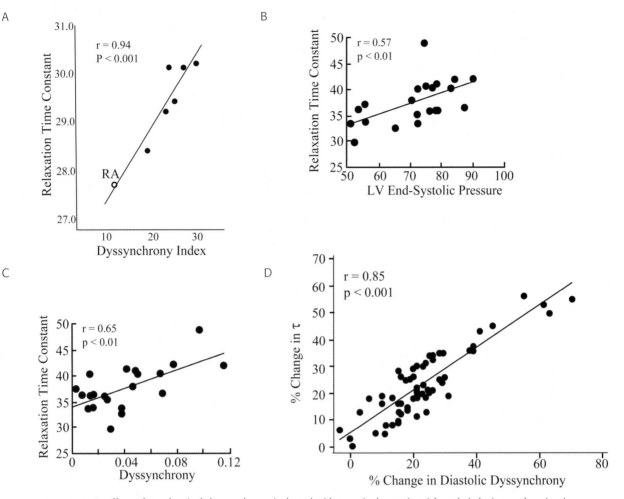

FIG. 1.2. **A**: Effect of mechanical dyssynchrony induced with ventricular pacing (closed-circles) on relaxation in a normal canine as compared with baseline synchronous contraction (right atrial pacing, open circle). Ventricular pacing was performed from various LV and RV sites. **B** and **C**: Cardiac dyssynchrony and delay in chamber relaxation induced by increasing afterload (systolic end-systolic pressure) by aortic occlusion. **D**: Percent change in relaxation and diastolic dyssynchrony after improving cardiac loading with pharmacologic therapy. (A, Adapted from Aoyagi T, Iizuka M, Takahashi T, et al. Wall motion asynchrony prolongs time constant of left ventricular relaxation. *Am J Physiol.* 1989;257:H883–H890. B and C, adapted from Yano M, Kohno M, Konishi M, et al. Influence of left ventricular regional nonuniformity on afterload-dependent relaxation in intact dogs. *Am J Physiol.* 1994;267:H148–H154. D, adapted from Wang J, Kurrelmeyer KM, Torre-Amione G, et al. Systolic and diastolic dyssynchrony in patients with diastolic heart failure and the effect of medical therapy. *J Am Coll Cardiol.* 2007;49:88–96.)

decrease in the early-activated septum was observed. Local stress-strain plots illustrate these findings (Fig. 1.3B). Early shortening under low external load and late-systolic stretching under higher load creates a "figure-8" shaped stress-strain plot. The workload (loop area) for this territory is consequently low. In contrast, in the late-activated lateral wall, which functions at higher initial stretch and contracts against higher stress, the workload is much greater. These regional differences in work correlate with regional blood flow and metabolic demands.[25-27] Total myocardial oxygen consumption (MVO_2) is unaltered despite a striking decline in LV stroke work correlating with a marked decline in LV efficiency (work / MVO_2 consumption).[28, 29, 30]

Gross Pathologic Changes Associated with LV Dyssynchrony

Chronic dyssynchrony leads to maladaptive ventricular remodeling. Vernooy et al.[26] assessed structural and functional changes 16 weeks after ablating the left-bundle branch in dogs to create cardiac dyssynchrony. A decline in LV EF (−25%) paralleled an increase in chamber diameter by +23%. As previously discussed, RV pacing also generates LV dyssynchrony, and Thambo et al.[31] studied the long-term effects of RV pacing at physiologic heart rates in 23 patients with congenital heart block undergoing pacer implantation. Combined thinning of the early-activated septum and thickening in

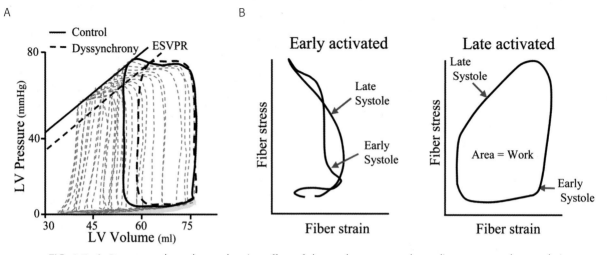

FIG. 1.3. **A:** Pressure-volume loops showing effect of dyssynchrony on end-systolic pressure-volume relation (ESPVR) and resting cardiac cycle (loop). The ESPVR shifts rightward, end-systolic volume increases, and stroke volume and work declines. **B:** Stress-strain loops from early- versus late-activated regions in a dyssynchronous heart. Whereas these loops would normally appear the same, with dyssynchrony the early-activated region first contracts at low load and is then stretched generating a figure-8 shaped loop with little area (reduced work). The late contracting lateral wall operates at higher preload and stress, requiring greater work. (A, adapted from Park, RC, Little WC, O'Rourke RA. Effect of alteration of left ventricular activation sequence on the left ventricular end-systolic pressure volume relation in closed-chest dogs. *Circ Res.* 1985;57:706–717.)

late-activated posterior wall resulted in a 30% increase in the ratio of posterior to septal wall thickness. In addition, LV chamber diameter increased by 20%.

Dyssynchrony induces regional changes in underlying cardiac fiber architecture. In a canine model of dyssynchronous heart failure (LBB ablation followed by 3 weeks of atrial tachypacing), Helm et al.[32] used high-resolution MRI and computational anatomical registering to show that, while the primary fiber orientation (epicardium downward, endocardium upward, and mid-myocardial circumferential) was not significantly altered, the transmural fiber gradient was markedly increased in the septal region owing largely to wall thinning. In addition, they found that the orientation of laminar sheets (planes of muscle fibers that constitute the myocardium) were oriented more vertically in the early-activated septum but not changed in the lateral wall. Such regional alterations in fiber architecture could affect the local biophysical/mechanical properties of tissue and impact propagation of electrical excitation.

Biochemical Consequences of Dyssynchrony

The combined effect of dyssynchrony and heart failure alters expression and activity of various proteins beyond that observed with heart failure alone. In the first study to test for such effects, Spragg et al.[33] contrasted regional molecular changes in failing canine hearts with and without dyssynchrony (eg, right ventricular versus right atrial tachypacing). Sarcoplasmic reticulum (SR) Ca^{2+}-ATPase, which actively transfers Ca^{2+} from the cytosol into the SR, and phospholamban, a coregulator of the latter protein, were down-regulated (~20-30%) in the lateral endocardium versus other territories.

The extracellular response kinase (ERK1/2), a mitogen-activated kinase that is associated with stress stimulation pathways modulating cell survival and differentiation, was highly activated in the lateral endocardium versus other regions. Connexin 43 (Cx43), a gap-junction protein that allows for rapid cell-to-cell depolarization, was marked downregulated. Importantly, these molecular changes in the lateral endocardium were not observed in failing myocardium without dyssynchrony. Recently Chakir et al. [34] showed differential activation of stress response proteins, such as tumor necrosis factor-alpha, Ca^{2+}-calmodulin-dependent kinase II, and p38 MAP kinase. Interestingly, these changes were only observed when dyssynchrony was combined with heart failure and not with dyssynchrony alone[35]—indicating that dyssynchrony interacts specifically with underlying heart failure substrate to trigger molecular alterations. Finally, Bilchick et al.[36] similarly observed regional expression of genes involved with growth and hypertrophy, stress signaling, and matrix remodeling in normal mice after only 7 to 10 days of RV (dyssynchrony) pacing. Regional molecular polarization in the dyssynchronous failing heart may contribute to heterogeneous electromechanical coupling and enhanced arrhythmia susceptibility.

Dyssynchrony Alters Regional Electrical Heterogeneity and Arrhythmia Susceptibility

Heart failure and QRS prolongation[11-37] are powerful and independent predictors of mortality due to ventricular arrhythmias in heart failure patients. Two prerequisites for reentrant arrhythmia are 1) unidirectional conduction block and 2) either sufficiently long circuit path-length or regionally delayed conduction allowing for adequate time to regain excitability in the blocked limb. Selective prolongation of APD within mid-myocardial cells due to remodeling of delayed rectifier K current and possibly Ca^{2+} currents have been implicated in causes for QT-interval prolongation, transmural heterogeneity of repolarization, and susceptibility to conduction block (the first prerequisite for arrhythmia induction) observed in dyssynchronous HF.[38, 39] In addition, dyssynchrony alone (without HF) alters regional myocardial conduction and has been implicated in arrhythmia susceptibility, fulfilling the second prerequisite for reentry. Myocardial con-

duction is anisotropic with more rapid cell-to-cell conduction occurring along the myocardial fiber direction owing to gap junction protein coupling at intercalated discs. Spragg et al.[35] compared regional myocardial conduction in canine hearts with chronic mechanical dyssynchrony (LBB ablation) without superimposed heart failure to normal control dogs. Normal dogs with synchronous contraction had faster endocardial versus epicardial conduction in both anterior and lateral territories (Fig. 1.4A). However, in hearts with a chronic LBBB, the transmural pattern of conduction

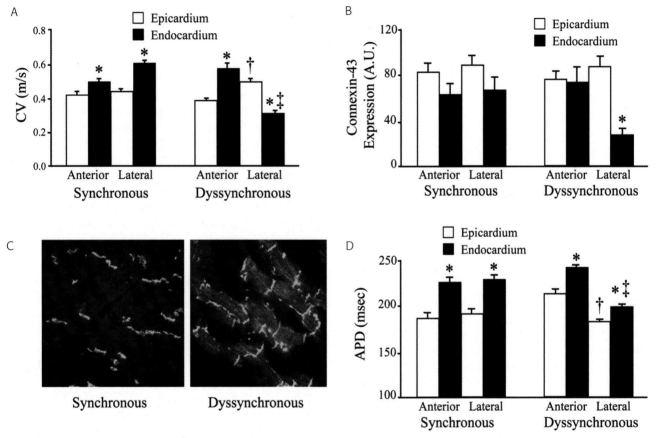

FIG. 1.4. **A**: Epicardial and endocardial conduction velocity in normal and dyssynchronous (LBBB) canine ventricular wedge preparations isolated from anterior and lateral regions. The normal pattern shows faster endocardial conduction throughout. However, with chronic dyssynchrony, there is reversal of this pattern in the lateral wall, but maintenance of the pattern in the earlier activated anterior wall. *p <0.001 versus corresponding epicardial value; † p = 0.001 versus all other epicardial values; ‡ P = 0.001 versus all other endocardial values. **B**: Expression of connexin-43 in synchronous controls is slightly reduced in endocardium overall, though these changes were not statistically significant. However, with chronic LBBB, expression fell markedly solely in the lateral epicardium, with a marked transmural gradient in this territory (*p <0.001). **C**: Con-focal imaging of connexin-43 in myocytes from normal synchronous versus dyssynchronous hearts. Normal localization at the terminal intercalated discs was altered, as connexin-43 appeared more prevalent in the lateral margins of the cells (remodeling). **D**: Epicardial and endocardial action potential durations (APD) in normal synchronous and dyssynchronous (LBBB) canine ventricular wedge preparations isolated from anterior and lateral regions. The normal pattern shows prolonged APD in endocardium versus epicardium in both regions. However, with chronic dyssynchrony, there is a reduction in APD in both layers with maintenance of the endocardial to epicardial pattern. *p <0.05 versus corresponding epicardial value; †p<0.05 versus corresponding anterior epicardium; ‡P = 0.05 versus corresponding anterior endocardium. (Data from Spragg DD, Akar FG, Helm RH, et al. Abnormal conduction and repolarization in late-activated myocardium of dyssynchronously contracting hearts. *Cardiovasc Res.* 2005;67:77–86.)

speed was flipped in the lateral wall (epicardium faster than endocardium), but was unchanged from normal in the anterior wall. This was accompanied by both a reduction in the expression of the gap protein (Cx43) in lateral epicardium (Fig. 1.4B) and its redistribution away from intercalated discs to the lateral wall of the myocyte (Fig. 1.4C). Both lateral wall myocardial layers had similar Cx43 redistribution, so altered Cx43 trafficking was unlikely the only basis for reduced endocardial conduction velocity. Altered Cx43 phosphorylation and the formation of heterotypic and heteromeric gap junction channels (Cx43 + Cx45) with reduced conductance have been implicated in reduced velocity of propagation. Finally, Spragg et al. observed significant reductions in action potential duration and relative refractory period in the lateral compared to anterior wall, whereas both time periods were regionally similar in normal (synchronous) controls (Fig. 1.4D). The combination of shortened refractoriness and slowed conduction would seem a potential substrate for arrhythmia.[39]

ACUTE EFFECTS OF CARDIAC RESYNCHRONIZATION THERAPY
Mechanics and Energetics

The mechanical and hemodynamic effects of CRT occur rapidly—essentially within a beat. Figure 1.5A shows the abrupt hemodynamic effects (increase in dP/dt_{max} and aortic pulse pressure) of CRT in a patient with dilated cardiomyopathy (DCM). Pressure-volume analysis (Fig. 1.5B) shows a marked increase in stroke volume and decline in end-systolic stress, with little change in end-diastolic volume or pressure. Improved chamber contraction is accompanied by enhanced efficiency.[40] Figure 1.5C compares myocardial oxygen consumption per beat during dobutamine infusion versus CRT. While both similarly enhanced dP/dt_{max}, a fall in O_2 consumption was observed with CRT. The finding of negligible energetic cost despite improved systolic function from CRT has been supported by other studies,[41,42] and is a particularly unique feature of CRT among current HF therapies. Thus far, inotropic drugs that acutely enhance systolic function have been found to worsen mortality when employed chronically. This likely relates to the precise mechanism of action, and the success of CRT indicates that if done the right way, chronic systolic improvement with enhanced survival is possible. Finally, CRT improves functional reserve both acutely[43] and following chronic therapy.[44,45] Figure 1.5D shows an example of how the systolic disparity between dyssynchronous and resynchronized hearts is amplified at faster heart rates. The force-frequency relationship during acute LV-only or BiV pacing (compared to RV pacing - dyssynchrony baseline) increased more with both modes of CRT.

Contractile synchrony from CRT can be best documented using regional circumferential strain maps (Fig. 1.6A and Fig. 1.6B).[46] CRT reduces the out-of-phase reciprocal stretch and shortening in anteroseptal versus lateral walls. These data were also used to generate the first temporal plot of the evolution and resolution of dyssynchrony (Fig. 1.6C). A vector index that increases not only if regions of the heart are contracting out of phase, but particularly if they are geographically clustered (i.e., lateral wall),[46] was used to quantify dyssynchrony, and a color cine is available on line.[46] Dyssynchrony increases throughout systole peaking shortly after end-systole and then declining in diastole. CRT reduces both systolic and diastolic dyssynchrony.

CHRONIC EFFECTS OF CARDIAC RESYNCHRONIZATION THERAPY
Reverse Chamber Remodeling

Chronic CRT induces further changes in LV remodeling.[47–50] End-systolic and end-diastolic volumes decline in most studies by an average of 10% over a 6-month period. As first shown by Yu et al.[50] this reduction of heart volumes is not an acute effect of CRT. When pacing is temporarily suspended after chronic CRT, the observed reduction in chamber volumes persists in the short term (Fig. 1.7A). In contrast, suspension of pacing in this setting results in an abrupt fall in dP/dt_{max} (Fig. 1.7B). Reduction of end-systolic volume has been used as a surrogate for mortality in heart failure patients receiving CRT,[51] and marker of response,[15] whereas acute hemodynamic changes have not generally predicted long-term response to therapy.[52]

CRT Alters Gene Expression

CRT improves excitation-contraction coupling and calcium handling, both of which are impaired in heart failure, and consequently enhances cardiac reserve. As previously discussed, acute CRT improves cardiac reserve or force-frequency relationship (FFR), (Fig. 1.5D), owing to improved diastolic filling rather than gene modulation. In contrast, chronic CRT therapy upregulates gene expression of calcium handling proteins involved in excitation-contraction coupling. With endomyocardial biopsies from the left interventricular apical septum in heart failure patients, Mullens et al.[44] compared the gene expression of key calcium-handling proteins at the time of CRT implant to 4 months follow-up. Significant up regulation in the expression of the sarcoplasmic reticular ATPase (SERCA2α), phospholamban, and β1- adrenergic receptor were observed after chronic CRT, and the SERCA2α/PLB ratio was found to increase. The latter is associated with improving calcium uptake into the SR and FFR. There was also a trend toward increased sodium calcium exchange (NCX) gene expression, which has also been associated with an improved FFR.[53] The authors found that these chronic gene expression changes were accompanied by an increase in the FFR at the time of follow-up compared to pre-implant.

Other investigators have similarly shown altered gene expression in CRT patients. Iyengar et al.[54] obtained endomyocardial biopsies from the RV septum in patients with nonischemic cardiomyopathy undergoing CRT implantation and compared gene expression of various proteins after

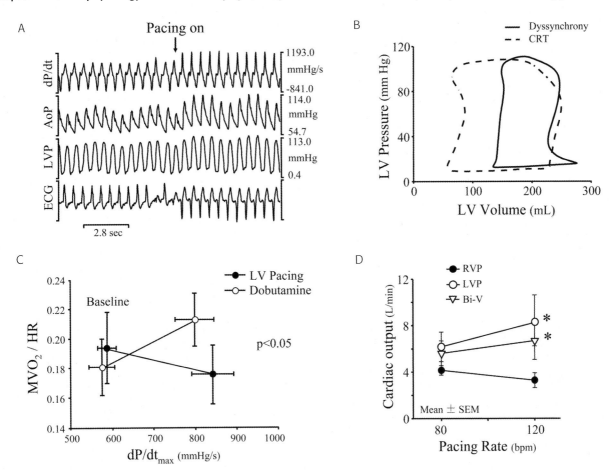

FIG. 1.5. **A**: Acute hemodynamic effects of CRT in a patient, assessed by peak rate of pressure rise (dP/dt$_{max}$), aortic pressure (AoP) pulse (indicating enhanced cardiac output), and LV pressure (LVP). Changes occur abruptly upon initiating CRT (note change in QRS morphology). **B**: Pressure-volume loops showing the acute effect of CRT (dashed line) compared with baseline dyssynchronous contraction (solid line). Resynchronization induces a left shift of the entire loop, with increased stroke volume and reduced end-diastolic filling pressures. **C**: CRT improves LV energetics. Data shows comparison to intravenous dobutamine. Both interventions raised dP/dt$_{max}$ over baseline, but dobutamine increased myocardial oxygen consumption (MVO$_2$) whereas CRT reduced it. **D**: CRT enhances cardiac output with increasing heart rates. Data from patients with complete AV block undergoing RV, LV, or BiV pacing. Output was lowest with RV pacing (LBBB-type dyssynchrony) and was improved by LV-only and Bi V pacing at heart rate of 80 bpm. These disparities became enhanced at the faster pacing rate due to improved diastolic filling with CRT (*p < 0.05). (B, from Kass DA, Chen CH, Curry C, et al. Improved left ventricular mechanics from acute VDD pacing in patients with dilated cardio myopathy and ventricular conduction delay. *Circulation*. 1999;99:1567–1573. C, from Nelson GS, Berger RD, Fetics BJ, et al. Left ventricular or biventricular pacing improves cardiac function at diminished energy cost in patients with dilated cardiomyopathy and left bundle-branch block. *Circulation*. 2000;102:3053–3059. D, from Hay I, Melenovsky V, Fetics, BJ, et al. Short-term effects of right-left heart sequential cardiac resynchronization in patients with heart failure, chronic atrial fibrillation, and atrioventricular nodal block. *Circulation*. 2004;110:3404–3410.)

6 months of CRT. Resynchronization increased the expression of α–myosin heavy chain (MHC) with a trend toward decreasing β–MHC, an isoform switch that is the reversal of that observed in heart failure (fetal gene recapitulation pattern).[55] The authors also found a rise in phospholamban and trend toward increased SERCA2α expression. Recently, Vanderheyden et al.[45] reported similar changes in gene expression, and further showed this occurred only in clinical "responders" to

the therapy and not "non responders." However, these data may be confounded by apparent baseline differences in the two groups, with nonresponders having expression levels at baseline often equal to those in the responder group after CRT.

To study the molecular and cellular remodeling effects of CRT in more detail, we have developed a canine model of dyssynchronous failure (DHF) and examined effects of CRT. All dogs are first atrially tachypaced in the presence of a LBBB to

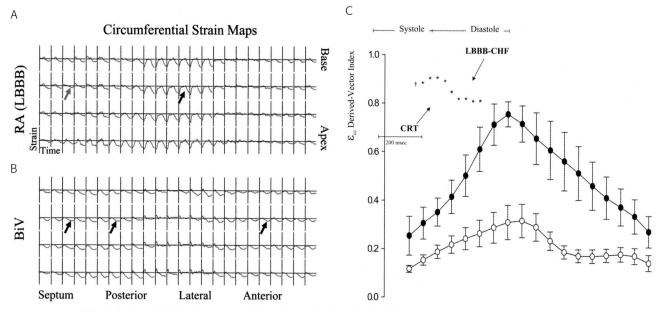

FIG. 1.6. A and **B**: Regional circumferential strain plots derived from tagged-MRI data. Plots are shown for dyssynchronous (LBBB) failing heart with right atrial (RA) pacing and with BiV pacing at similar heart rate. Marked heterogeneity of strain, with reciprocal shortening/stretch of septal and then lateral walls, was reduced by CRT. **C:** Time course of dyssynchrony development and resolution during a single cardiac cycle in failing heart with LBBB. Dyssynchrony peaks near end-systole, and CRT markedly reduces both systolic and diastolic dyssynchrony. (Adapted from Helm RH, Leclercq C, Faris OP, et al. Cardiac dyssynchrony analysis using circumferential versus longitudinal strain: implications for assessing cardiac resynchronization. *Circulation.* 2005;111:2760–2767.)

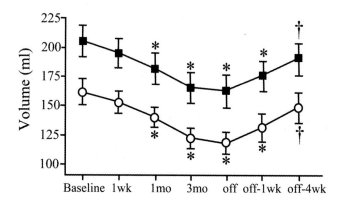

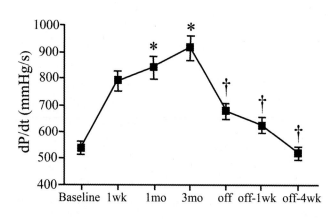

FIG. 1.7. A and **B**: Changes in LV end-diastolic (EDV, square), end-systolic (ESV, circle) volumes and dP/dt$_{max}$ before (baseline), after (1 week, 1 month, 3 months), and with suspension of (off, off-1 week, off-4 weeks) biventricular pacing. *p $<$ 0.05 versus baseline. †p $<$ 0.05 versus biventricular pacing for 3 months. Unlike dP/dt$_{max}$ the changes in volumes were not acute. Suspension of pacing showed a gradual return to baseline (increased) volumes. (Data from Yu CM, Chau E, Sanderson JE, et al. Tissue Doppler echocardiographic evidence of reverse remodeling and improved synchronicity by simultaneously delaying regional contraction after biventricular pacing therapy in heart failure. *Circulation.* 2002;105:438–445.)

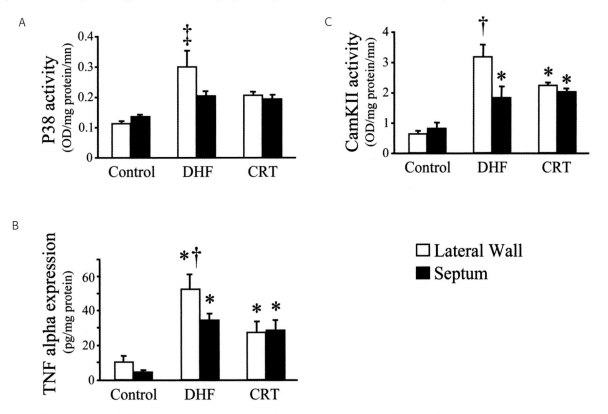

FIG. 1.8. **A** and **B**: Regional polarization of stress kinase activity in dyssynchronous failing heart is ameliorated by CRT. Data for p38 mitogen-activated kinase and calcium-calmodulin dependent kinase II (CAMKII) in septal and lateral regions are shown. $^{\dagger}P<0.001$ vs. control and CRT, $P<0.05$ vs. septum; $^{*}P<0.001$ vs. control; $P<0.05$ vs. septum, $^{\dagger}P<0.05$ vs. CRT. **C**: Regional expression of tumor necrosis factor-alpha (TNF-α). Enhanced total and particularly alteral wall expression in DHF hearts was ameliorated by CRT. $^{*}P<0.05$ vs. control; $P<0.05$ vs. septum; $P<0.05$ vs. CRT. (From Chakir K, Daya SK, Tunin RS, et al. Reversal of Global Apoptosis and Regional Stress Kinase Activation by Cardiac Resynchronization. *Circulation.* 2008;117:1369–1377.)

generate DHF, and this is either continued or switched to CRT (tachypaced-biventricular stimulation) for an additional 3 weeks. Chakir et al.[34] found regional amplification of stress kinase expression and activation (p38 MAP kinase and calcium-calmodulin dependent kinase II) in the late-activated lateral wall of DHF animals (Fig. 1.8A and Fig 1.8B). Both proteins are linked to maladaptive changes in heart failure, contributing to fibrosis and myocyte dysfunction as well as arrhythmia.[56, 57] In addition, the cytokine tumor necrosis factor-α (TNF-α) was markedly increased in the lateral wall (Fig. 1.8C). Upregulation of TNF-α itself induces dilated cardiomyopathy.[58] In the resynchronized (CRT) failing dogs, however, these regional increases were reduced achieving a more homogeneous activation and expression. Limited clinical data on stress kinase modulation exists to date. D'Ascia et al.[59] have reported similar suppression of TNF-α in LV biopsies from a small group of patients studied before and after receiving CRT.

Even more intriguing, Chakir et al.[34] observed a global improvement in cell survival signaling associated with CRT. Increased myocyte apoptosis associated with DHF, confirmed by TUNEL staining, caspase-3 activity (a key pro-apoptotic enzyme; Fig. 1.9A and Fig. 1.9B) was reduced with CRT. These data are consistent with clinical studies showing reduced

TUNEL positive myocytes in LV myocardial biopsies of CRT patients.[59] Unlike stress kinase signaling, however, Chakir et al.[34] showed that the decline in apoptosis was global owing to a global normalization of activated (phosphorylated) Akt kinase and BAD, regulators of cell survival pathways to suppress apoptosis (Fig. 1.9C and Fig. 1.9D).

Alterations in Arrhythmia Susceptibility and Electrophysiologic Properties with CRT

Several studies have assessed the effect of CRT on arrhythmia susceptibility and electrical remodeling. While a few small clinical studies have shown reduced ventricular tachycardia (VT),[60–61] there have been case reports to the contrary[62–63] with the latter thought to relate to epicardial LV stimulation.[64] However, meta-analyses of CRT trials indicate the incidence of arrhythmia does not increase,[65] and long-term follow-up analysis of the CARE-HF study suggests improved mortality was due both to a reduction in heart failure and sudden death.[66] Whether this reflects a primary effect on arrhythmia substrate or reduction in heart failure progression remains difficult to discern.[67]

The impact of CRT on acute myocardial repolarization is controversial. Medina-Ravel et al.[64] showed an increase in QT

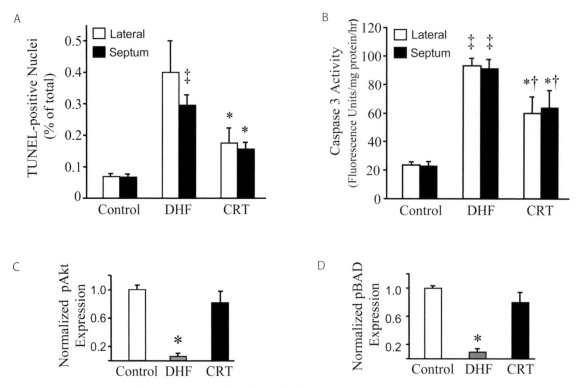

FIG. 1.9. **A**: CRT reduces apoptosis throughout the heart. Data summarized TUNEL positive nuclei in myocardium from both DHF and CRT hearts. Positive nuclei were more prevalent in DHF than in CRT or controls. *p < 0.05 vs. control and DHF, ‡ p < 0.01 vs. control. **B**: Caspase-3 activity (pro-apoptotic) is globally increased in DHF, and significantly reduced by CRT dogs. *p ≤ 0.05 vs. DHF, † p ≤ 0.01 vs. control, ‡ p ≤ 0.0003 vs. control. **C** and **D**: Phosphorylation of AKT and BAD in control, DHF and CRT dogs. Reduced phosphorylation was observed with DHF and essentially normalized by CRT. * p < 0.001 vs. control and CRT. (Reproduced from Chakir K, Daya SK, Tunin RS, et al. Reversal of Global Apoptosis and Regional Stress Kinase Activation by Cardiac Resynchronization. *Circulation.* 2008;117:1369–1377.)

interval with CRT, particularly with LV-only pacing. In rabbit wedge preparations, they further showed epicardial pacing prolonged repolarization. They postulated that this might increase arrhythmia susceptibility in some patients receiving CRT. In contrast, Berger et al.[68] used a high-resolution ECG mapping system on 25 patients undergoing CRT implantation and found BiV pacing significantly decreased all metrics of repolarization including root mean square T peak-to-end interval and interlead QT dispersion.

The chronic effect of CRT on electrical remodeling has not been well investigated. In a small clinical study, Henrikson et al.[69] showed QRS duration declined nearly 10% after 6 months of CRT therapy (with pacing temporarily suspended), suggesting improved intramyocardial conduction in HF patients. In cardiac myocytes isolated from dyssynchronous failing dog hearts, prolonged action potential durations (APD, at 50% and 90% repolarization) are observed (as compared with normal controls).[70] but when these dogs were subject to chronic CRT, Nishijima et al.[70] found APD similar to normal controls. They similarly found a reversal in resting membrane potentials associated with chronic CRT with reduced potentials in dyssynchronous

failing cells increasing and approaching that of normal controls. Ongoing studies aim to understand molecular signaling and mechanisms responsible for electrical remodeling.

Optimizing CRT

Several parameters determine the efficacy of CRT, including timing intervals between atrial-ventricular (AV) and right-left ventricular stimulation, the location of the left ventricular lead, and whether one stimulates both ventricles or only the LV. The last issue attracted attention early on, when it was found that LV-only pacing could enhance systolic function as well if not slightly better than BiV pacing.[71–73] While both modes similarly enhance LV function as reflected in parameters such as dP/dt$_{max}$, stroke work, and cardiac output,[72] LV-only pacing does not typically shorten the QRS duration nor generate electrical synchrony.[73–74] This was also revealed in studies in which there was no possibility of a fusion complex as patients had complete AV blockade,[75] leading to the conclusion that mechanical synchrony was more important to achieve CRT effects.[22, 46, 73, 76, 77] Increasing evidence suggests that BiV stimulation may better impact diastolic relaxation and early filling.[75]

AV timing delay influences both the interaction of atrial systole on cardiac preload and mitral valve function, and determines if sufficient pre-excitation has been achieved for BiV stimulation. While many studies have examined how this delay can be optimized,[78–79] clinical findings indicate that it has only minor impact in most patients and that a standard delay of near 120 msec is generally effective.[72, 76] The RV-LV delay similarly has been shown to be a parameter that can influence CRT efficacy in some subjects, with LV advanced being the usually preferred mode. However, the phase delay is short (≤ 20 msec in most patients) and simultaneous stimulation results in similar effects on average.[75] Furthermore, op-

timization of these delays has always been performed in subjects at rest, and it remains unclear if these values remain "optimal" under stress.

Response to CRT is dependent on LV lead placement. This was first reported by Butter et al.[80] in patients but more comprehensively tested in experimental animals by Helm et al.[22] Dogs with dyssynchronous heart failure were subject to BiV pacing where the LV stimulation site was randomly varied across the LV by means of a multi-electrode epicardial shock. In this manner, more than 90 different LV pacing sites were tested. 3-D functional response maps were generated to characterize the geographic extent of efficacious sites. Figures 1.10A to 1.10D show representative functional maps depicting response to CRT measured with various hemodynamic

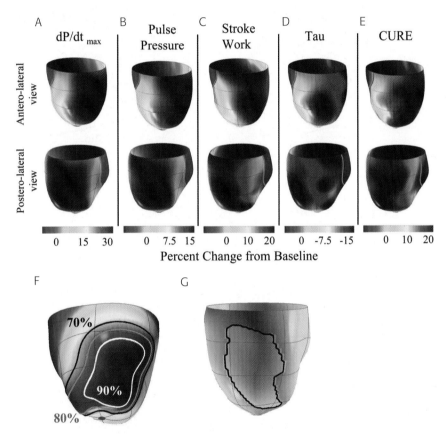

FIG. 1.10. A-E: Representative global heart function maps showing percent change in various hemodynamic (dP/dt$_{max}$, pulse pressure, stroke work, tau – relaxation) and dyssynchrony (CURE) indices with CRT as a function of LV pacing site. Color coding indicates magnitude of response. Dark orange/red indicates the most optimal response to CRT. Data are shown for dyssynchronous failing dog heart and are displayed in anterolateral and posterolateral orientations. The size and relative location of optimal LV-pacing region was generally similar between parameters and dyssynchronous (LBBB) dogs without heart failure (data not shown). **F:** Identification of response iso-regions defined by territories achieving 70%, 80%, or 90% of the maximal CRT response. **G:** Global functional response (stroke work, 10C) maps correlated with mechanical synchrony maps (CURE index, 10E) for the various LV pacing sites. This was further demonstrated by their overlay (green region) showing generally similar pacing region on the LV free wall that generated optimal mechanical synchrony and global work. (Adapted from Helm RH, Byrne M, Helm PA, et al. Three-dimensional mapping of optimal left ventricular pacing site for cardiac resynchronization. *Circulation.* 2007;115:953–961.)

indices plotted as a function of LV pacing site. The region of efficacious sites (dark orange/red) was similarly localized independent of which hemodynamic index (systolic or diastolic) was being represented, and was fairly broad. Similar maps were generated in dyssynchronous dogs without heart failure demonstrating that the anatomical extent and location of this region was not influenced by heart failure despite the

underlying myocardial abnormalities in the latter, suggesting the result was more dependent on the geographic location of LV stimulation than electrical dispersion. The region of efficacious sites similarly enhanced mechanical synchrony. To assess this, strain maps (e.g., Fig. 1.6A) derived from tagged MRI were used to assess mechanical synchrony for each pacing site tested. The strain maps were analyzed using the CURE

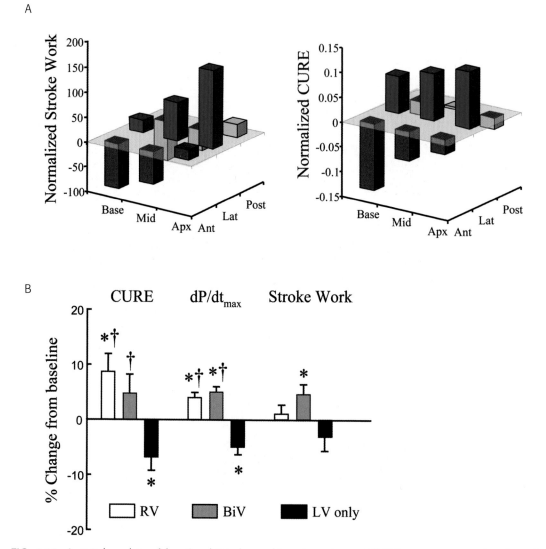

FIG. 1.11. **A:** 3-D bar plots of functional (stroke work) and synchrony (CURE) response as a function of the base-apex and anterior-posterior positioning of the LV lead during BiV pacing. Lateral mid-apical sites achieved the best response. **B:** Effect of CRT in canine model of heart failure with a right bundle branch block. Responses for three different pacing modes—RV only, LV only, and BiV stimulation—are shown as percent change relative to right-atrial paced baseline. *p < 0.007 compared to baseline; †p < 0.047 compared with baseline; ‡p < 0.005 compared with left ventricular (LV)-only pacing; p = 0.015 compared with LV-only pacing. CURE, circumferential uniformity ratio estimate (metric of mechanical synchrony); dP/dt$_{max}$, maximum time derivative of left ventricular pressure; RV, right ventricle. RV and BiV pacing resulted in similar improvements, and both were quantitatively less than reported in HF and LBBB studies.[46, 72–73] (A, Data from Helm RH, Byrne M, Helm PA, et al. Three-dimensional mapping of optimal left ventricular pacing site for cardiac resynchronization. *Circulation.* 2007;115:953–961. B, Data from Byrne MJ, Helm, RH, Daya, S, et al. Diminished left ventricular dyssynchrony and impact of resynchronization in failing hearts with right versus left bundle branch block. *J Am Coll Cardiol.* 2007;50:1484–1490.)

index for dyssynchrony (CURE = 1 for pure synchrony, 0 for pure dyssynchrony)[46, 73] and synchrony maps were generated plotting CURE value as a function of LV pacing site tested (Fig. 1.10E). A region of efficacious pacing sites that enhanced mechanical synchrony was similar to that generated using hemodynamic indices to assess response to CRT.

While we observed a large region of efficacious sites, it is important to define the optimal zone for lead placement. In this regard we developed a cost-function based on the ratio of mean CRT response in a given region to the size of region involved. A region that yielded a big response to CRT but was very small (i.e., would be difficult for directed LV lead placement) would be less advantageous than a region with somewhat less response but greater geographic expanse. On the downside, too broad a territory would include sites that yielded little CRT effect. Using this cost function, we determined that the 70% response territory was optimal and a representative map is shown in Figure 1.10F. This optimal region extends over about 40% of the lateral free wall surface providing reassurance to the clinician responsible for implanting a lead in this region. An overlap map of optimal functional response (indexed with stroke work) and mechanical synchrony (indexed with CURE) demonstrated rather good concordance but with a shift away from basal regions (Fig. 1.10G). This was confirmed with regression analysis. Finally, we examined the impact of altering pacing site (base to apex; anterior-lateral-posterior) for function (stroke work) and wall motion synchrony (CURE). The best results were pacing in the lateral and somewhat more apical regions for both types of parameter. Anterior pacing particularly at the base could worsen both synchrony and function (Fig. 1.11A).

The optimal pacing site certainly depends upon the specifics of the conduction delay, and while most patients have late lateral wall activation others have right-sided delay due to RBBB. Interestingly, dyssynchrony generated from a pure RBBB is significantly less than that associated with LBBB,[14] and the corresponding impact of CRT is less (Fig. 1.11B). Furthermore, RV-pacing alone achieves the same benefit as traditional biventricular activation mode. In this setting LV-only pacing had no benefit—but rather actually decreased function.

CONCLUSION

Dyssynchronous heart failure is characterized by marked abnormalities of regional and global molecular signaling and cellular dysfunction resulting in altered excitation-contraction coupling, myocyte-survival, and enhanced arrhythmia susceptibility. Furthermore, dyssynchrony reduces global pump function and energetic efficiency. CRT not only improves global heart function and energetics, but also has a profound beneficial effect on molecular and cellular phenotype. Understanding the critical link between such reverse remodeling and clinical response to CRT may provide insight into how to best integrate pharmacotherapy with pacing the heart and who is most likely to benefit.

PRACTICAL POINTS

1. Cardiac dyssynchrony occurs when one portion of the wall contracts at a later time than another. It can be the consequence of electrical conduction delay, but also can be produced by increases in ventricular afterload or regional differences in contraction function.
2. The mechano-energetic consequence of dyssynchrony is a decline in net cardiac systolic function with a relative increase in myocardial oxygen consumption.
3. Dyssynchrony due to conduction delay results in changes in the transmural distribution of conduction velocity, alterations in gap junction protein expression and distribution, and alterations in repolarization.
4. Chronic resynchronization treatment results in reversal of chamber remodeling, or a decline in cardiac end-systolic volumes, which are not related to the acute therapy, but rather due to reversal of pathologic chamber dilation.
5. Dyssynchrony results in regional disparities in stress kinase and other protein expression/activation, which is reversed and rendered more homogeneous by cardiac resynchronization therapy.
6. CRT has a beneficial effect on cardiac cell survival signaling—reducing apoptosis coupled with enhancement of activated Akt kinase signaling.
7. The region of LV pacing, which achieves >70% of peak CRT benefit, is fairly large. It is located in the midlateral wall and covers about 40% of the LV free wall. This territory is similar when defined by the area that produces the most resynchronization based on wall motion as well as global chamber function (e.g., stroke work).

REFERENCES

1. Mudd JO, Kass DA. Tackling heart failure in the twenty-first century. *Nature.* 2008;451:919–928.
2. Hill JA, Olson EN, Cardiac plasticity. *N Engl J Med.* 2008;358: 1370–1380.
3. Zou Y, Akazawa H, Qin Y, et al. Mechanical stress activates angiotensin II type 1 receptor without the involvement of angiotensin II. *Nat Cell Biol.* 2004;6:499–506.
4. Zheng M, Han QD, Xiao RP. Distinct beta-adrenergic receptor subtype signaling in the heart and their pathophysiological relevance. *Sheng Li Xue Bao.* 2004;56:1–15.
5. Bers DM. Altered cardiac myocyte Ca regulation in heart failure. *Physiology* (Bethesda). 2006;21:380–387.
6. Bers DM. Calcium cycling and signaling in cardiac myocytes. *Annu Rev Physiol.* 2008;70:23–49.
7. McKinsey TA, Kass DA. Small-molecule therapies for cardiac hypertrophy: moving beneath the cell surface. *Nature Reviews Drug Discovery.* 2007;6:1–18.
8. Heineke J, Molkentin JD. Regulation of cardiac hypertrophy by intracellular signalling pathways. *Nat Rev Mol Cell Biol.* 2006;7:589–600.
9. Neubauer S. The failing heart—an engine out of fuel. *N Engl J Med.* 2007;356:1140–1151.

10. Linke WA. Sense and stretchability. The role of titin and titin-associated proteins in myocardial stress-sensing and mechanical dysfunction. *Cardiovasc Res.* 2008;77:637–648.

11. Baldasseroni S, Opasich C, Gorini M, et al. Left bundle-branch block is associated with increased 1-year sudden and total mortality rate in 5517 outpatients with congestive heart failure: a report from the Italian network on congestive heart failure. *Am Heart J.* 2002;143:398–405.

12. Wilensky RL, Yudelman P, Cohen AI, et al. Serial electrocardiographic changes in idiopathic dilated cardiomyopathy confirmed at necropsy. *Am J Cardiol.* 1988;62:276–283.

13. Akar FG, Spragg DD, Tunin RS, et al. Mechanisms underlying conduction slowing and arrhythmogenesis in nonischemic dilated cardiomyopathy. *Circ Res.* 2004;95:717–725.

14. Byrne MJ, Helm RH, Daya S, et al. Diminished left ventricular dyssynchrony and impact of resynchronization in failing hearts with right versus left bundle branch block. *J Am Coll Cardiol.* 2007;50:1484–1490.

15. Bleeker GB, Mollema SA, Olman ER, et al. Left ventricular resynchronization is mandatory for response to cardiac resynchronization therapy. *Circulation.* 2007;116:1140–1148.

16. Yu CM, Zhang Q, Fung JW, et al. A novel tool to assess systolic asynchrony and identify responders of cardiac resynchronization therapy by tissue synchronization imaging. *J Am Coll Cardiol.* 2005;45:677–684.

17. Aoyagi T, Iizuka M, Takahashi T, et al. Wall motion asynchrony prolongs time constant of left ventricular relaxation. *Am J Physiol.* 1989; 257:H883–H890.

18. Yano M, Kohno M, Konishi M, et al. Influence of left ventricular regional nonuniformity on afterload-dependent relaxation in intact dogs. *Am J Physiol.* 1994;267:H148–H154.

19. Wang J, Kurrelmeyer KM, Torre-Amione G, et al. Systolic and diastolic dyssynchrony in patients with diastolic heart failure and the effect of medical therapy. *J Am Coll Cardiol.* 2007;49:88–96.

20. Kass DA. An epidemic of dyssynchrony: but what does it mean? *J Am Coll Cardiol.* 2008;51:12–17.

21. Park RC, Little WC, O'Rourke RA. Effect of alteration of left ventricular activation sequence on the left ventricular end-systolic pressure-volume relation in closed-chest dogs. *Circ Res.* 1985;57:706–717.

22. Helm RH, Byrne M, Helm PA, et al. Three-dimensional mapping of optimal left ventricular pacing site for cardiac resynchronization. *Circulation.* 2007;115:953–961.

23. Suga H, Goto Y, Yaku H, et al. Simulation of mechanoenergetics of asynchronously contracting ventricle. *Am J Physiol.* 1990;259: R1075–R1082.

24. Prinzen FW, Hunter WC, Wyman BT, et al. Mapping of regional myocardial strain and work during ventricular pacing: experimental study using magnetic resonance imaging tagging. *J Am Coll Cardiol.* 1999;33:1735–1742.

25. van Oosterhout. MF, Arts T, Bassingthwaighte JB, et al. Relation between local myocardial growth and blood flow during chronic ventricular pacing. *Cardiovasc Res.* 2002;53:831–840.

26. Vernooy K, Verbeek XA, Peschar M, et al. Left bundle branch block induces ventricular remodelling and functional septal hypoperfusion. *Eur Heart J.* 2005;26:91–98.

27. Nowak B, Sinha AM, Schaefer WM, et al. Cardiac resynchronization therapy homogenizes myocardial glucose metabolism and perfusion in dilated cardiomyopathy and left bundle branch block. *J Am Coll Cardiol.* 2003;41:1523–1528.

28. Owen CH, Esposito DJ, Davis JW, et al. The effects of ventricular pacing on left ventricular geometry, function, myocardial oxygen consumption, and efficiency of contraction in conscious dogs. *Pacing Clin Electrophysiol.* 1998;21:1417–1429.

29. Baller D, Wolpers HG, Zipfel J, et al. Unfavorable effects of ventricular pacing on myocardial energetics. *Basic Res Cardiol.* 1981;76:115–123.

30. Baller D, Wolpers HG, Zipfel J, et al. Comparison of the effects of right atrial, right ventricular apex and atrioventricular sequential pacing on myocardial oxygen consumption and cardiac efficiency: a laboratory investigation. *Pacing Clin Electrophysiol.* 1988;11:394–403.

31. Thambo JB, Bordachar P, Garrigue S, et al. Detrimental ventricular remodeling in patients with congenital complete heart block and chronic right ventricular apical pacing. *Circulation.* 2004;110:3766–3772.

32. Helm PA, Younes L, Beg MF, et al. Evidence of structural remodeling in the dyssynchronous failing heart. *Circ Res.* 2006;98:125–132.

33. Spragg DD, Leclercq C, Loghmani M, et al. Regional alterations in protein expression in the dyssynchronous failing heart. *Circulation.* 2003;108:929–932.

34. Chakir K, Daya SK, Tunin RS, et al. Reversal of Global Apoptosis and Regional Stress Kinase Activation by Cardiac Resynchronization. *Circulation.* 2008;117:1369–1377.

35. Spragg DD, Akar FG, Helm RH, et al. Abnormal conduction and repolarization in late-activated myocardium of dyssynchronously contracting hearts. *Cardiovasc Res.* 2005;67:77–86.

36. Bilchick KC, Saha SK, Mikolajczyk E, et al. Differential regional gene expression from cardiac dyssynchrony induced by chronic right ventricular free wall pacing in the mouse. *Physiol Genomics.* 2006;26: 109–115.

37. Iuliano S, Fisher SG, Karasik PE, et al. QRS duration and mortality in patients with congestive heart failure. *Am Heart J.* 2002;143: 1085–1091.

38. Akar FG, Rosenbaum DS. Transmural Electrophysiological Heterogeneities Underlying Arrhythmogenesis in Heart Failure. *Circ Res.* 2003;93:638–645.

39. Akar FG, Spragg DD, Tunin RS, et al. Mechanisms underlying conduction slowing and arrhythmogenesis in nonischemic dilated cardiomyopathy. *Circ Res.* 2004;95:717–725.

40. Nelson GS, Berger RD, Fetics BJ, et al. Left ventricular or biventricular pacing improves cardiac function at diminished energy cost in patients with dilated cardiomyopathy and left bundle-branch block. *Circulation.* 2000;102:3053–3059.

41. Lindner O, Sorensen J, Vogt J, et al. Cardiac efficiency and oxygen consumption measured with 11C-acetate PET after long-term cardiac resynchronization therapy. *J Nucl Med.* 2006;47:378–383.

42. Ukkonen H, Beanlands RS, Burwash IG, et al. Effect of cardiac resynchronization on myocardial efficiency and regional oxidative metabolism. *Circulation.* 2003;107:28–31.

43. Vollmann D, Luthje L, Schott P, et al. Biventricular pacing improves the blunted force-frequency relation present during univentricular pacing in patients with heart failure and conduction delay. *Circulation.* 2006;113:953–959.

44. Mullens W, Bartunek J, Wilson Tang WH, et al. Early and late effects of cardiac resynchronization therapy on force-frequency relation and contractility regulating gene expression in heart failure patients. *Heart Rhythm.* 2008;5:52–59.

45. Vanderheyden M, Mullens W, Delrue L, et al. Myocardial gene expression in heart failure patients treated with cardiac resynchronization therapy responders versus nonresponders. *J Am Coll Cardiol.* 2008;51: 129–136.

46. Helm RH, Leclercq C, Faris OP, et al. Cardiac dyssynchrony analysis using circumferential versus longitudinal strain: implications for assessing cardiac resynchronization. *Circulation.* 2005;111: 2760–2767.

47. St. John Sutton MG, Plappert T, Abraham WT, et al. Effect of cardiac resynchronization therapy on left ventricular size and function in chronic heart failure. *Circulation.* 2003;107:1985–1990.

48. Steendijk P, Tulner SA, Bax J J, et al. Hemodynamic effects of long-term cardiac resynchronization therapy: analysis by pressure-volume loops. *Circulation.* 2006;113:1295–1304.

49. Sutton MG, Plappert T, Hilpisch KE, et al. Sustained reverse left ventricular structural remodeling with cardiac resynchronization at one year is a function of etiology: quantitative Doppler echocardiographic evidence from the Multicenter InSync Randomized Clinical Evaluation (MIRACLE). *Circulation.* 2006;113:266–272.

50. Yu CM, Chau E, Sanderson J E, et al. Tissue Doppler echocardiographic evidence of reverse remodeling and improved synchronicity by simultaneously delaying regional contraction after biventricular pacing therapy in heart failure. *Circulation.* 2002;105:438–445.

51. Yu CM, Bleeker GB, Fung JW, et al. Left ventricular reverse remodeling but not clinical improvement predicts long-term survival after cardiac resynchronization therapy. *Circulation.* 2005;112:1580–1586.

52. Stellbrink C, Breithardt OA, Franke A, et al. Impact of cardiac resynchronization therapy using hemodynamically optimized pacing on left ventricular remodeling in patients with congestive heart failure and ventricular conduction disturbances. *J Am Coll Cardiol.* 2001; 38:1957–1965.

53. Schillinger W, Lehnart SE, Prestle J, et al. Influence of SR Ca(2+)-ATPase and Na(+)- Ca(2+)-exchanger on the force-frequency relation. *Basic Res Cardiol.* 1998;93 Suppl 1:38–45.

54. Iyengar S, Haas G, Lamba S, et al. Effect of cardiac resynchronization therapy on myocardial gene expression in patients with nonischemic dilated cardiomyopathy. *J Card Fail.* 2007;13:304–311.

55. Abraham WT, Gilbert EM, Lowes BD, et al. Coordinate changes in Myosin heavy chain isoform gene expression are selectively associated with alterations in dilated cardiomyopathy phenotype. *Mol Med.* 2002;8:750–760.

56. Liao P, Georgakopoulos D, Kovacs A, et al. The in vivo role of p38 MAP kinases in cardiac remodeling and restrictive cardiomyopathy. *Proc Natl Acad Sci U S A.* 2001;98:12283–12288.

57. Zhang R, Khoo MS, Wu Y, et al. Calmodulin kinase II inhibition protects against structural heart disease. *Nat Med.* 2005;11:409–417.

58. Kubota T, McTiernan CF, Frye CS, et al. Dilated cardiomyopathy in transgenic mice with cardiac-specific overexpression of tumor necrosis factor-alpha. *Circ Res.* 1997;81:627–635.

59. D'Ascia C, Cittadini A, Monti MG, et al. Effects of biventricular pacing on interstitial remodelling, tumor necrosis factor-alpha expression, and apoptotic death in failing human myocardium. *Eur Heart J.* 2006;27:201–206.

60. Kies P, Bax JJ, Molhoek SG, et al. Effect of cardiac resynchronization therapy on inducibility of ventricular tachyarrhythmias in cardiac arrest survivors with either ischemic or idiopathic dilated cardiomyopathy. *Am J Cardiol.* 2005;95:1111–1114.

61. Ermis C, Seutter R, Zhu AX, et al. Impact of upgrade to cardiac resynchronization therapy on ventricular arrhythmia frequency in patients with implantable cardioverter-defibrillators. *J Am Coll Cardiol.* 2005; 46:2258–2263.

62. Di CA, Bongiorni MG, Arena G, et al. New-onset ventricular tachycardia after cardiac resynchronization therapy. *J Interv Card Electrophysiol.* 2005;12:231–235.

63. Guerra JM, Wu J, Miller JM, et al. Increase in ventricular tachycardia frequency after biventricular implantable cardioverter defibrillator upgrade. *J Cardiovasc Electrophysiol.* 2003;14:1245–1247.

64. Medina-Ravell VA, Lankipalli RS, Yan GX, et al. Effect of epicardial or biventricular pacing to prolong QT interval and increase transmural dispersion of repolarization: does resynchronization therapy pose a risk for patients predisposed to long QT or torsade de pointes? *Circulation.* 2003;107:740–746.

65. McSwain RL, Schwartz RA, Delurgio DB, et al. The impact of cardiac resynchronization therapy on ventricular tachycardia/fibrillation: an analysis from the combined Contak-CD and InSync-ICD studies. *J Cardiovasc Electrophysiol.* 2005;16:1168–1171.

66. Cleland JG, Daubert JC, Erdmann E, et al. Longer-term effects of cardiac resynchronization therapy on mortality in heart failure [the CArdiac REsynchronization-Heart Failure (CARE-HF) trial extension phase]. *Eur Heart J.* 2006;27:1928–1932.

67. Rivero-Ayerza M, Theuns DA, Garcia-Garcia HM, et al. Effects of cardiac resynchronization therapy on overall mortality and mode of death: a meta-analysis of randomized controlled trials. *Eur Heart J.* 2006;27:2682–2688.

68. Berger T, Hanser F, Hintringer F, et al. Effects of cardiac resynchronization therapy on ventricular repolarization in patients with congestive heart failure. *J Cardiovasc Electrophysiol.* 2005;16:611–617.

69. Henrikson CA, Spragg DD, Cheng A, et al. Evidence for electrical remodeling of the native conduction system with cardiac resynchronization therapy. *Pacing Clin Electrophysiol.* 2007;30:591–595.

70. Tomaselli GF, Beuckelmann DJ, Calkins HG, et al. Sudden cardiac death in heart failure. The role of abnormal repolarization. *Circulation.* 1994;90:2534–2539.

71. Blanc JJ, Etienne Y, Gilard M, et al. Evaluation of different ventricular pacing sites in patients with severe heart failure: results of an acute hemodynamic study. *Circulation.* 1997;96:3273–3277.

72. Kass DA, Chen CH, Curry C, et al. Improved left ventricular mechanics from acute VDD pacing in patients with dilated cardiomyopathy and ventricular conduction delay. *Circulation.* 1999;99:1567–1573.

73. Leclercq C, Faris O, Tunin R, et al. Systolic improvement and mechanical resynchronization does not require electrical synchrony in the dilated failing heart with left bundle-branch block. *Circulation.* 2002; 106:1760–1763.

74. Bordachar P, Lafitte S, Reuter S, et al. Biventricular pacing and left ventricular pacing in heart failure: similar hemodynamic improvement despite marked electromechanical differences. *J Cardiovasc Electrophysiol.* 2004;15:1342–1347.

75. Hay I, Melenovsky V, Fetics BJ, et al. Short-term effects of right-left heart sequential cardiac resynchronization in patients with heart failure, chronic atrial fibrillation, and atrioventricular nodal block. *Circulation.* 2004;110:3404–3410.

76. Auricchio A, Stellbrink C, Block M, et al. Effect of pacing chamber and atrioventricular delay on acute systolic function of paced patients with congestive heart failure. The Pacing Therapies for Congestive Heart Failure Study Group. The Guidant Congestive Heart Failure Research Group. *Circulation.* 1999;99:2993–3001.

77. Kawaguchi M, Murabayashi T, Fetics BJ, et al. Quantitation of basal dyssynchrony and acute resynchronization from left or biventricular pacing by novel echo-contrast variability imaging. *J Am Coll Cardiol.* 2002;39:2052–2058.

78. Vernooy K, Verbeek XA, Cornelussen RN, et al. FW. Calculation of effective VV interval facilitates optimization of AV delay and VV interval in cardiac resynchronization therapy. *Heart Rhythm.* 2007; 4:75–82.

79. Dupuis JM, Kobeissi A, Vitali L, et al. Programming optimal atrioventricular delay in dual chamber pacing using peak endocardial acceleration: comparison with a standard echocardiographic procedure. *Pacing Clin Electrophysiol.* 2003;26:210–213.

80. Butter C, Auricchio A, Stellbrink C, et al. Effect of resynchronization therapy stimulation site on the systolic function of heart failure patients. *Circulation.* 2001;104:3026–3029.

Clinical Predictors of Improvement in Left Ventricular Performance with Cardiac Resynchronization Therapy

Luis A. Pires

Heart failure (HF) is characterized by progressive dilatation of the left ventricle (LV) and loss of contractile performance, together referred to as LV remodeling. It is not surprising, therefore, that the extent of LV remodeling[1] and treatments aimed at reversing its course[2–5] have a significant impact on the outcome of HF patients. Despite recent advances in the pharmacologic therapy of HF, morbidity and mortality remain high.[6] This plus the increasing incidence of HF[6] has recently led to a search for new treatment modalities, most notably the role of cardiac resynchronization therapy (CRT), precisely because it is thought to reverse the course of LV remodeling.[7,8] Although the precise mechanism by which CRT improves patient outcome is not completely understood, but is beginning to be elucidated,[9,10] a likely explanation is thought to be its significant impact on systolic and, perhaps to a lesser extent, diastolic LV performance observed both acutely and over several months.[11] The results of several observational and randomized clinical trials have established CRT (via biventricular pacing), as a major breakthrough in the treatment of patients with moderate-to-severe HF, impaired LV systolic function, and intraventricular conduction delay.[12] CRT improves quality of life and exercise capacity, reduces severity of mitral regurgitation (MR), reduces HF hospitalizations, and improves overall survival in patients who are already receiving optimal pharmacologic therapy.[13] Despite the impressive results obtained from CRT in terms of both symptom improvement and reversal of LV remodeling, however, as many as 20% to 50% of patients do not respond to such therapy.[14] None of the established CRT selection criteria (NYHA class, LV ejection fraction, and QRS duration) are able to adequately predict either acute or long-term response to CRT.[15–23] On the other hand, improvement in LV performance, quantified primarily as reversal of LV remodeling, appears to be a strong predictor of patient outcome,[24–26] similar to what is observed with drug therapy.[2–5] Although far less is known about CRT and right ventricular (RV) performance, CRT also acutely improves RV performance,[27–29] which, in turn, predicts adverse events.[30] The focus of this chapter, however, will be on the effect of CRT on LV performance.

This chapter reviews predictors of acute and long-term improvement in LV performance in patients with chronic systolic HF and established indications for CRT. The latter part of the chapter will focus on patient groups for whom indications (and results) of CRT are less well established.

IMPROVEMENT IN LEFT VENTRICULAR SYSTOLIC PERFORMANCE WITH CRT

Improvement in LV systolic performance has been quantified, most commonly, in terms of changes in dP/dt_{max}, pulse pressure, stroke volume, LV ejection fraction (EF), LV end-systolic (LVESV) and end-diastolic (LVEDV) volumes. Though earlier reports focused on invasive tools (pressure-volume analysis), echocardiography has now become the preferred method to assess global and regional changes in LV performance before and after CRT.[31] Determination of the impact of CRT on LV systolic (and diastolic) performance, both acutely and long-term, greatly enhances our understanding of the potential mechanism(s) of action of CRT and the relationship between such improvement (and its absence) and long-term patient outcome. Yu et al.[26] recently reported that, unlike improvements in clinical parameters such as NYHA functional class and exercise capacity, a reduction in LVESV (by ≥10%) was the only independent predictor of all-cause and cardiovascular mortalities over 3 to 6 months of follow-up in CRT-treated HF patients.[27] The 87 (62%) CRT responders (i.e., those with a ≥10% reduction in LVESV) had significantly lower all-cause mortality (6.9% versus 30.6%, p = 0.0003), cardiovascular mortality (2.3% versus 24.1%, p < 0.0001), and heart failure events (11.5% versus 33.3%, p = 0.0032) than nonresponders (i.e., those with a <10% reduction in LVESV). From this and other studies,[24–26] it is becoming clear that reduction in LV volumes and increase in LVEF are not only surrogate markers of a favorable response to CRT but may also be used as objective measures to predict long-term clinical outcome, thereby facilitating selection of patients who are most likely to respond to and benefit from therapy.

Acute Improvement in LV Systolic Performance

Several acute hemodynamic studies have shown that CRT results in immediate and sustained improvement in LV performance,[32–38] which served as the background for subsequent clinical trials confirming the substantial benefits of CRT. CRT acutely enhances systolic function while modestly lowering energy cost,[38] an important feature considering the adverse impact of pharmacologic therapies that enhance LV function at increased myocardial oxygen consumption.[39, 40] Improvement in stroke volume and cardiac output, expressed usually as changes in aortic pulse pressure, range from 7% to 15%.[9, 11, 32–38] An acute increase of 13% to 21% in dP/dt_{max}, a reflection of global LV performance, has been reported.[9, 11, 32–35] Similarly, acute reductions in LVESV and to a lesser degree LVEDV have been observed, often in parallel with changes in pulse pressure and dP/dt_{max}.[9, 11, 13, 38] Acute absolute (relative) increases of 4% to 10% (15% to 36%) in LVEF have been reported.[11, 13, 28, 29, 37, 41] Acute improvement in LV performance is maintained chronically,[11, 29, 42] but such improvement disappears to a substantial degree with cessation of pacing.[11,42] Yu et al.[42] elegantly showed that several measures of LV performance progressively increased after both one week and three months of biventricular pacing. These measures of improvement gradually declined with cessation of pacing (Fig. 2.1). Moreover, such changes were paralleled by concordant changes in LV volumes, severity of MR, exercise capacity, and quality of life score. The fact that CRT-mediated gains in LV performance are lost with termination of pacing indicates that some of the derived benefits are purely pacing dependent ("electrical" phenomenon), and not the result of reversal of remodeling, which would imply actual structural changes.[43] It should also be noted that the acute impact of CRT on LV performance noted in resting conditions, typical of the reported results,[32–38] is not maintained under "stress" conditions,[44] which raises the interesting possibility that, in some cases, this may account for the lack of response to CRT during long-term follow-up.[14] The settings under which LV performance is determined should be taken into account in data analysis.

Predictors of Acute Improvement in LV Systolic Performance

Predictors of acute improvement in LV performance with CRT have been reported by several investigators.[28, 45–51] Using various measures to define improvement in LV performance, responders (46% to 91%) were identified with sensitivities of up to 100% and similar specificities (Table 2.1). In general, traditional, readily available clinical variables, or patient demographics, have not proven useful. In one of the earlier reports involving 22 patients, Nelson et al.[45] found baseline QRS duration and dP/dt_{max} to be weak predictors of increases in dP/dt_{max} ($\geq$25%) and pulse pressure ($\geq$10%) individually, but strong predictors when combined. The majority of studies, however, focused on various measures of interventricular and intraventricular dyssynchrony to identify predictors of acute improvements in LV performance (Table 2.1). Using radial strain imaging to quantify LV dyssynchrony and a cut-off value of $\geq$130 ms, Dohi et al.[49] found a close relationship between improvement in stroke volume and baseline dyssynchrony (Fig. 2.2A) and change (reduction) in dyssynchrony after CRT (Fig. 2.2B). Suffoletto et al.[51] reported similar results, including high sensitivity and specificity in predicting an immediate $\geq$15% increase in stroke volume with CRT. Moreover, these investigators found that in the 22 patients whose LV leads were positioned concordant with the site of latest mechanical activation by radial strain had a greater increase in LVEF from baseline ($10\pm5\%$) than the 14 patients with discordant LV lead positions ($6\pm5\%$, p < 0.05). These results emphasize the importance of proper LV lead position in determining CRT response.[52, 53] An excellent correlation between speckle-tracking and tissue Doppler determined dyssynchrony, defined as the time difference between septal and posterior wall peak strain,[51] was observed. This is potentially an important finding given that the more commonly used tissue Doppler method may be more susceptible to passive translational motion or tethering,[54] and thus subject to interpretive errors.[31]

The extent of myocardial viability in patients with ischemic cardiomyopathy appears to play an important role in both acute and long-term (see below) CRT response. Hummel et al.[55] found a close relationship between acute (the day after CRT implantation) improvement in LVEF and stroke volume and extent of myocardial viability (perfusion score index) quantified by contrast echocardiography. These investigators showed that baseline intraventricular dyssynchrony and degree of resynchronization only weakly predicted acute LVEF improvement; resynchronization resulted in improvement in LVEF only in patients with significant tissue viability.[55] These findings suggest that largely nonviable akinetic or dyskinetic LV segments contribute little to LV systolic performance, whether or not they are resynchronized. In an acute hemodynamic study involving 53 patients with moderate-to-severe HF, Van Gelder et al.[56] found a significantly lower percent increase in dP/dt in patients whose LV lead tips were placed where transmural scar (MRI-detected hyperenhancement involving >50% of wall thickness) was present (14.5 ± 10.4) compared with sites remote from scar (27.5 ± 18.4) or where there was no scar (32.0 ± 20). They also found that the optimal V-V interval was significantly longer in patients with scar tissue, perhaps a reflection of scar-mediated slowing of conduction.

Other investigators have used combinations of arguably simpler baseline (LV contractility and mechanical dyssynchrony) and procedural (position and electrical delay of LV leads relative to RV leads) variables to construct a "response score" to predict hemodynamic improvement (and clinical outcome) of CRT-treated patients.[57] These investigators found a highly significant association between response score (0 to 4 points) and the proportion of hemodynamic

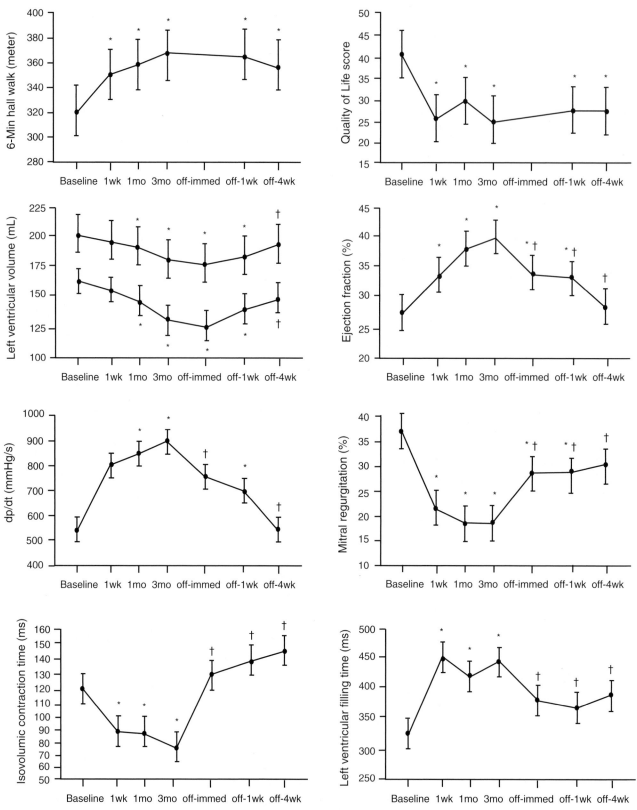

FIG. 2.1. Changes in 6-minute hall-walk distance, Minnesota Living With Heart Failure quality of life score, LV end-diastolic (top) and end-systolic (bottom) volumes, ejection fraction, dP/dt, mitral regurgitation, isovolumic contraction time, and LV filling time before and after biventricular pacing as well as when pacing was suspended for 4 weeks. *Significant difference vs. baseline. †Significant difference vs. biventricular pacing for 3 months. (Reprinted with permission from Yu, CM, et al. Tissue Doppler Echocardiographic Evidence of Reverse Remodeling and Improved Synchronicity by Simultaneously Delaying Regional Contraction After Biventricular Pacing Therapy in Heart Failure. *Circulation.* 2002;105:438.)

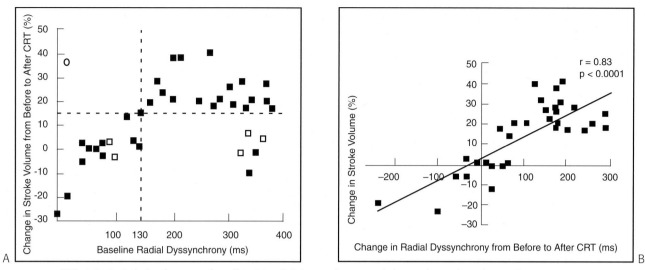

FIG. 2.2. **A:** Relation between baseline LV radial dyssynchrony and change in stroke volume after CRT. A cut-off of 130 ms of radial dyssynchrony was predictive of a 15% increase in stroke volume. Closed squares, posterior or lateral lead position; open squares, anterior lead position; open circle, patient with heart rate change from 86 to 52 beats/min after CRT. **B:** Relation between change in LV radial dyssynchrony and change in stroke volume the day after resynchronization therapy. (Reprinted with permission from Dohl K., et al. Utility of Echocardiogram Radial StrainIMaging to Quantify Left Ventricular Dyssynchrony and Predict Acute Response to Cardiac Resynchronization Therapy. *Am J Cardiol.* 2005;(96) 1:114.)

responders to CRT ($\geq$25% increase in dP/dt with pacing), with one point given to each of four analyzed variables: LV/RV lead distance >10cm; LV lead electrical delay >50% of QRS; dP/dt_{max} <600 mm Hg/s; and LV dyssynchrony >100 ms delay. They also observed a significant link between response score and overall patient survival. As pointed out by the authors, such response score was generated retrospectively; therefore its utility in predicting CRT response (acutely and chronically) must be validated prospectively.

The results of these studies (Table 2.1) are not without limitations, including relatively small number of patients, single-center enrollments, different definitions of measures of response, heavy focus on echocardiographic predictors, and, of course, lack of randomization of CRT. Moreover, other investigators did not identify any reliable predictor, among several potential parameters, of an acute improvement in stroke volume with CRT.[44] None of these studies addressed whether or not these acute results can be used to predict or determine long-term clinical outcome. Limited data, on a small number of patients, suggest that acute improvement in LV performance (stroke volume and LVEF) leads to further short-term increase in LVEF[29] as well as improvements in exercise duration[58] and NYHA functional class.[47, 59] There exists no large-scale data on the significance of acute improvement in LV performance and long-term outcome of CRT-treated patients.

Short- and Long-Term Improvement in LV Systolic Performance

Enthusiasm regarding the role of CRT as an adjunctive treatment modality in patients with chronic systolic HF grew when randomized clinical trials confirmed its substantial benefit on LV performance and reversal of LV remodeling.[12] It is now widely believed that the overall positive impact of CRT on short- (3 months) and long-term (6 months or longer) patient outcome is attributed to its sustained, progressive enhancement in LV performance[7, 8, 11, 25, 29, 42] through retiming (resynchronization) of dyssynchronous LV contraction.[10] Aside from its immediate hemodynamic effect,[11, 32–38] CRT results in improvement in LV performance starting as early as one week,[29, 42] and maintained over several years.[60]

Predictors of Improvement in Short- and Long-Term LV Performance

Several predictors of improvement in short- and long-term LV performance have been identified.[29, 61–69] Relying on various changes in LVEF or LV volumes to define response, the authors reported response rates of 40% to 85% with sensitivities of 72% to 100%, and specificities of 55% to 100% (Table 2.2). Non echocardiographic factors have not been particularly helpful as predictors. On a multivariate model of the combined data from MIRACLE and MIRACLE-ICD trials, in which 60% of the patients experienced a decrease in LVEDV, and 40% had an increase in LVEDV, Cappola et al.[61] identified male gender, baseline BNP level, severity of MR, and baseline (smaller) LVEDV each as independent predictors of LV enlargement (remodeling).[61] This suggests that female gender, lower BNP levels, less-severe MR, and larger LVEDV might be protective against LV enlargement. The observation that male gender attenuated the decline in LVEDV might explain, in part, the higher mortality rate in men with HF compared with

TABLE 2.1   Rates and Predictors of Acute Improvement in Left Ventricular Systolic Performance with CRT

Authors	No. of patients*	Measured response	Response rate (%)	Independent predictors of response	Sensitivity/ Specificity (%)
Nelson[45]	22	≥25% ↑ dP/dt $_{max}$ ≥ 10 % ↑ PP	91	QRS ≥ 155 and dP/dt $_{max}$ ≤700 mm Hg/s	100/100 90/100
Sogaard[46]	25	↑ LVEF	-	LV dyssynchrony, DLC	Response related to improved dyssynchrony
Kerwin[28]	13	↑ LVEF		Interventricular dyssynchrony	Response related to improved dyssynchrony
Bax[47]	25	≥ 5% ↑ LVEF	68	LV dyssynchrony, >60 ms cutoff†	76/89
Gorcsan III[48]	29	≥ 15% ↑ SV	52	LV dyssynchrony, >65 ms cutoff†	87/100
Dohi[49]	38	≥ 15% ↑ SV	55	LV dyssynchrony, ≥130 ms cutoff‡	95/88
Breithardt[50]	34	↑ dP/dt $_{max}$	-	LV dyssynchrony, >25% phase delay	Response related to improved dyssynchrony
Suffoletto[51]	48	≥ 15% ↑ SV	67	LV dyssynchrony, ≥130ms cutoff‡	91/75
Heist[57]	39	≥ 25% ↑ dP/dt $_{max}$	46	"Response Score" (0–4)¶ 4 points	100/100

DLC, delayed longitudinal contraction; LV, left ventricular; LVEF, left ventricular ejection fraction; PP, pulse pressure; SV, stroke volume; ↑, increase
*Only alive patients who had complete follow-up.
†Opposing two-wall delay.
‡Septal to posterior wall delay, radial strain
¶One point for each factor: LV/RV lead distance >10 cm; LV lead electrical delay >50% of QRS; dP/dt $_{max}$ <600 mm Hg/s; LV dyssynchrony (maximum wall delay) >100 ms.

TABLE 2.2   Rates and Predictors of Long-Term Improvement in Left Ventricular Systolic Performance with CRT

Authors	Number of Patients*	Follow-Up (Months)	Measured Response	Response Rate (%)	Independent Predictors of Response	Sensitivity/ Specificity (%)
Mangiavacchi[62]	156	12	>10% absolute ↑ LVEF	40	Nonischemic etiology	-
Toussaint[29]	34	20	>5% ↑ LVEF	-	LVEF >15%, interventricular delay >60 ms	78/79
Sogaard[20]	20	12	↑ in LVEF	-	LV dyssynchrony, DLC	Close relationship
Yu[64]	30	3	>15% ↓ LVESV	57	LV dyssynchrony, 32.6 ms cutoff†	100/100
Bax[21]	80	6	≥ 15% ↓ LVESV	74	LV dyssynchrony, >65 ms cutoff‡	92/92
Penicka[65]	49	6	≥25% ↑ LVEF	55	LV dyssynchrony, >102 ms cutoff¶	96/77
Yu[66]	56	3	≥15% ↓ LVESV	54	LV dyssynchrony, >34.4 ms cutoff†	87/81
Pitzalis[22]	51	6	>5% ↑ LVEF	47	SPWD ≥130 ms (m-Mode echo)	92/78
Notobartolo[67]	49	3	≥15% ↓ LVESV	59	LV dyssynchrony, ≥100 ms**	97/55
Van de Veire[68]	60	6	≥15% ↓ LVESV	53	LV dyssynchrony, >65 ms cutoff‡	81/89
Suffoletto[51]	50	8	≥15% ↑ LVEF	76	LV dyssynchrony, >130 ms cutoff#	89/83
Bleeker[10]	100	6	>10% ↓ LVEDV	85	>20% immediate resynchronization	100/93
Kapetanakis[63]	26	10	↑ LVEF, ↓ LVEDV	-	Reduction in SDI (3-D echo)	Close relationship
Gorcsan III[69]	176	6	≥15% ↑ LVEF	66	LV dyssynchrony, ≥60 ms‡ radial strain, ≥130 ms# both parameters	72 / 77 84 / 73 88 / 80

DLC, delayed longitudinal contraction; LVEDV, left ventricular end-diastolic volume; LVEF, left ventricular ejection fraction; LVESV; left ventricular end-systolic volume; SDI, systolic dyssynchrony index; SPWD, septal to posterior wall delay.
*Only alive patients who had complete follow-up.
†Yu index (SD maximum wall delay, 12 sites.)
‡Opposing two-wall delay.
¶Delay in onset of systolic velocity.
#Septal to posterior wall delay.
**Maximum wall delay, 12 sites.

women.[70] Mangiavacchi et al.[62] identified nonischemic etiology of HF as the only independent predictor of a marked improvement in LV performance, defined as an increase of >10 absolute percentage points in LVEF (observed in 39.7% of patients). This finding is in agreement with other studies in which a better improvement in LV performance was observed among patients with nonischemic LV systolic dysfunction who were treated with either beta-blockers[71] or CRT.[17,18,72,73] Similarly, mortality appears to be lower among HF patients with nonischemic cardiomyopathy treated either medically[6] or with CRT.[73] The better CRT-induced improvement in LV performance (and overall outcome) in patients with nonischemic etiology probably reflects the fact that CRT may not be able to resynchronize scar-laden myocardial segments, a finding in agreement with the reduced benefit of CRT in patients with substantial scarring or reduced tissue viability.[41,55,74–76] Bleeker et al.[74] found that patients with MRI-detected extensive posterolateral scarring, a favored site of LV lead placement, are unlikely to show improvement in LV performance regardless of the extent of baseline LV dyssynchrony. A higher overall scar burden, a larger number of severely scarred segments, greater scar density near the LV tip,[75,76] or reduced tissue viability[42,55] portend an unfavorable response to CRT in terms of changes in LV performance and in functional improvement (Fig. 2.3). Other investigators, however, found that, as long as acceptable LV pacing was achieved, placement of the LV lead at an akinetic (scarred) segment did not adversely impact acute hemodynamic or 12-month clinical response to CRT.[77]

Extensive LV wall scarring may prevent "resynchronization," a prerequisite for CRT benefit.[10] LV resynchronization occurs immediately after CRT and is directly related to CRT response, defined as >10% reduction in LVESV.[10] Patients with <20% acute reduction in LV dyssynchrony did not respond to CRT.[10] Responders showed a significant reduction in LV dyssynchrony from 115 ± 37 to 32 ± 23 ms, whereas nonresponders showed no significant reduction in dyssynchrony (from 106 ± 29 to 79 ± 44 ms). Except for rare reports,[55] response to CRT is closely linked to correction or substantial reduction in the degree of interventricular[28,29,65] and intraventricula[22,26,47–51,63–69] LV dyssynchrony. Figure 2.4 shows an example of a patient whose LVEF increased (21% to 56%) and LVEDV decreased (164 ml to 121 ml) substantially 6 months after CRT, accompanied by complete elimination of LV dyssynchrony determined by both M-mode (septal-to-posterior wall delay, 0 from 159 ms) and tissue Doppler (septal to lateral wall delay, 0 from 70 ms) images.

Except for two earlier reports,[61,62] identification of predictors of improvement in LV performance has focused on measures of intraventricular and, to a lesser extent interventricular,[28,29,65] LV dyssynchrony, predicated on the close relationship between extent of baseline dyssynchrony with improvement in LVEF (Fig. 2.5)[22] and overall patient outcome.[21] In other words, as one might expect, CRT imparts no benefit to HF patients unless there is substantial dyssynchrony to correct.[10,21,22] It should be noted, however, that even when

patients were preselected *based* on presence of dyssynchrony,[10] the rate of response to CRT ($\geq$10% reduction in LVESV) is 85%, suggesting that there must exist other unidentified predictive factors[14,30,44] and other mechanisms[9,30] responsible for CRT benefit. Interventricular dyssynchrony, though simpler to determine, appears to be a nonspecific predictor of CRT response.[31]

Furthermore, as in the case of predictors of acute improvement in LV performance (See Table 2.1 on page 20), the investigators relied, except in rare reports,[69,78] on single echocardiographic parameters to identify predictors of response in a relatively small number of highly select patients evaluated at single centers. Given the potential limitations of echocardiographic assessment of LV dyssynchrony,[31] plus the ultimate clinical meaning of dyssynchrony,[79] the shortcomings of the reported results (Table 2.2) call for a reassessment of the methods used to identify CRT response. The Predictors of Response to CRT (PROSPECT) trial was designed to answer some of these issues.[80] The study prospectively tested whether published parameters of mechanical dyssynchrony can identify patients who improve with CRT. While some parameters predicted statistically significant improvement in LV performance ($\geq$15% increase in LVESV), sensitivity and specificities were only modest. Moreover, and perhaps more important, interobserver variability for TDI and M-mode measures of dyssynchrony were quite high, thus precluding their predictive capability. Additional work is required before any of the echocardiographic parameters, alone or in combination,[69,78] can be recommended to improve patient selection for CRT.

IMPROVEMENT IN LEFT VENTRICULAR DIASTOLIC PERFORMANCE WITH CRT

Diastolic dysfunction contributes significantly to morbidity and mortality of patients with systolic HF.[81,82] There has been a greater focus on the effect of CRT on LV systolic performance, but the benefit of CRT also extends to LV diastolic performance.[7–9,11,23,28,65,83–85] Accumulating evidence indicates overall outcome of CRT-treated HF patients depends to some extent on concomitant improvement of diastolic LV performance.[9,65,83–89] Indeed some have proposed that the reduction of diastolic ventricular interaction with CRT may be the dominant mechanism by which LV pacing improves LV systolic performance in patients with chronic HF.[9,86,87] This explanation has considerable merit given that LV pacing alone, whereby arguably there is no "resynchronization" of opposing LV segments, is in most cases as effective as biventricular pacing in terms of hemodynamic benefit.[32,34,36,39,45,86–89] A thorough discussion of diastolic dysfunction and its evaluation is beyond the scope of this chapter, but is available elsewhere.[90] Briefly, assessment of diastolic function reported in any setting, including following CRT, rests on the following two broad categories: LV filling and LV relaxation. CRT seems to consistently increase diastolic filling,[7–9,42,64,65]

LV diastolic function (increased LV filling and lowered LV filling pressure) after CRT were closely coupled to improvements in systolic performance[91] and pulse-wave Doppler (PWD) determined LV filling characteristics prior to CRT.[92] In a study involving 50 patients with chronic HF, only those patients whose LVEF increased by >5% (responders, 56%) after CRT demonstrated improvements in diastolic function. Moreover, LV relaxation remained either unchanged or worsened regardless of the LVEF response after CRT.[91] The same investigators also showed that improvements in LV diastolic performance only occurred in patients with pre-CRT mitral E/A ratio >1.0.[92] Others have shown reversal of abnormal, restrictive filling pattern with CRT, which in turn portends favorable prognosis.[83] Such observations are important considering the close relationship between the presence[93] and resolution[94] of restrictive filling pattern and prognosis of medically treated HF patients.

The extent of myocardial viability, an important determinant of improvement in LV systolic performance,[41, 55, 75, 76] also seems to play a role in LV diastolic function. Hummel et al.[55] reported a close link between myocardial perfusion score index (a measure of extent of viability) and early diastolic LV relaxation (r = 0.50, p <0.05) and global myocardial performance (r = 0.63, p = 0.003), both acutely and after 6 months of CRT. The fact that these findings occurred acutely, before any significant LV remodeling, suggest that they were secondary to improvement in LV systolic performance, in agreement with the findings by other investigators.[91]

We are also beginning to understand the role of diastolic asynchrony and its correction (resynchronization) with CRT on patient outcome. Schuster et al. identified LV diastolic asynchrony, defined as the time difference between the shortest and longest electromechanical delay (timed based on onset of diastolic E-wave relative to QRS), in a third of patients with systolic HF.[95] CRT resulted in a greater decrease in LV systolic asynchrony (71% to 33%, p <0.0001) than in diastolic asynchrony (81% to 55%, p <0.0002). The authors concluded that

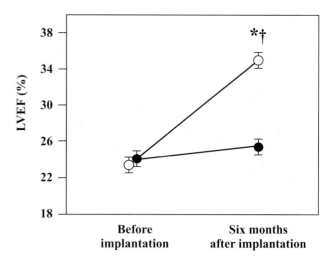

FIG. 2.5. Left ventricular ejection fraction (LVEF) at baseline and after six months in patients with a septal-to-posterior wall motion delay (SPWMD) of 130 ms **(open circles)** and < 130 ms **(closed circles)**. Date expressed as mean values ±SEM. *p < 0.05 vs. baseline; †p <0.05 vs. patients with an SPWMD of <130ms. (Reprinted with permission from Pitzalis et al. Ventricular Asynchrony Predicts a Better Outcome in Patients with Chronic Heart Failure Receiving Cardiac Resynchronization Therapy. *J Am Coll Cardiol.* 2005 (45) 1:68.)

persistent (i.e., incomplete reduction) in diastolic asynchrony might explain lack of response to CRT despite apparent systolic resynchronization.[95]

LEFT VENTRICULAR PERFORMANCE IN SPECIAL CATEGORIES

The previous comments and much of the data on the overall benefit of CRT pertain to those patients with cardiomyopathy (LVEF ≤35%) and other established criteria: normal sinus

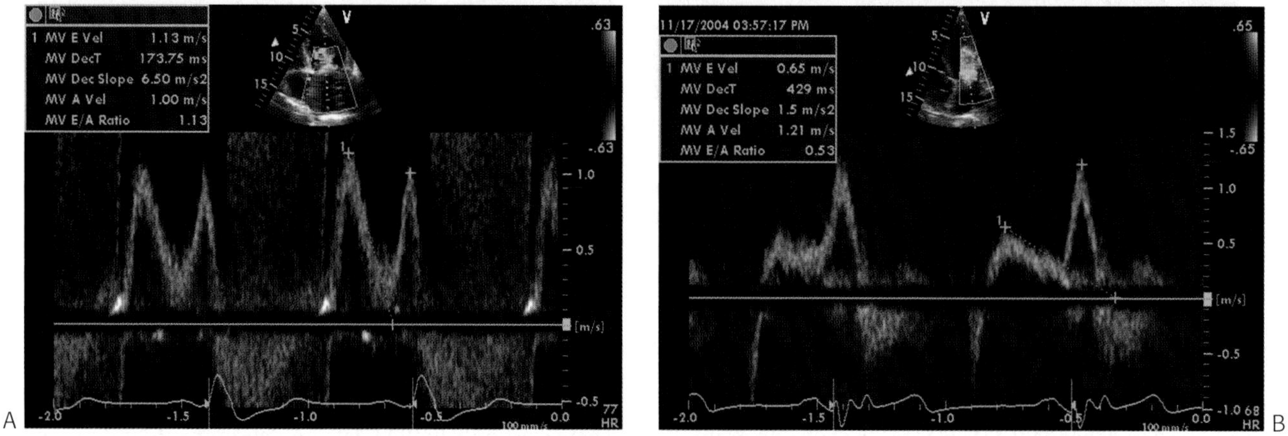

FIG. 2.6. Pulse-wave Doppler images depicting significant improvement in LV diastolic function (reduced E:A ratio and longer E-wave deceleration time) from baseline (A) to 6 months after CRT (B). Results were obtained from patient shown in Figure 2.4.

CRT.[129] In a
lation, chron
chrony in 33
post-pacing
velop dyssyn
and LV volur
nificant dete
p <0.001) ar
p <0.001). /
grade showe
ment in LV
responders (
itive change
tion) among
150 ms. Alth
LVEF along v
tricular dyss
identify any
line demogra
eral randomi
of biventricu
quire RV pac

SUMMAR

CRT has bee
diastolic per
some cases,
factors have
dictors of, or
performance
provement d
in LV perfor
tion of such
who are mos
been identifie
diographic p
applicable ir
need for sim
identify patie
LV performa

PRACTI

1. CRT ha
   improv
   perforn
   by retir
   wall seg
2. Improv
   terms o
   volume
   import
   patient

rhythm, NYHA class III and IV HF, nonpaced QRS >120 ms. However, CRT has been applied and evaluated, albeit in far fewer patients, in other groups. Since the results may not be applicable to those with traditional indications for CRT, we will briefly explore the role of CRT on LV performance of some of these other patient groups.

Patients with Atrial Fibrillation

Atrial fibrillation (AF) and HF often coexist and AF prevalence increases with the severity of HF.[96] The development of AF in HF patients is associated with increased morbidity and mortality.[96–98] There exists limited data on the impact of CRT in HF patients with AF, in terms of both functional and LV performance improvement. Except for a relatively small, randomized crossover substudy of the MUSTIC trial,[99] which did not analyze LV performance, all other randomized CRT trials were restricted to patients in sinus rhythm.[12] Although CRT does not appear to reduce the incidence of AF, the development of AF in CRT-treated patients does not preclude improved patient outcome.[100] In nonrandomized studies, CRT seems to equally improve LV systolic (and in some cases diastolic) performance in patients with AF versus sinus rhythm both acutely[101–102] and long term,[103–105] provided there is adequate ventricular rate control and consistent LV pacing. [60, 106]

In a large observational study, Gasparini et al.[60] compared the outcome, including changes in LV performance, of 162 patients with permanent AF and 511 patients with sinus rhythm treated with CRT—with emphasis on the importance of atrioventricular (AV) junction ablation on the AF patients (performed in those who failed to achieve >85% biventricular pacing with drug therapy). Both groups experienced significant and sustained (up to 4 years) improvement in LVEF and reduction in LVESV after CRT. The proportion of responders (≥10% reduction in LVESV from baseline) to CRT at one year was similar for both groups (sinus rhythm 69% versus AF 60%). Within the AF group, however, only the ablated group (114 of 162, 70%) showed a significant increase in LVEF and reduction in LVESV over the follow-up period.[60] The authors attributed the results to consistent and predictable biventricular pacing achieved with AV junction ablation, a plausible explanation given the harmful effects of rate irregularity[106] and interruption of LV pacing.[11, 42] AV junction ablation was not allocated randomly and, therefore, whether or not *all* patients with AF who require CRT based on established criteria should undergo AV junction ablation (to facilitate consistent LV capture) requires randomized trials. Interestingly, like patients with sinus rhythm, correction of LV dyssynchrony created by RV pacing in ablated patients with AF[107] may explain improvement in LV performance in such patients.

Patients with Mild Heart Failure

The fact that CRT improves LV performance in patients with advanced (NYHA class III and IV) HF is well established.[7–8, 12] Since asymptomatic (NYHA class I) or mildly symptomatic

patients (NYHA class II) with LV systolic dysfunction often become symptomatic over time despite optimal medical therapy, the role of (prophylactic) CRT is clinically relevant. To date only two CRT trials,[108, 109] involving patients with LVEF ≤35%, QRS >120–130 ms, and class I indications for defibrillator therapy, have included NYHA class I and II patients. In the Contak CD trial, Higgins et al.[108] found that CRT resulted in significant reduction in LV dimensions but no improvement in LVEF in Class I and Class II patients. On the other hand, in the randomized MIRACLE-ICD II trial involving 186 patients, Abraham et al. reported a significant increase in LVEF plus parallel reductions in LV dimensions after six months of CRT.[109] Neither study evaluated predictors of improvement in LV performance.[108–109] The impact of prophylactic CRT on overall mortality (and LV performance) of patients with no symptoms or mild symptoms of HF is currently being evaluated in a large (nearly 2,000 patient) prospective, randomized trial (MADIT CRT).

Patients with Narrow QRS Duration

Only about a third of patients with systolic HF have QRS duration >120 ms,[110] currently the cutoff for CRT prescription. This combined with the fact that QRS duration is a weak indicator of the presence of mechanical LV dyssynchrony,[111–114] and the close link between extent of dyssynchrony and CRT response[14, 21, 22, 47–51, 65–69] have led to a great interest in the role of CRT in patients with narrow QRS. Very little is known about the acute effect of CRT on hemodynamic variables in patients with narrow QRS. In a small study involving 20 patients, temporary LV pacing resulted in an increase in cardiac output and a decrease in pulmonary capillary wedge pressure (PCWP) only in patients (n = 10) with baseline PCWP >15 mmHg.[58] The authors attributed this response to a reduction in diastolic ventricular interaction present in those with PCWP >15 mmHg but not in those with PCWP <15 mmHg, a mechanism similar in patients with wide QRS durations.[9.]

As for long-term outcome, in nonrandomized, single-center studies,[115,116] CRT has been shown to significantly improve LV performance in patients with QRS <120 ms and intraventricular dyssynchrony on TDI. Yu et al.[115] reported that a similar response (>15% reduction in LVESV rate) (45% vs. 63%, p = 0.07) to CRT in patients with narrow QRS and a second group of patients with QRS >120 ms and similar clinical characteristics. Moreover, they found a close relationship between baseline asynchrony index and reduction in LVESV after 6 months of CRT, and by multivariate analysis, asynchrony index was the only independent predictor of LV reverse remodeling in both patient groups.[115] A cutoff value of 32.7 ms, remarkably similar for both groups, predicted response with similar sensitivities (96% and 97%) and specificities (82% and 84%). Interestingly, as previously observed,[42] when pacing was withheld for 4 weeks, the improvements in LV performance (increase in LVEF and reduction in LVESV) disappeared equally in both groups.[115]

18. Reuter S, Garrigue S, Barold SS, et al. Comparison of characteristics in responders versus nonresponders with biventricular pacing for drug-resistant congestive heart failure. *Am J Cardiol*. 2002;89:346–350.

19. Alonso C, Leqlercq C, Victor F, et al. Electrocardiographic predictive factors of long-term clinical improvement with multisite pacing in advanced heart failure. *Am J Cardiol*. 1999;84:1417–1421.

20. Sogaard P, Egeblad H, Kim WY, et al. Tissue Doppler imaging predicts improved systolic performance and reversed left ventricular remodeling during long-term cardiac resynchronization therapy. *J Am Coll Cardiol*. 2002;40:723–730.

21. Bax JJ, Bleeker GB, Marwick TH, et al. Left ventricular dyssynchrony predicts response and prognosis after cardiac resynchronization therapy. *J Am Coll Cardiol*. 2004;44:1834–1840.

22. Pitzalis MV, Iacoviello M, Romito R, et al. Ventricular asynchrony predicts a better outcome in patients with chronic heart failure receiving cardiac resynchronization therapy. *J Am Coll Cardiol*. 2005;45:65–69.

23. Yu CM, Fung JWH, Chan CK, et al. Comparison of efficacy of reverse remodeling and clinical improvement for relatively narrow and wide QRS complexes after cardiac resynchronization therapy for heart failure. *J Cardiovasc Electrophysiol*. 2004;15:1058–1065.

24. Bleeker GB, Bax JJ, Fung JWH, et al. Clinical versus echocardiographic parameters to assess response to cardiac resynchronization therapy. *Am J Cardiol*. 2006;97:260–263.

25. Davis DR, Krahn AD, Tang AS, et al. Long-term outcome of cardiac resynchronization therapy in patients with severe congestive heart failure. *Can J Cardiol*. 2005;21:413–417.

26. Yu CM, Bleeker GB, Fung JWH, et al. Left ventricular reverse remodeling but not clinical improvement predicts long-term survival after cardiac resynchronization therapy. *Circulation*. 2005;112:1580–1586.

27. Donal E, Vignat N, De Place C, et al. Acute effects of biventricular pacing on right ventricular function assessed by tissue Doppler imaging. *Europace*. 2007;9:108–112.

28. Kerwin WF, Botvinick EH, O'Connell JW, et al. Ventricular contraction abnormalities in dilated cardiomyopathy: effect of biventricular pacing to correct interventricular dyssynchrony. *J Am Coll Cardiol*. 2000;35:1221–1227.

29. Toussaint JP, Lavergne T, Kerrou K, et al. Basal asynchrony and resynchronization with biventricular pacing predict long-term improvement of LV function in heart failure patients. *PACE*. 2003;26:1815–1823.

30. Tedrow UB, Kramer DB, Stevenson LW, et al. Relation of right ventricular peak systolic pressure to major adverse events in patients undergoing cardiac resynchronization therapy. *Am J Cardiol*. 2006;97:1737–1740.

31. Gorcsan J III, Abraham T, Agler DA, et al. Echocardiography for cardiac resynchronization therapy: Recommendations for performance and reporting—a report from the American Society of Echocardiography Dyssynchrony Writing Group. *J Am Soc Echo*. 2008;21:191–213.

32. Auricchio A, Stellbrink C, Sack S, et al. Long-term clinical effect of hemodynamically optimized cardiac resynchronization therapy in patients with heart failure and ventricular conduction delay. *J Am Coll Cardiol*. 2002;39:2026–2033.

33. Auricchio A, Stellbrink C, Block M, et al. Effect of pacing chamber and atrioventricular delay on acute systolic function of paced patients with congestive heart failure: the PATH-CHF Study group. *Circulation*. 1999;99:2993–3001.

34. Kass DA, Chen CH, Curry C, et al. Improved left ventricular mechanics from acute VDD pacing in patients with dilated cardiomyopathy and ventricular conduction delay. *Circulation*. 1999;99:1567–1573.

35. Auricchio A, Ding J, Spinelli JC, et al. Cardiac resynchronization therapy restores optimal atrioventricular mechanical timing in heart failure patients with ventricular conduction delay. *J Am Coll Cardiol*. 2002;39:1163–1169.

36. Breithardt OA, Stellbrink C, Franke A, et al. Acute effects of cardiac resynchronization therapy on left ventricular Doppler indices in patients with congestive heart failure. *Am Heart J*. 2002;143:34–44.

37. Ukkonen H, Beanlands RS, Burwash IG, et al. Effect of cardiac resynchronization on myocardial efficiency and regional oxidative metabolism. *Circulation*. 2003;107:28–31.

38. Nelson GS, Berger RD, Fetics BJ, et al. Left ventricular or biventricular pacing improves cardiac function at diminished energy cost in patients with dilated cardiomyopathy and left bundle-branch block. *Circulation*. 2000;102:3053–3059.

39. O'Connor CM, Gattis WA, Uretsky BF, et al. Continuous intravenous dobutamine is associated with an increased risk of death in patients with advanced heart failure: insights from the Flolan International Randomized Survival Trial (FIRST). *Am Heart J*. 1999;138:78–86.

40. Packer M, Carver JR, Rodeheffer RJ, et al. Effect of oral milrinone on mortality in severe chronic heart failure: PROMISE Study Research Group. *N Engl J Med*. 1991;325:1468–1475.

41. Da Costa A, Thevenin J, Roche F, et al. Prospective validation of stress echocardiography as an identifier of cardiac resynchronization therapy responders. *Heart Rhythm*. 2006;3:406–413.

42. Yu CM, Chau E, Sanderson JE, et al. Tissue Doppler echocardiographic evidence of reverse remodeling and improved synchronicity by simultaneously delaying regional contraction after biventricular pacing therapy in heart failure. *Circulation* 2002;105:438–445.

43. Dizon J, Horn E, Neglia J, et al. Loss of left bundle branch block following biventricular pacing therapy for heart failure: Evidence for electrical remodeling? *J Interv Card Electrophysiol*. 2004;10:47–50.

44. Sundell J, Engblom E, Koistinen J, et al. The effects of cardiac resynchronization therapy on left ventricular function, myocardial energetic, and metabolic reserve in patients with dilated cardiomyopathy and heart failure. *J Am Coll Cardiol*. 2004;43:1027–1033.

45. Nelson GS, Curry CW, Wyman BT, et al. Predictors of systolic augmentation from left ventricular preexcitation in patients with dilated cardiomyopathy and intraventricular conduction delay. *Circulation*. 2000;101:2703–2709.

46. Sogaard P, Kim WY, Jensen HK, et al. Impact of acute biventricular pacing on left ventricular performance and volumes in patients with severe heart failure. *Cardiology*. 2001;95:173–182.

47. Bax JJ, Marwick TH, Molhoek SG, et al. Left ventricular dyssynchrony predicts benefit of cardiac resynchronization therapy in patients with end-stage heart failure before pacemaker implantation. *Am J Cardiol*. 2003;92:1238–1240.

48. Gorcsan JIII, Kanzaki H, Bazaz R, et al. Usefulness of echocardiographic tissue synchronization imaging to predict acute response to cardiac resynchronization therapy. *Am J Cardiol*. 2004;93:1178–1181.

49. Dohi K, Suffoletto MS, Schwartzman D, et al. Utility of echocardiographic radial strain to quantify left ventricular dyssynchrony and predict acute response to cardiac resynchronization therapy. *Am J Cardiol*. 2005;96:112–116.

50. Breithardt OA, Stellbrink C, Kramer AP, et al. Echocardiographic quantification of left ventricular asynchrony predicts an acute hemodynamic benefit of cardiac resynchronization therapy. *J Am Coll Cardiol*. 2002;40:536–545.

51. Suffoletto MS, Dohi K, Canneson M, et al. Novel speckle-tracking radial strain from routine black-and-white echocardiographic images to quantify dyssynchrony and predict response to cardiac resynchronization therapy. *Circulation*. 2006;113:960–968.

52. Butter C, Auricchio A, Stellbrink C, et al. Effect of resynchronization therapy stimulation site on the systolic function of heart failure patients. *Circulation*. 2001;104:3026–3029.

53. Ansalone G, Giannantoni P, Ricci R, et al. Doppler myocardial imaging to evaluate the effectiveness of pacing sites in patients receiving biventricular pacing. *J Am Coll Cardiol*. 2002;39:489–499.

54. Helm RH, Leclercq C, Faris OP, et al. Cardiac dyssynchrony analysis using circumferential versus longitudinal strain: implications for assessing cardiac resynchronization. *Circulation*. 2005;111:2760–2767.

55. Hummel JP, Lindner JR, Becik JT, et al. Extent of myocardial viability predicts response to biventricular pacing in ischemic cardiomyopathy. *Heart Rhythm*. 2005;2:1211–1217.

56. Van Gelder BM, Janssen AH, Bracke FA, et al. Electrophysiological and hemodynamic consequences of myocardial scar tissue in cardiac resynchronization therapy. *Heart Rhythm*. 2006;3: S24.

57. Heist EK, Taub C, Fan D, et al. Usefulness of a novel "response score" to predict hemodynamic and clinical outcome from cardiac resynchronization therapy. *Am J Cardiol*. 2006;97:1732–1736.

58. Kim WY, Sogaard P, Mortensen PT, et al. Three dimensional echocardiography documents haemodynamic improvement by biventricular pacing in patients with severe heart failure. *Heart*. 2001;85:514–520.

59. Oguz E, Dgdeviren B, Bilsel T, et al. Echocardiographic prediction of long-term response to biventricular pacemaker in severe heart failure. *Eur J Heart Fail*. 2001;4:83–90.

60. Gasparini M, Auricchio A, Regoli F, et al. Four-year efficacy of cardiac resynchronization therapy on exercise tolerance and disease progression: the importance of performing atrioventricular junction ablation in patients with atrial fibrillation. *J Am Coll Cardiol*. 2006;48:734–743.

In an
group),
was note
substanti
was obse
Yu et al.[1]
chrony a
of CRT.[1]

Despi
lead to i
other pa
mension
and QRS
to date.[1]
chemic o
toward a
a subgr
consider
ipated su
results b
domized
measure:
the issue

Patient

Long-ter
with dete
clinical
pacing (
LBBB,[12]
duration

TABL

Acute Pe

QRS ≥15
dP/dt$_{max}$<
≤700
Extent of
dyssyn
Separatio
LV lead e

LV, left ven
* Factors v
† In genera

61. Cappola TP, Harsch MR, Jessup M, et al. Predictors of remodeling in the CRT era: influence of mitral regurgitation, BNP, and gender. *J Card Fail.* 2006;12:182–188.

62. Mangiavacchi M, Gasparini M, Faletra F, et al. Clinical predictors of marked improvement in left ventricular performance after cardiac resynchronization therapy in patients with chronic heart failure. *Am Heart J.* 2006;151:477–482.

63. Kapetanakis S, Kearny MT, Silva A, et al. Real-time three-dimensional echocardiography: a novel technique to quantify global left ventricular mechanical dyssynchrony. *Circulation.* 2005;112:992–1000.

64. Yu CM, Fung WH, Lin H, et al. Predictors of left ventricular reverse remodeling after cardiac resynchronization therapy for heart failure secondary to idiopathic or ischemic cardiomyopathy. *Am J Cardiol.* 2002;91:684–688.

65. Penicka M, Bartunek J, De Bruyne B, et al. Improvement of left ventricular function after cardiac resynchronization therapy is predicted by tissue Doppler imaging echocardiography. *Circulation.* 2004;109:978–983.

66. Yu CM, Zhang Q, Fung JWH, et al. A novel tool to assess systolic asynchrony and identify responders of cardiac resynchronization therapy by synchronization imaging. *J Am Coll Cardiol.* 2005;45:677–684.

67. Notobartolo D, Merlino JD, Smith AL, et al. Usefulness of the peak velocity difference by tissue Doppler imaging technique as an effective predictor of response to cardiac resynchronization therapy. *Am J Cardiol.* 2004;94:817–820.

68. Van de Veire NR, Bleeker GB, De Sutter J, et al. Tissue synchronization imaging accurately measures left ventricular dyssynchrony and predicts response to cardiac resynchronization therapy. *Heart.* 2007; 93:1034–1039.

69. Gorcsan J III, Tanabe M, Bleeker GB, et al. Combined longitudinal and radial dyssynchrony predicts ventricular response after resynchronization therapy. *J Am Coll Cardiol.* 2007;50:1476–1483.

70. Ghali JK, Krause-Steinrauf HJ, Adams KF, et al. Gender differences in advanced heart failure: insights from the BEST study. *J Am Coll Cardiol.* 2003;42:2128–2134.

71. Shelman KA, Lindenfeld JA, Lowes BD, et al. Predicting response to carvedilol for the treatment of heart failure: a multivariate retrospective analysis. *J Card Fail.* 2001;7:4–12.

72. Sutton MG, Plappert T, Hilpisch KE, et al. Sustained reverse left ventricular structural remodeling with cardiac resynchronization at one year is a function of etiology: quantitative Doppler echocardiographic evidence from the MIRACLE trial. *Circulation.* 2006;113:266–272.

73. Yeim S, Bordachar P, Reuter S, et al. Predictors of a positive response to biventricular pacing in patients with severe heart failure and ventricular conduction delay. *PACE.* 2007;30:970–975.

74. Bleeker GB, Kaandorp TA, Lamb HJ, et al. Effect of posterolateral scar tissue on clinical and echocardiographic improvement after cardiac resynchronization therapy. *Circulation.* 2006;113:969–976.

75. Adelstein EC, Saba S. Scar burden by myocardial perfusion imaging predicts echocardiographic response to cardiac resynchronization therapy in ischemic cardiomyopathy. *Am Heart J.* 2007;153:105–112.

76. Ypenburg C, Schalij MJ, Bleeker GB, et al. Impact of viability and scar tissue on response to cardiac resynchronization therapy in ischemic heart failure patients. *Eur Heart J.* 2007;28:33–41.

77. Arzola-Castaner D, Taub C, Heist EK, et al. Left ventricular lead proximity to an akinetic segment and impact on outcome of cardiac resynchronization therapy. *J Cardiovasc Electrophysiol.* 2006;17:623–627.

78. Yu CM, Fung JWH, Zhang Q, et al. Tissue Doppler imaging is superior to strain rate imaging and postsystolic shortening on the prediction of reverse remodeling in both ischemic and nonischemic heart failure after cardiac resynchronization therapy. *Circulation.* 2004;110:66–73.

79. Kass DA. An epidemic of dyssynchrony: But what does it mean? *J Am Coll Cardiol.* 2008;51:12–17.

80. Chung E, Leon AR, Tavazzi L. Results of the Predictors of Response to CRT (PROSPECT) Trial. *Circulation.* 2008;17:2608–2616.

81. Vanoverschelde JJ, Raphael DA, Robert AR, et al. Left ventricular filling in dilated cardiomyopathy: relation to functional class and hemodynamics. *J Am Coll Cardiol.* 1990;15:1288–1295.

82. Rihal CS, Nishimura RA, Hatle LK, et al. Systolic and diastolic dysfunction in patients with clinical diagnosis of dilated cardiomyopathy: relation to symptoms and prognosis. *Circulation.* 1994;90: 2772–2779.

83. Porciani MC, Valsecchi S, Demarchi G, et al. Evolution and prognostic significance of diastolic filling in cardiac resynchronization therapy. *Intern J Cardiol.* 2006;112:322–328.

84. Agacdiken A, Vural A, Ural D, et al. Effect of cardiac resynchronization therapy on left ventricular diastolic filling pattern in responder and nonresponder patients. *PACE.* 2005;28:654–660.

85. Soliman OII, Theuns DA. MJ, ten Cate FJ, et al. Baseline predictors of cardiac events after cardiac resynchronization therapy in patients with heart failure secondary to ischemic or nonischemic etiology. *Am J Cardiol.* 2007;100:464–469.

86. Morris-Thurgood J, Turner M, Nightingale A, et al. Pacing in heart failure: improved ventricular interaction in diastole rather than systolic resynchronization. *Europace.* 2002;2:271–275.

87. Turner MS, Bleasdale RA, Mumford CE, et al. Left ventricular pacing improves haemodynamic variable in patients with heart failure with a normal QRS duration. *Heart.* 2004;90:502–505.

88. Touiza A, Etienne Y, Gilard M, et al. Long-term left ventricular pacing: assessment and comparison with biventricular pacing in patients with severe congestive heart failure. *J Am Coll Cardiol.* 2001;38: 1966–1970.

89. Leclercq C, Faris O, Tunin R, et al. Systolic improvement and mechanical resynchronization does not require electrical synchrony in the dilated failing heart with left bundle-branch block. *Circulation.* 2002; 106:1760–1763.

90. Lester SJ, Tajik AJ, Nishimura RA, et al. Unlocking the mysteries of diastolic function: deciphering the Rosetta Stone 10 years later. *J Am Coll Cardiol.* 2008;51:679–689.

91. Waggoner AD, Faddis MN, Gleva MJ, et al. Improvements in left ventricular diastolic function after cardiac resynchronization therapy are coupled to response in systolic performance. *J Am Coll Cardiol.* 2005; 46:2244–2249.

92. Waggoner AD, Faddis MN, Gleva MJ, et al. Cardiac resynchronization therapy acutely improves diastolic function. *J Am Soc Echocardiogr.* 2005;18:216–220.

93. Pinamonti B, Di Lenarda A, Sinagra G, et al. Restrictive left ventricular filling pattern in dilated cardiomyopathy assessed by Doppler echocardiography: clinical, echocardiographic and hemodynamic correlations and prognostic implications. *J Am Coll Cardiol.* 1993;22: 808–815.

94. Pinamonti B, Zecchin M, DiLenarda A, et al. Persistence of restrictive left ventricular filling pattern in dilated cardiomyopathy: an ominous prognostic sign. *J Am Coll Cardiol.* 1997;29:604–612.

95. Schuster I, Habib G, Jego C, et al. Diastolic asynchrony is more frequent than systolic asynchrony in dilated cardiomyopathy and is less improved by cardiac resynchronization therapy. *J Am Coll Cardiol.* 2005; 46:2250–2257.

96. Maisel WH, Stevenson LW. Atrial fibrillation in heart failure: epidemiology, pathophysiology, and rationale for therapy. *Am Heart J.* 2003;91: 2D–8D.

97. Wang TJ, Larson MG, Levy D, et al. Temporal relations of atrial fibrillation and congestive heart failure and their joint influence on mortality: the Framingham Heart Study. *Circulation.* 2003;107:2920–2925.

98. Dries DL, Exner DV, Gersh BJ, et al. Atrial fibrillation is associated with an increased risk for mortality and heart failure progression in patients with asymptomatic and symptomatic left ventricular dysfunction: a retrospective analysis of the SOLVD trials. *J Am Coll Cardiol.* 1998;32: 695–703.

99. Leclercq C, Walker S, Linde C, et al. Comparative effects of permanent biventricular and right-univentricular pacing in heart failure patients with chronic atrial fibrillation. *Eur Heart J.* 2002;23:1780–1787.

100. Hope UC, Casares JM, Eiskjaer H, et al. Effect of cardiac resynchronization on the incidence of atrial fibrillation in patients with severe heart failure. *Circulation.* 2006;144:18–25.

101. Etienne Y, Mansourati J, Gilard M, et al. Evaluation of left ventricular based pacing in patients with congestive heart failure and atrial fibrillation. *Am J Cardiol.* 1999;83:1138–1140.

102. Garrigue S, Bordachar P, Reuter S, et al. Comparison of permanent left ventricular and biventricular pacing in patients with heart failure and chronic atrial fibrillation. *Card Electrophysiol Rev.* 2003;7: 315–324.

103. Hay I, Melenovsky V, Fetics BJ, et al. Short-term effects of right-left heart sequential cardiac resynchronization in patients with heart failure, chronic atrial fibrillation, and atrioventricular nodal block. *Circulation.* 2004;110:3404–3410.

104. Molhoek SG, Bax JJ, Bleeker GB, et al. Comparison of response to cardiac resynchronization therapy in patients with sinus rhythm versus atrial fibrillation. *Am J Cardiol.* 2004;94:1506–1509.

105. Delnoy PP, Ottervanger JP, Luttikhuis HO, et al. Comparison of usefulness of cardiac resynchronization therapy in patients with atrial fibrillation and heart failure versus patients with sinus rhythm and heart failure. *Am J Cardiol.* 2007;99:1252–1257.

106. Melenovsky V, Hay I, Fetics BJ, et al. Functional impact of rate irregularity in patients with heart failure and atrial fibrillation receiving cardiac resynchronization therapy. *Eu Heart J.* 2005;26:705–711.

107. Tops LF, Schalij MJ, Holman ER, et al. Right ventricular pacing can induce ventricular dyssynchrony in patients with atrial fibrillation after atrioventricular node ablation. *J Am Coll Cardiol.* 2006;48:1642–1648.

108. Higgins SL, Hummel JD, Niazi IK, et el. Cardiac resynchronization therapy for the treatment of heart failure in patients with intraventricular conduction delay and malignant ventricular tachyarrhythmias. *J Am Coll Cardiol.* 2003;42:1454–1459.

109. Abraham WT, Young JB, Leon AR, et al. Effects of cardiac resynchronization on disease progression in patients with left ventricular systolic dysfunction, an indication for implantable cardioverter-defibrillator, and mildly symptomatic chronic heart failure. *Circulation.* 2004;110:2864–2868.

110. Aaronson KD, Schwartz JS, Chen TM, et al. Development and prospective validation of a clinical index to predict survival in ambulatory patients referred for cardiac transplant evaluation. *Circulation.* 1997;95:2660–2667.

111. Yu CM, Lin H, Zhang Q, et al. High prevalence of left ventricular systolic asynchrony and diastolic asynchrony in patients with normal QRS duration. *Heart.* 2003;89:54–60.

112. Ghio S, Constantin C, Klersy C, et al. Interventricular and intraventricular dyssynchrony are common in heart failure patients, regardless of QRS duration. *Eur Heart J.* 2004;25:571–578.

113. Fauchier L, Marie O, Casset-Senson D, et al. Reliability of QRS duration and morphology on surface electrocardiogram to identify ventricular dyssynchrony in patients with idiopathic dilated cardiomyopathy. *Am J Cardiol.* 2003;92:341–344.

114. Turner MS, Bleasdale RA, Vinereaunu D, et al. Electrical and mechanical components of dyssynchrony in heart failure patients with normal QRS duration and left bundle-branch block: impact of left biventricular pacing. *Circulation.* 2004;109:2544–2549.

115. Yu CM, Chan YS, Zhang Q, et al. Benefits of cardiac resynchronization therapy for heart failure patients with narrow QRS complexes and coexisting systolic asynchrony by echocardiography. *J Am Coll Cardiol.* 2006;48:2251–2257.

116. Bleeker GB, Holman ER, Steendijk P, et al. Cardiac resynchronization therapy in patients with a narrow QRS complex. *J Am Cardiol.* 2006;48:2243–2250.

117. Beshai J, Grimm RA, Nagueh SF, et al. Cardiac-resynchronization therapy in heart failure with narrow QRS complexes. *N Engl J Med.* 2007;357:2461–2471.

118. Willkoff BL, Cook JR, Epstein AE, et al. Dual-chamber pacing or ventricular backup pacing in patients with an implantable defibrillator: the DAVID Trial. *JAMA.* 2002;288:3115–3123.

119. Sweeney MO, Helkamp AS, Ellenbogen KA. Adverse effects of ventricular pacing on heart failure and atrial fibrillation among patients with a normal baseline QRS duration in a clinical trial of pace-maker therapy for sinus node dysfunction. *Circulation.* 2003;107:2932–2937.

120. Sukhija R, Aronow WS, Sorbera C, et al. Mortality, left ventricular ejection fraction, and prevalence of new left ventricular wall motion abnormality at long-term follow-up in patients with implantable defibrillators treated with biventricular versus right ventricular pacing. *Am J Therapeutics.* 2007;14:328–330.

121. Little WC, Reeves RC, Arciniegas J, et al. Mechanism of abnormal interventricular septal motion during delayed left ventricular activation. *Circulation.* 1982;65:1486–1491.

122. Rosenqvist M, Brandt J, Schuller H. Long term pacing in sinus node disease: effects of stimulation mode on cardiovascular morbidity and mortality. *Am Heart J.* 1988;116:16–22.

123. Bordachar P, Garrigue S, Lafitte S, et al. Interventricular and intra-left ventricular electromechanical delays in right ventricular paced patients with heart failure: implications for upgrading to biventricular stimulation. *Heart.* 2003;89:1401–1405.

124. Horwich T, Foster E, De Marco T, et al. Effects of resynchronization therapy on cardiac function in pacemaker patients "upgraded" to biventricular devices. *J Cardiovasc Electrophysiol.* 2004;15:1284–1289.

125. Valls-Bertault V, Fatemi M, Gilard M, et al. Assessment of upgrading to biventricular pacing in patients with right ventricular pacing and congestive heart failure after atrioventricular junctional ablation for chronic atrial fibrillation. *Europace.* 2004;6:438–443.

126. Baker CM, Christopher TJ, Smith PF, et al. Addition of a left ventricular lead to conventional pacing systems in patients with congestive heart failure. *PACE.* 2002;25:1166–1171.

127. Leon AR, Greenberg JM, Kanuru N, et al. Cardiac resynchronization in patients with congestive heart failure and chronic atrial fibrillation: effect of upgrading to biventricular pacing after chronic right ventricular pacing. *J Am Colll Cardiol.* 200239:1258–1263.

128. Eldadah ZA, Rosen B, Hay I, et al. The benefit of upgrading chronically right ventricle-paced heart failure patients to resynchronization therapy demonstrated by strain rate imaging. *Heart Rhythm.* 2006;3:435–442.

129. Wittte KKA, Pipes RR, Nanthakumar K, et al. Biventricular pacemaker upgrade in previously paced heart failure patients—Improvements in ventricular dyssynchrony. *J Card Fail.* 2006;12:199–204.

130. Laurenzi F, Achilli A, Avella A, et al. Biventricular upgrading in patients with conventional pacing system and congestive heart failure: results and response predictors. *PACE.* 2007;30:1096–1104.

131. Yannopoulos D, Lurie KG, Sakaguchi S, et al. Reduced atrial tachyarrhythmia susceptibility after upgrade of conventional implanted pulse generator to cardiac resynchronization therapy in patients with heart failure. *J Am Coll Cardiol.* 2007;50:1246–51.

132. Leclercq C, Cazeau S, Lellouche D, et al. Upgrading from single chamber right ventricular to biventricular pacing in permanently paced patients with worsening heart failure: the RD-CHF Study. *PACE.* 2007;30:S23–S30.

133. Lin G, Rea RF, Hammill SC, et al. Effect of cardiac resynchronization therapy on occurrence of ventricular arrhythmia in patients with implantable cardioverter defibrillators undergoing upgrade to cardiac resynchronization therapy devices. *Heart.* 2008;94:186–190.

134. Voigt A, Barrington W, Ngwu O, et al. Biventricular pacing reduces ventricular arrhythmic burden and defibrillator therapies in patients with heart failure. *Clin Cardiol.* 2006;29:74–77.

135. Tops LF, Suffoletto MS, Bleeker GB, et al. Speckle-tracking radial strain reveals left ventricular dyssynchrony in patients with permanent right ventricular pacing. *J Am Coll Cardiol.* 2007;50:1180–1188.

136. Fung JW, Chan JY, Omar R, et al. The Pacing to Avoid Cardiac Enlargement (PACE) trial: background, rationale, design, and implementation. *J Cardiovasc Electrophysiol.* 2007;18:735–739.

137. de Teresa E, Gomez-Doblas JJ, Lamas G, et al. Preventing ventricular dysfunction in pacemaker patients without advanced heart failure: rational and design of the PREVENT-HF study. *Europace* 2007;9:442–446.

138. Hamdan MH, Freedman RA, Gilbert EM, et al. Atrioventricular junction ablation followed by resynchronization therapy in patients with congestive heart failure and atrial fibrillation (AVERT-AF) study design. *PACE* 2006;29:1081–1088.

Importance of Left Ventricular Diastolic Function and Prediction of Clinical Outcomes Following Cardiac Resynchronization Therapy

Alan D. Waggoner • Lisa de las Fuentes • Victor G. Davila-Roman

Diastolic function is invariably impaired in patients with symptomatic heart failure (HF). In those with HF secondary to systolic dysfunction, left ventricular (LV) diastolic dysfunction is a major contributor to symptoms of heart failure and has been reported to predict long-term outcomes. Although cardiac resynchronization therapy (CRT) is directed at improvement in LV dyssynchrony and systolic function, its effects on diastolic function and whether diastolic function may be a predictor of clinical outcomes has been less well-characterized.[1–3] This chapter will review the results of studies that have evaluated LV diastolic function for patients treated with CRT immediately after device implant, and at early and intermediate follow-up after CRT. Furthermore, the authors discuss indices of LV diastolic function that predict clinical outcomes after CRT.

Diastolic Function in Heart Failure

Abnormalities in diastolic function are known to play a major role in symptoms of heart failure.[4] For example, increases in preload (i.e., increased LV end-diastolic volume and/or end-diastolic pressures) result in an upward shift of the diastolic pressure/volume relationship with reduced LV compliance (i.e., a "stiff" left ventricle). Decreased LV compliance in systolic heart failure is often due to myocardial fibrosis (i.e., a result of long-standing hypertension and hypertrophy) and/or myocardial scarring (resulting from prior myocardial infarction). Increased LV end-systolic volume alters elastic recoil and results in prolonged LV relaxation. Increased afterload (i.e., increased blood pressure and/or increased wall stress) due to LV dilatation, particularly in the absence of a compensatory increase in wall thickness (i.e., eccentric LV hypertrophy), may cause subendocardial ischemia, and the combination results in decreased LV contractility and prolongation of LV relaxation. Two additional issues play an important role in the systolic/diastolic interactions in candidates for CRT. First, the presence of abnormal ventricular conduction (i.e., left bundle branch block) causes discordant LV contractility, which further exacerbates LV systolic and diastolic performance. Second, increased left atrial volumes and impaired left atrial function play an important role in compromising diastolic function.[5]

Stages of LV Diastolic Dysfunction

One approach for staging the severity of LV diastolic dysfunction in HF patients with LV systolic dysfunction is based on patterns of LV diastolic filling determined by pulsed-wave Doppler mitral inflow velocities, as shown in Figure 3.1. It is important to recognize that mitral inflow velocities are influenced by the combined effects of changes in LV relaxation, instantaneous changes in left atrial and LV diastolic pressures, and LV compliance.[6,–7] Impaired relaxation is universally present in HF patients. Early diastolic LV filling pressures may be relatively normal in some patients with LV systolic dysfunction, but LV end-diastolic pressure is usually elevated. The pulsed-wave Doppler mitral inflow pattern of impaired relaxation in this setting demonstrates a low mitral E-wave velocity and E/A ratio, and prolonged deceleration time (DT). An intermediate stage of LV diastolic dysfunction, described as a "pseudonormalized pattern," occurs when early LV filling pressures are elevated and increases mitral E-wave velocity and the E/A ratio with normalization or shortening of DT. LV relaxation, however, typically remains abnormally prolonged. Restrictive LV filling in HF patients is a result of markedly increased LV filling pressures and the LVEDP. The mitral E-wave velocity and E/A ratio are increased, the A-wave velocity is diminished, and the mitral DT is shortened. Several studies have reported that these patterns of pulsed-wave Doppler-derived mitral inflow velocities predict clinical outcomes in patients with HF and LV systolic dysfunction.[8–13] The cumulative results of these studies indicate that a restrictive LV filling pattern is associated with higher morbidity and mortality, regardless of the impairment in LV systolic dysfunction (determined by the LV ejection fraction), compared

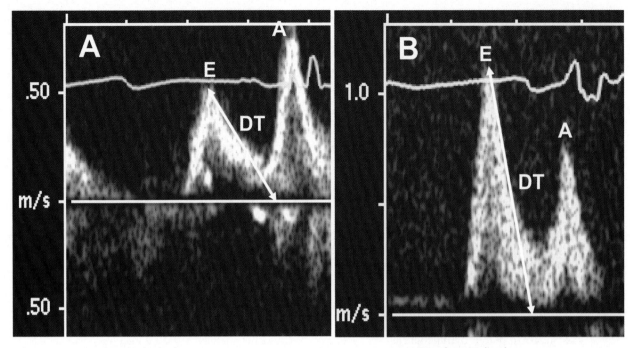

Impaired relaxtion   Pseudonormalized

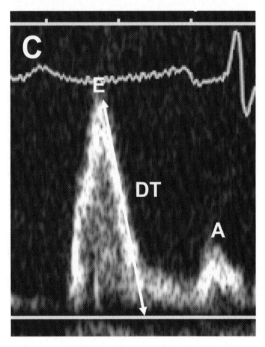

FIG. 3.1. Pulsed-wave Doppler left ventricular diastolic filling patterns of **(A)** impaired relaxation: mitral E/A velocity ratio is decreased (0.7), and deceleration time (DT) is prolonged (235 ms); **(B)** pseudonormalized filling: mitral E/A ratio is normal (1.5), but DT is 160 ms; **(C)** restrictive filling: the mitral E/A ratio is increased (2.8), and DT is 140 ms.

Restrictive

to patients with an impaired relaxation, or a "pseudonormalized" filling pattern.

Assessment by Tissue Doppler Imaging

Another method for assessing LV diastolic function includes tissue Doppler imaging (TDI) measurements of early diastolic mitral annular velocities (E') that are a relatively load-independent determinant of LV relaxation.[14] TDI measurements of E' are obtained by placement of a sample volume in the myocardial wall, adjacent or superior to the mitral annulus, in the apical four-chamber and two-chamber views as shown in Figure 3.2. Impaired LV relaxation results in a decrease in the E' velocity but is relatively unaffected by the changes in early LV filling pressure. Importantly, the ratio of the mitral E-wave/E' velocity at the lateral and/or at the

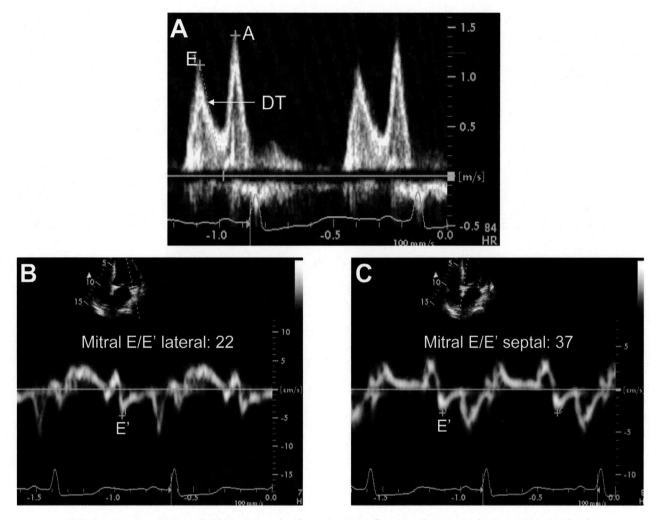

FIG. 3.2. Representative pulsed-wave Doppler-derived mitral inflow E and A-wave velocities, E/A ratio, deceleration time (DT), and diastolic filling time (DFT) in a patient with a nonischemic cardiomyopathy and severe LV systolic dysfunction prior to CRT (A). The mitral inflow pattern is consistent with pseudonormalized LV filling with a mitral DT of 109 ms. Tissue Doppler mitral annular early diastolic velocities (E') at the lateral (B) and septal base (C). The E' is decreased at both sites but mitral E/E' ratios are increased, consistent with impaired LV relaxation and elevated LV filling pressures, respectively.

septal annulus can be used to accurately estimate LV filling pressures.[15–16] As early LV filling pressures increase, with an accompanying increase in mitral E-wave velocity, E' remains low due to the underlying myocardial relaxation abnormality. One study reported that a reduced E' and a mitral E/E' ratio >20 provides incremental value to predict cardiac related events, in addition to mitral E-wave deceleration time.[17]

TDI-derived measurements of the timing of E' have been used to determine LV diastolic dyssynchrony in HF patients and the response to CRT.[18–20] Diastolic dyssynchrony is determined by measurements of the time from onset of the QRS to the onset, or to peak E' velocities, at several mitral annular sites (Fig. 3.3). The extent of diastolic dyssynchrony is expressed as the maximal difference of the time intervals between sites in the apical views. The maximal difference between individual LV segments in normal subjects is <40 ms.[19]

Acute Effects of CRT on LV Diastolic Function

Invasive studies performed at the time of device implant have shown variable effects of CRT on LV diastolic function. In separate single-center studies that included 41 patients (32% ischemic), pulmonary artery capillary wedge pressure and/or LV end-diastolic pressure (LVEDP) immediately after CRT decreased or remained relatively unchanged.[21–22] Another single center study reported that, in subjects with a high LVEDP, significant decreases can occur immediately after CRT; conversely, if LVEDP is normal, minimal or no changes are observed.[23] The programmed atrioventricular (AV) delay during CRT also affects LV diastolic function.[24–25] While relatively short programmed AV delays (i.e., <100 ms) decrease LVEDP, this reduction may occur at the expense of decreased stroke volume and cardiac output.[24, 26] These findings may be

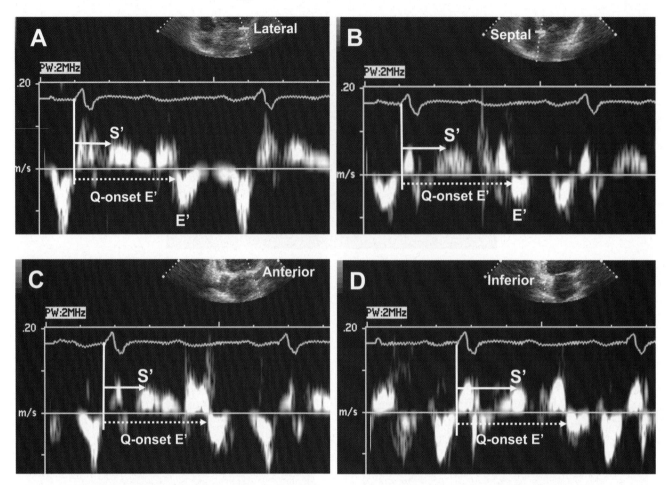

FIG. 3.3. Determination of LV systolic and diastolic dyssynchrony by tissue Doppler annular velocities recorded at the lateral **(A)**, septal **(B)**, anterior **(C)** and inferior **(D)** base. Measurements of the time intervals from Q-wave to peak systolic (S') velocity (solid line) and Q-wave to onset of early diastolic (E') velocity (dashed line) are shown at each site. The time from Q-peak S' is significantly longer at the inferior base; the time from Q-onset of E' is relatively similar between sites.

explained by the fact that patients with HF due to LV systolic dysfunction require increased LV filling pressures for optimal systolic performance.[1] Invasive studies have also shown that, despite significant increases in peak-positive LV dP/dt immediately after CRT, these are not accompanied by significant changes in LV relaxation, determined by peak-negative LV dP/dt or Tau (the time constant of LV relaxation).[27–29] However, left ventricular diastolic filling time usually increases during CRT, regardless of changes in LV filling pressures or relaxation, as a result of improved atrio-ventricular (AV) synchrony with programming the AV delay of the CRT device.

Two-dimensional and Doppler echocardiography has also been used to assess the acute effects of CRT on measurements of systolic and diastolic function.[30–32] Although significant reductions in LV volumes and increases in LV ejection fraction (LVEF) occur immediately after CRT, the responses in PWD- and TDI-derived indices of diastolic function may depend on the pre-CRT diastolic filling pattern. In patients with a pattern of impaired LV relaxation, CRT did not result in significant changes in PWD-derived E-wave velocity, A-wave velocity, the

E/A ratio, or the deceleration time, although diastolic filling time increased significantly.[33] TDI-derived E' velocities remain unchanged or may actually decrease; the E/E' ratio also remains unchanged.[31–32] In patients with pseudonormalized or restrictive LV filling patterns, however, the PWD-derived E-wave velocity decreases, DT increases, and the E/E' ratio decreases, suggesting reduction in LV filling pressures (Fig 3.4). Thus, the results obtained by two-dimensional and Doppler echocardiography, immediately after CRT, are similar to those reported by invasive measurements. It is not known whether the acute response in left ventricular diastolic function immediately after CRT predicts functional improvement and/or clinical outcomes during long-term follow-up.

Effects of CRT on LV Diastolic Function at Early Follow-Up

Invasive studies of diastolic function at 3 to 6 months following CRT are limited. One study of 22 patients (64% ischemic) reported that the LVEDP decreased and peak-negative

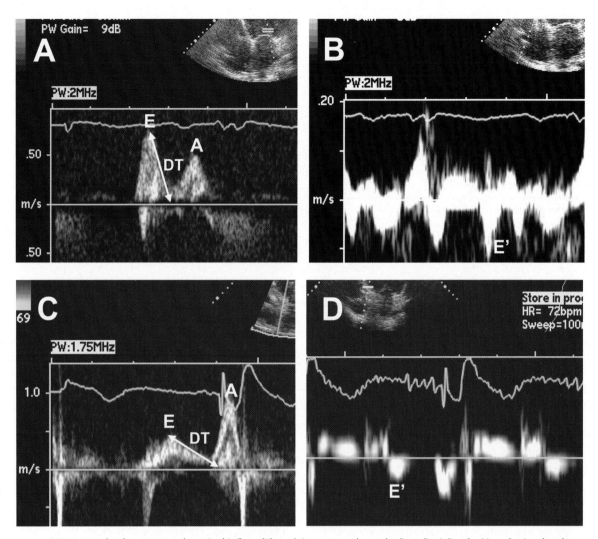

FIG. 3.4. Pulsed-wave Doppler mitral inflow (A) and tissue Doppler early diastolic (E') velocities obtained at the septal annulus (B) prior to CRT in a patient with nonischemic cardiomyopathy. The pre-CRT mitral E/A ratio is 1.6, deceleration time (DT) is 110 ms, and mitral E/E' ratio is 10.0, consistent with pseudonormalized LV filling. After 5 months of CRT, LV end-systolic volume decreased by 15%, and the LV ejection increased from 17% to 24%. The mitral E/A ratio decreased to 0.5, DT increased to 240 ms, (C) and mitral E/E' decreased to 8.0 (D), consistent with improvement in diastolic function to an impaired relaxation pattern.

LV dP/dt increased, although Tau remained unchanged at 6-month follow-up.[34] Significant reductions in LV end-diastolic volume after CRT were observed and may have influenced the response in both LVEDP and peak-negative LV dP/dt, which are preload-dependent measurements.[35]

Results of early follow-up studies after CRT assessed by two-dimensional and Doppler echocardiography have shown variable findings (Table 3.1). LV diastolic filling time invariably increases at early follow-up after CRT.[36–45] In a large CRT multicenter clinical trial of 172 patients, LV diastolic function was evaluated by PWD-derived measurements at baseline and at 3 months, and 6 months after CRT. There were significant decreases in mitral E-wave velocity and increase in DT and DFT, but the mitral E/A ratio remained unchanged from pre-CRT levels.[37] The results demonstrated that CRT had a ben-

eficial effect on diastolic function, manifested by improved LV diastolic filling and/or decreased LV filling pressures (i.e., decreased E and increased DT). Significant improvement in LVEF and decrease in LV volumes in the CRT group were observed, although evident to a greater extent in the nonischemic group. It was not reported, however, whether HF etiology (i.e., ischemic vs. nonischemic) was a factor in the improvement in LV diastolic filling indices. Thus, the results suggest that improvements in LV diastolic function after CRT are coupled to the beneficial effects on systolic performance and/or reverse remodeling.

Some studies have evaluated whether improvements in LV diastolic function are coupled to the response in LV systolic performance after CRT. One study reported that the mitral E/A ratio decreased in patients (n = 49, 47% ischemic HF eti-

TABLE 3.1   **Response in LV Systolic and Diastolic Function after CRT at 3-to-6 Month Follow-up**

Author (ref)	n	LVEF	LVESV	MV E	E/A	DT	DFT	TDI E'	E/E'
Saxon (34)	53	↔	↓	NR	↔	↑	NR	NR	NR
St. John Sutton (35)	172	↑	↓	↓	↔	↑	↑	NR	NR
Penicka (37)*	49	↑,↔	↓,↔	NR	↓	↑,↔	↑	NR	NR
Yu (36)**	30	↑,↔	↓,↔	↔	NR	↔	↑	NR	NR
Vidal (43)***	64	↑,↔	↓,↔	NR	↔	↑,↔	NR	↔	NR
Agacdiken (38)	23	↑	↓	↓	↓	↑	NR	NR	NR
Jansen (39)**	52	↑,↔	↓,↔	↔	↓,↔	↑,↔	↑	↑,↔	↓,↔
Waggoner (18)*	50	↑,↔	↓	↓,↔	↓,↔	↑,↔	↑,↔	↓,↔	↓,↔
Yu (20)	76	↑	↓	↓	↔	↔	↑	↓	↔

Abbreviations: LVEF, left ventricular ejection fraction; LVESV, left ventricular end-systolic volume; NR, not reported; MV E, mitral early filling velocity; E/A, mitral early filling/atrial filling velocity ratio; DT, deceleration time; DFT, diastolic filling time; TDI E', tissue Doppler early diastolic annular velocities; E/E', ratio of mitral E-wave velocity/tissue Doppler early diastolic annular velocity.

Notes: ↑, increased; ↓, decreased; ↔, no change based on changes in individual variables by significant increase, or lack of increase in LVEF,* respectively; changes in individual variables defined by significant decrease, or no change in LV end systolic volume,** respectively, changes in individual variable defined by significant increase, or no change in 6-minute walk distance,*** respectively.

ology) regardless of the improvement in LVEF (defined as a relative increase >25% after CRT), but mitral DT improved only in the group whose LVEF improved by >25%.[39] Another study (n = 23, 39% ischemic HF etiology) reported that the mitral E/A ratio remained unchanged regardless of the LVEF response, but the mitral E-wave velocity decreased, and DT improved in the group with increases in LVEF >25%.[40] A study from the authors' group (n = 50, 28% ischemic HF etiology) reported that mitral inflow indices (i.e., decreases in mitral E-wave velocity and the E/A ratio, increases in DT) improved only in the group who had an absolute increase in LVEF by >5% after CRT.[18]

Other investigators have evaluated the response in LV diastolic function based on the reduction in LVESV (i.e., defined as <15% vs. ≥15% decrease compared to baseline) at early follow-up after CRT.[20, 41] In one study (n = 76, 49% ischemic HF etiology), the mitral E-wave velocity decreased regardless of the response in LVESV, but the mitral E/A ratio and DT were unchanged.[20] A separate study (n = 52, 48% ischemic HF etiology) reported the mitral E-wave and mitral E/A ratio decreased, and DT increased only in the group that had a reduction in LVESV >15% after CRT.[41] Interestingly, several studies have reported that a pre-CRT mitral inflow pattern of restrictive LV filling was frequently present in nonresponders when defined by 2D echocardiographic evidence of no significant improvement in either LVEF or LVESV compared to pre-CRT and in patients with an ischemic etiology of HF.[18, 20, 39, 41–42, 44]

Several studies have evaluated the effects of CRT on LV diastolic function determined by TDI-derived E' velocities to assess LV relaxation, and both the E' and E/E' ratio variables for estimation of LV filling pressure, have shown discrepant findings.[18, 20, 41–45] In a study from the authors' laboratory, E' was unchanged regardless of the response in LVEF, but the E/E' ratio at the septal annulus decreased in the group who exhibited improvement in LVEF >5% after CRT.[18] Another

study demonstrated that E' velocities increased (i.e., improved LV relaxation) and the E/E' decreased in the group that had a reduction in LVESV by 15% after CRT but remained unchanged in the group without reverse remodeling.[41] A separate study reported that E' remained unchanged in the group with a reduction in LVESV by 15%, but decreased (i.e., worse LV relaxation) in the group without reverse remodeling, and that E/E' remained unchanged regardless of the response in LVESV.[20] Another investigation from the authors' laboratory revealed that the etiology of HF was also responsible for the response in E' and E/E' ratio after CRT.[42] E' remained unchanged and E/E' decreased after CRT in the group with a nonischemic HF etiology (Fig. 3.5). In the ischemic HF etiology group, the E' decreased and the mitral E/E' ratio remained unchanged after CRT, despite significant reductions in LVESV and improvement in LVEF (Fig. 3.5).

In summary, the improvement in LV diastolic function early after CRT, whether determined by Doppler mitral inflow indices (i.e., E-wave velocity, E/A ratio, DT), tissue Doppler E' velocities or the mitral E/E' ratio, are therefore influenced by several factors: (a) the extent of LV volume reduction, (b) the improvement in LV systolic performance, and (c) the etiology of HF (ischemic vs. non ischemic). Although reduction in LV volumes and increases in LVEF should result in an improvement in LV diastolic function this may be mediated to some extent by an ischemic HF etiology. The TDI-derived E' velocity is relatively unchanged after CRT and reflects the underlying relaxation abnormality associated with LV systolic dysfunction, LV enlargement, and/or eccentric LV hypertrophy. LV relaxation may be further impaired in patients with an ischemic HF etiology and likely will not improve after CRT potentially due to the amount of scarring. The decrease (or no change) in the mitral E/E' ratio is therefore primarily a result of a reduced mitral E-wave velocity relative to the decrease (or no change) in LV volume and/or increase (or lack thereof) in LVEF after CRT.

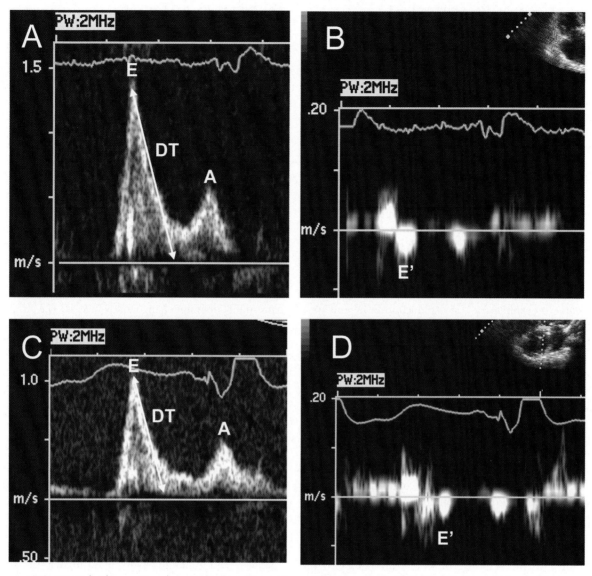

FIG. 3.5. Pulsed-wave Doppler mitral inflow (A) and tissue Doppler early diastolic (E') velocities obtained at the septal annulus (B) in a patient with an ischemic cardiomyopathy. The pre-CRT mitral E/A ratio is 2.3, deceleration time (DT) is 155 ms, and mitral E/E' ratio is 32 consistent with restrictive LV filling. After 4 months of CRT, the LV end-systolic volume and LV ejection fraction were unchanged. Pulsed-wave Doppler mitral inflow (C) and tissue Doppler early diastolic (E') velocities obtained at the septal annulus (D) remained also unchanged (mitral E/A: 2.25, DT: 150 ms, mitral E/E' is 25.5).

Diastolic Dyssynchrony and the Effects of CRT

In patients with LV systolic dyssynchrony, diastolic dyssynchrony is also typically present and may contribute to diastolic dysfunction (see Assessment by Tissue Doppler Imaging section on page 33 and Figure 3.3 on page 34 for assessment of diastolic dyssynchrony). The effects of CRT on LV diastolic dyssynchrony have reported differing findings.[18–20, 42–43] In one study of 42 patients, it was reported that immediately following CRT there was a reduction in the extent of LV diastolic dyssynchrony from 81% to 55% (p <.001).[19] However, other studies reported no significant improvements in diastolic dyssynchrony at short-term follow-up, regardless of the response in LVEF or LVESV.[18, 20] Other studies from our laboratory reported significant reductions in diastolic dyssynchrony at short-term follow-up after CRT in patients with a nonischemic etiology of HF and in patients with the LV lead positioned in a lateral versus an anterolateral coronary vein.[42, 43] Further studies regarding the clinical significance of the presence of LV diastolic dyssynchrony prior to and after CRT represents an area of research that may have clinically important implications.

Diastolic Function after CRT: Serial Echocardiographic Studies Performed at Early and at Intermediate Follow-up

Several studies have evaluated the effects of CRT on LV diastolic function at early stages (i.e., 3 to 6 months) and at 12 months of follow-up (Table 3.2). The results from the MIRACLE trial, a multicenter study of 228 patients with equal distribution of HF etiology, reported that the mitral E-wave and the E/A ratio decreased significantly 6 months after CRT and remained decreased at 12 months of follow-up. Although the mitral DT increased at 6 months after CRT, it was similar to pre-CRT at 12 months of follow-up.[47] Other studies have shown that the mitral E/A ratio did not change early after CRT or at 12 months of follow-up, and DT increased significantly only at the 12 month follow-up.[45–46] One study reported that decreases in mitral E-wave velocities and E/A ratio including increased mitral DT at early follow-up after CRT remains sustained at 12 months, but occurred only in patients who exhibited a >15% reduction in LV end systolic volumes.[41]

There are two studies that reported the TDI-derived E' velocity remains unchanged at early follow-up and after 12 months of CRT.[45–46] However, a separate investigation reported that E' improved in a patient group who had a reduction in LVESV >15% after CRT and remained sustained at the 12-month follow-up.[41] The mitral E/E' ratio was unchanged at the early and the 12-month follow-up after CRT in one study.[46] However, a separate study reported that the E/E' ratio decreased significantly in the group that had significant reductions in LV end-systolic volumes after CRT.[41] The pre-CRT mitral E/E' ratio differed in these studies and likely were an additional factor that influenced the results.

In summary, the results of these studies suggest that the effects of CRT on improvement in LV diastolic function are coupled to the response in LVEF and reduction in LV end-systolic volumes, regardless of the follow-up time interval. Furthermore, the effects of CRT on LV diastolic function remains sustained (i.e., unchanged) at 12 months compared to the results at short-term follow-up (i.e., 3 to 6 months).

Pre-CRT Indices of Diastolic Function Predict Clinical Outcomes

Both PWD- and TDI-derived measurements of diastolic function have been shown to predict clinical outcomes after CRT. In a single center study of 65 patients who received CRT, those who exhibited a restrictive filling pattern (n = 25) prior to CRT (defined as a mitral E/A ratio ≥2, or ≥1 and DT ≤140 ms) were compared to the group (n = 40) without a restrictive filling pattern.[48] The etiology of HF (i.e., ischemic vs. nonischemic) was similar between groups. A restrictive filling pattern was associated with higher all-cause mortality or rehospitalization for a cardiovascular event at the 12-month follow-up after CRT. Furthermore, among patients with a pre-CRT restrictive filling pattern that improved to nonrestrictive pattern at 12 months, clinical event rates were similar to those who had a pre-CRT nonrestrictive filling pattern. The results indicate that reversal of restrictive filling after CRT may result in a better outcome compared to a restrictive LV filling pattern that does not change following CRT (i.e., irreversible restrictive LV filling). An irreversible restrictive filling pattern has also been associated with higher mortality in non-CRT patients with heart failure.[13]

The authors' group reported long-term clinical outcomes after CRT (mean follow-up: 20±11 months) based on a single-center study of 57 patients grouped by HF etiology (33% ischemic). The pre-CRT mitral E-wave and E/A ratio were higher in the ischemic group, while the DT, E' and E/E' were similar between groups.[42] At 4 months after CRT, the ischemic group exhibited a decrease in the mitral E-wave velocity, whereas the E' decreased significantly; the mitral E/A ratio, DT, and mitral E/E' remained unchanged. Conversely, in the nonischemic group, LV diastolic function improved to a greater extent, including decreased E-wave, E/A ratio and E/E', and increased DT, although the E' velocities remained unchanged. The ischemic group had a higher prevalence of cardiac-related events (i.e., rehospitalization for HF exacerbation and/or cardiac-related death) compared to the non-ischemic group (53% vs. 26%, p <.05) at long-term follow-up. Multivariate analysis demonstrated that the pre-CRT mitral DT and the E/E' ratio (at the septal annulus) were

TABLE 3.2 Response in LV Systolic and Diastolic Function at 3 to 6 months and at 12 Month Follow-up after CRT

Author (ref)	n	LVEF	LVESV	MV E	E/A	DT	DFT	TDI E'	E/E'
Waggoner (44)	46	↑, ↔	↔, ↓	↔, ↓	↔	↔, ↑	↑, ↔	↔	↔
St. John Sutton (45)	228	↑, ↑	↓, ↔	↓, ↔	↓, ↔	↑, ↓	NR	NR	NR
Vidal (43)	64	↑, ↔	↓, ↔	NR	↔	↔	NR	↔	NR
Jansen (39)*	30	↑, ↔	↓, ↔	↔	↓, ↔	↑, ↑	↑, ↔	↑, ↔	↓, ↔
Jansen (39)**	22	↔	↔	↔	↔	↔	↑, ↔	↔	↔

Abbreviations: LVEF, left ventricular ejection fraction; LVESV, left ventricular end-systolic volume; NR, not reported; MV E, mitral early filling velocity; E/A, mitral early filling/atrial filling velocity ratio; DT, deceleration time; DFT, diastolic filling time; TDI E', tissue Doppler early diastolic annular velocities; E/E', ratio of mitral E-wave velocity/tissue Doppler early diastolic annular velocity.

Note: ↑, increased; ↓, decreased; or ↔, no change by changes in individual variables at 3 to 6-month follow-up and at 12-month follow-up, respectively; * decrease in LV end systolic volume > 15% after CRT, ** decrease in LV end systolic volume <15% after CRT.

predictive of cardiac-related events at long-term follow-up.

A single-center study of 74 patients (36 with ischemic HF etiology) who were followed up at 24 months after CRT, evaluated whether pre-CRT indices of LV diastolic function were predictive of cardiac events (i.e., cardiac-related death, cardiac transplantation, and/or rehospitalization due to HF).[44] In the group with clinical events after CRT (n = 21, 28%), the pre-CRT mitral E-wave and E/A ratio were higher, DT was shorter, and the E/E' ratio was higher compared to the group without events. A restrictive LV filling pattern was present in 67% of patients with events versus 20% without events. Although the prevalence of an ischemic HF etiology was significantly higher in the group with clinical events, univariate analysis demonstrated a higher mitral E/A and E/E' ratio were significant predictors of clinical events; multivariate analysis disclosed the E/E' ratio (at the lateral annulus) was the most significant predictor of long-term clinical events.

Future Challenges Regarding Echocardiographic Assessment of LV Diastolic Function after CRT

Two-dimensional (2D)-Doppler echocardiography and TDI have been widely used to identify HF patients who may be candidates for CRT and to determine the response in LV systolic performance and diastolic function at follow-up. However, important issues limit the widespread acceptance and applicability of these findings. First, the majority of studies have been conducted at single sites. Second, many studies have included a relatively small number of subjects. Third, the end-points used to define CRT responders have varied between studies. For example, some studies used functional response end-points (i.e., NYHA class, HF questionnaire scores), which have raised the issue of the placebo effect of CRT, or the 6-minute walk distance, while others have used 2D echocardiographic-determined changes in LV volumes and/or systolic function. Fourth, large multicenter trials to determine whether pre-CRT measurements of ventricular dyssynchrony are predictors of response at short-term follow-up are now emerging but it is not known whether diastolic indices will be analyzed.[49, 50] Fifth, most of the reported echo-Doppler studies have been limited by a relatively short-term follow-up (i.e., ≤12 months), and clinical outcomes at long-term follow-up after CRT remain to be determined. Finally, the value of pre-CRT measurements of LV diastolic function as a predictor of long-term clinical outcomes remains mostly unknown. Future clinical studies could include the selection of patients for CRT by a "clinical score" that could include a number of factors, such as HF etiology, myocardial viability and/or scar burden, pulmonary artery pressure, renal function, and the pre-CRT LV systolic and diastolic measurements (i.e., LV volume, mitral deceleration time, and E/E' ratio).

There are newer echo-derived methods that are also promising to further characterize patients who receive CRT. Strain and strain rate imaging (SRI) have been reported as an alternative approach to TDI-derived velocity measurements to assess LV dyssynchrony.[51-52] To the authors' knowledge, there are no studies that have evaluated the use of SRI to evaluate diastolic function in CRT patients. It may be that the signal-to-noise ratio may limit widespread applicability of strain rate imaging, and more studies are necessary to determine a role, if any, for this technique.[3, 51] Three-dimensional (3D) echocardiography is another promising method for measurements of LV volumes and systolic dyssynchrony in CRT patients.[53-54] Future investigations could define the role of 3D echocardiographic techniques for assessment of diastolic function in CRT patients.

CONCLUSION

The results of studies that have evaluated LV diastolic function prior to and after CRT can be summarized as follows: 1) there is physiologic coupling of the response in LV systolic performance and/or reversed LV remodeling after CRT with the improvement in LV diastolic function; 2) restrictive LV filling, characterized by short mitral E-wave deceleration time and/or increased E/E' ratio prior to CRT, are predictive of clinical outcomes, independent of LVEF response or changes in LV volumes after CRT; and 3) patients with an ischemic HF etiology and restrictive LV filling have worse clinical outcomes after CRT.

PRACTICAL POINTS

1. LV diastolic dysfunction is common in patients with severe LV systolic dysfunction and prolonged QRS interval with impaired LV relaxation and altered LV compliance.

2. Doppler-derived LV filling patterns are variable prior to CRT and may not change at early follow-up, particularly if LV filling pressures are normal.

3. Improvements in Doppler measurements of LV diastolic function are often coupled to response in LV systolic function and reversed LV remodeling after CRT.

4. Restrictive LV diastolic filling with a Doppler mitral inflow pattern of E/A ratio >2 and/or deceleration time < 60 ms prior to CRT is associated with higher morbidity and mortality after CRT.

5. Elevated LV filling pressures prior to CRT by tissue Doppler imaging of LV annular velocities (E') at the septal and/or lateral base combined with mitral inflow early filling (E) velocities (E/E' ratio) are predictive of worse clinical outcomes at follow-up.

6. Ischemic etiology of heart failure may influence the response in LV diastolic function after CRT.

ACKNOWLEDGMENTS

The authors extend their sincere thanks to Mitchell N. Faddis, MD, PhD, FACC, and Marye J. Gleva, MD, FACC, for referral of patients, and to Joann Reagan, RN, BSN, RVT and Sharon Heuerman, RN, for assistance with patient care.

REFERENCES

1. Leclercq C, Kass DA. Retiming the failing heart: Principles and current clinical status of cardiac resynchronization. *J Am Coll Cardiol.* 2002; 39:194–201.
2. Abraham WT, Hayes DL. Cardiac resynchronization therapy for heart failure. *Circulation.* 2003;346:2596–2603.
3. Bax JJ, Ansalone G, Breithardt OA, et al. Echocardiographic evaluation of cardiac resynchronization therapy: Ready for routine clinical use? *J Am Coll Cardiol.* 2004;44:1–9.
4. Nishimura RA, Tajik AJ. Evaluation of diastolic filling of left ventricle in health and disease: Doppler echocardiography is the clinician's Rosetta stone. *J Am Coll Cardiol.* 1997;30:8–18.
5. Yu CM, Fang F, Zhang Q, et al. Improvement of atrial function and atrial reverse remodeling after cardiac resynchronization therapy for heart failure. *J Am Coll Cardiol.* 2007;50:778–785.
6. Oh JK, Appleton CP, Hatle LK, et al. The non-invasive assessment of left ventricular diastolic function with two-dimensional and Doppler echocardiography. *J Am Soc Echocardiogr.* 1997;10:246–270.
7. Thomas JD, Weyman AC. Echocardiographic Doppler evaluation of left ventricular diastolic function: Physics and physiology. *Circulation.* 1991;84:977–990.
8. Vanoverschelde J J, Raphael DA, Robert AR, Cosyns JR. Left ventricular filling in dilated cardiomyopathy: Relation to functional class and hemodynamics. *J Am Coll Cardiol.* 1990;15:1288–1295.
9. Xie G, Berk MR, Smith MD, et al. Prognostic value of Doppler transmitral flow patterns in patients with congestive heart failure. *J Am Coll Cardiol.* 1994;24:132–139.
10. Rihal CS, Nishimura RA, Hatle LK, et al. Systolic and diastolic dysfunction in patients with clinical diagnosis of dilated cardiomyopathy: relation to symptoms and prognosis. *Circulation.* 1994;90:2772–2779.
11. Hansen A, Haass M, Zugck C, et al. Prognostic value of Doppler echocardiographic mitral inflow patterns: Implications for risk stratification in patients with chronic congestive heart failure. *J Am Coll Cardiol.* 2001;37:1049–1055.
12. Bruch C, Gotzmann M, Stypmann J, et al. Electrocardiography and Doppler echocardiography for risk stratification in patients with chronic heart failure: Incremental prognostic value of QRS duration and a restrictive mitral filling pattern. *J Am Coll Cardiol.* 2005;45:1072–1075.
13. Whalley GA, Gamble GD, Doughty RN. The prognostic significance of restrictive diastolic filling associated with heart failure: A meta-analysis. *Int J Cardiol.* 2007;116:70–77.
14. Quinones MA, Otto CM, Stoddard M, et al. Recommendations for quantification of Doppler echocardiography: A Report from the Doppler Quantification Task Force of the Nomenclature and Standards Committee of the American Society of Echocardiography. *J Am Soc Echocardiogr.* 2002;15:167–184.
15. Nagueh SF, Middleton K J, Kopelen HA, et al. Doppler tissue imaging: A non-invasive technique for evaluation of left ventricular relaxation and estimation of filling pressures. *J Am Coll Cardiol.* 1997;30:1527–1533.
16. Ommen SR, Nishimura RA, Appleton CP, et al. Clinical utility of Doppler echocardiography and tissue Doppler imaging in the estimation of left ventricular filling pressures: A simultaneous Doppler-catheterization study. *Circulation.* 2000;102:1788–1794.
17. Wang M, Yip GWK, Wang AYM, et al. Peak early diastolic mitral annulus velocity by tissue Doppler imaging adds independent and incremental prognostic value. *J Am Coll Cardio.* 2003; 41: 820–826.
18. Waggoner AD, Faddis MN, Gleva MJ, et al. Improvements in left ventricular diastolic function after cardiac resynchronization therapy are coupled to response in systolic performance. *J Am Coll Cardiol.* 2005 46:2244–2249.
19. Schuster I, Habib G, Jego C, et al. Diastolic asynchrony is more frequent than systolic asynchrony in dilated cardiomyopathy and is less improved by cardiac resynchronization therapy. *J Am Coll Cardiol.* 2005;46: 2250–2257.
20. Yu CM, Zhang Q, Yip GWK, et al. Are left ventricular diastolic function and diastolic asynchrony important determinants of response to cardiac resynchronization therapy? *Am J Cardiol.* 2006;98:1083–1087.
21. LeClercq C, Cazeau S, Le Breton H, et al. Acute hemodynamic effects of biventricular DDD pacing in patients with end-stage-heart failure. *J Am Coll Cardiol.* 1998;32:1825–1831.
22. Blanc JJ, Etienne Y, Gilard M, et al. Evaluation of different ventricular pacing sites in patients with severe heart failure: Results of an acute hemodynamic study. *Circulation.* 1997;96:3273–3277.
23. Morris-Thurgood JA, Turner MS, Nightingale AK, et al. Pacing in heart failure: Improved ventricular interaction in diastole rather than systolic re-synchronization. *Europace.* 2000;2:271–275.
24. Auricchio A, Stellbrink C, Block M, et al. Effect of pacing chamber and atrioventricular delay on acute systolic function of paced patients with congestive heart failure. *Circulation.* 1999;99:2993–3001.
25. Auricchio A, Ding J, Spinelli JC, et al. Cardiac resynchronization therapy restores optimal atrioventricular timing in heart failure patients with ventricular conduction delay. *J Am Coll Cardiol.* 2002;39:1163–1169.
26. Perego GB, Chianca R, Facchini M, et al. Simultaneous vs. sequential biventricular pacing in dilated cardiomyopathy: an acute hemodynamic study. *Eur J Heart Failure.* 2003;5:305–513.
27. Kass DA, Chen C, Curry C, et al. Improved left ventricular mechanics from acute VDD pacing in patients with dilated cardiomyopathy and ventricular conduction delay. *Circulation.* 1999;99:1567–1573.
28. Bleasdale RA, Turner MS, Mumford CE, et al. Left ventricular pacing minimizes diastolic ventricular interaction, allowing improved preload-dependent systolic performance. *Circulation.* 2004;110: 2395–2400.
29. Nelson GS, Curry CW, Wyman BT, et al. Predictors of systolic augmentation from left ventricular preexcitation in patients with dilated cardiomyopathy and interventricular conduction delay. *Circulation.* 2000;101:2703–2709.
30. Breithardt OA, Stellbrink C, Franke A, et al. Acute effects of cardiac resynchronization therapy on left ventricular Doppler indices in patients with congestive heart failure. *Am Heart J.* 2002;143:34–44.
31. Yu CM, Lin H, Fung WH, et al. Comparison of acute changes in left ventricular volume, systolic and diastolic functions, and intraventricular synchronicity after biventricular and right ventricular pacing for heart failure *Am Heart J.* 2003;145:G1–G7.
32. Waggoner AD, Faddis MN, Gleva MJ, et al. Cardiac resynchronization therapy acutely improves diastolic function. *J Am Soc Echocardiogr.* 2005;18:216–220.
33. Ibid.
34. Steendijk P, Tulner SA, Bax JJ, et al. Hemodynamic effects of long-term cardiac resynchronization therapy: Analysis of pressure-volume loops. *Circulation.* 2006;113:1295–1304.
35. Ibid.
36. Saxon LA, De Marco T, Schafer J, et al. Effects of long-term biventricular stimulation for resynchronization on echocardiographic measures of remodeling. *Circulation.* 2002;105:1304–1310.
37. St. John Sutton MG, Plappert T, Abraham WT, et al. Effect of cardiac resynchronization therapy on left ventricular size and function in chronic heart failure. *Circulation.* 2003;107:1985–1990.
38. Yu CM, Fung WH, Lin HL, et al. Predictors of left ventricular reverse remodeling after cardiac resynchronization therapy for heart failure secondary to idiopathic or ischemic cardiomyopathy. *Am J Cardiol.* 2000;91:684–688.
39. Penicka M, Bartunek J, De Bruyne B, et al. Improvement in left ventricular function after cardiac resynchronization therapy is predicted by tissue Doppler imaging echocardiography. *Circulation.* 2004;109: 978–983.
40. Agacdiken A, Vural A, Ural D, et al. Effect of cardiac resynchronization therapy on left ventricular diastolic filling pattern in responder and non-responder patients. *PACE.* 2005;28:654–660.
41. Jansen AHM, van Dantzig JM, Bracke F, et al. Improvement in diastolic function and left ventricular filling pressure induced by cardiac resynchronization therapy. *Am Heart J.* 2007; 153: 843–849.
42. Waggoner A D, Rovner A, de las Fuentes L, et al. Clinical outcomes after cardiac resynchronization therapy: Importance of left ventricular diastolic function and etiology of heart failure. *J Am Soc Echocardiogr.* 2006;19:307–313.
43. Rovner A, de las Fuentes L, Faddis MN, et al. Relation of left ventricular lead placement in cardiac resynchronization therapy to left ventricular reverse remodeling and to diastolic dyssynchrony. *Am J Cardiol.* 2007;29:239–241.

44. Soliman O, Theuns DAMJ, ten Cate FJ, et al. Baseline predictors of cardiac events after cardiac resynchronization therapy in patients with heart failure secondary to ischemic or nonischemic etiology. *Am J Cardiol.* 2007; 100: 464–469.

45. Vidal B, Sitges M, Marigliano A, et al. Relation of response to cardiac resynchronization therapy to left ventricular reverse remodeling. *Am J Cardiol.* 2006;97:876–881.

46. Waggoner AD, Faddis MN, Gleva MJ, et al. Left ventricular diastolic function after cardiac resynchronization therapy: results at four-month and 12-month follow-up. *J Am Coll Cardiol.* 2005; 45 (Suppl 1):128A.

47. St. John Sutton MG, Plappert T, Hilpisch KE, et al. Sustained reverse left ventricular structural remodeling with cardiac resynchronization at one year is a function of etiology: Quantitative Doppler echocardiographic evidence from the Multicenter InSync Randomized Clinical Evaluation (MIRACLE). *Circulation.* 2006;113:266–272.

48. Porciani MC, Valsecchi S, Demarchi G, et al. Evolution and prognostic significance of diastolic filling pattern in cardiac resynchronization therapy. *Int J Cardiol.* 2006; 112: 322–328.

49. Cleland JGF, Abdellah AT, Khaleva O, et al. Clinical trials update from the European Society of Cardiology Congress 2007: 3CPO, ALOFT, PROSPECT and statins for heart failure. *Eur J Heart Fail.* 2007;9: 1070–1073.

50. Beshai JF, Grimm RA, Nagueh SF, et al. Cardiac resynchronization therapy in heart failure with narrow QRS complexes. *N Engl J Med.* 2007;357:2461–2471.

51. Popovic Z, Grimm RA, Perlic G, et al. Noninvasive assessment of cardiac resynchronization therapy for congestive heart failure using myocardial strain and left ventricular peak power as parameters of myocardial synchrony and function. *J Cardiovasc Electrophysiol.* 2002;13:1203–1208.

52. Yu CM, Gorcsan JIII, Bleeker GB, et al. Usefulness of tissue Doppler velocity and strain dyssynchrony for predicting left ventricular reverse remodeling response after cardiac resynchronization therapy. *Am J Cardiol.* 2007;100:1263–1270.

53. Kapetanakis S, Kearney MT, Siva MT, et al. Real-time three-dimensional echocardiography. A novel technique to quantify global left ventricular mechanical dyssynchrony. *Circulation.* 2005;112:992–1000.

54. Burgess MI, Jenkins C, Chan J, et al. Measurement of left ventricular dyssynchrony in patients with ischaemic cardiomyopathy: a comparison of real-time three-dimensional echocardiography and tissue Doppler echocardiography. *Heart.* 2007;93:1191–1196.

Selecting Patients for Cardiac Resynchronization Therapy: Electrical or Mechanical Dyssynchrony?

Nathaniel M. Hawkins • Mark C. Petrie • John J.V. McMurray

ardiac resynchronization therapy (CRT) improves functional status and reduces hospitalizations and mortality in patients with heart failure (HF). In the pivotal large, randomized trials, patients were selected on the basis of three main criteria: impaired functional status (New York Heart Association class III or IV), reduced left ventricular ejection fraction (≤ 0.35), and prolonged QRS duration (≥ 120 milliseconds). The latter was considered a marker of underlying ventricular dyssynchrony (so-called "electrical dyssynchrony") (Table 4.1). Consequently, international guidelines recommend CRT based on the electrocardiographic (ECG) inclusion criteria in those trials.[1]

Some have stated that around one-third of patients appear not to improve clinically or exhibit favorable echocardiographic remodeling (so-called "nonresponders"). It has been proposed that echocardiography may better identify those likely to respond to treatment by measuring actual mechanical dyssynchrony.[2] If correct, this alternate approach to patient selection has two important clinical consequences. First, nonresponders with a broad QRS would be spared an ineffective and invasive procedure, with resultant cost savings to health care providers. Conversely, patients with mechanical dyssynchrony but a narrow QRS complex, who were excluded from the landmark clinical trials, may benefit from CRT.

We review the meaning and measurement of electrical and mechanical dyssynchrony, the strengths and weaknesses of echocardiographic indices of dyssynchrony, and the controversial issue of predicting response to treatment. How valid is the concept of responders versus nonresponders? Should patients eligible for treatment based on inclusion criteria for clinical trials be excluded from that treatment in clinical practice? Why is such an approach advocated for devices but not for drug therapy?

ELECTRICAL DYSSYNCHRONY

What Is Electrical Dyssynchrony?

The QRS complex represents the vectorial sum of electrical forces generated by myocardial masses over time. Normal electrical activation propagates as a uniform high-velocity wavefront through the myocardial Purkinje network. In damaged myocardium, altered conduction properties impair the velocity and direction of electrical propagation. Abnormal ventricular depolarization, manifesting as QRS prolongation, generates regions of both early and delayed ventricular contraction. The delayed segments accommodate contractile force and volume, reducing systolic function.

Why Is Electrical Dyssynchrony Important?

A direct relationship exists between QRS duration and ejection fraction.[3-5] Prevalence of bundle branch block (BBB) varies from around 20% in the general HF population[3–4] to 35% among patients with more severely impaired systolic function.[5–6] BBB is a powerful independent predictor of mortality,[6] with no evidence of any threshold effect at 120 ms.[7] QRS duration has been the principal entry point to all major CRT trials to date (Table 4.1). International guidelines recommend CRT in patients with medically refractory, symptomatic (NYHA III/IV) heart failure, with prolonged QRS duration ≥ 120 msec, and ejection fraction ≤ 35%.[1] Simultaneous biventricular (BiV) pacing resynchronizes both intra- and interventricular contraction. The result is hemodynamic improvement,[8–11] reduced mitral regurgitation,[12] and reversal of maladaptive remodeling.[13–16] CRT improves symptoms, quality of life and functional class,[17] increases exercise tolerance,[17–20] and reduces hospitalizations and mortality.[21, 22]

Baseline QRS duration consistently fails to predict response (Table 4.2). However, change in QRS duration (ΔQRS) following CRT differs significantly between responders and

TABLE 4.1 Inclusion Criteria and Outcomes of CRT Trials

Study Acronym (Ref. No.)	n	Design	Follow-up (Months)	QRSd (msec)	Mean QRSd (msec)	LVEDD (mm)	Echo	LVEF (%)	NYHA class	SR/AF	ICD	End-points		
PATH-CHF[20]	41	Crossover	1	≥ 120	175 ± 32	No cut-off	No	No cut-off	III, IV	SR	No	6MWT +44m p<0.001	MLHFQ −19.3 p<0.001	Peak Vo$_2$ +1.8 p<0.001
PATH-CHF II[96]	86	Crossover	3	≥ 120	155 ± 20	No cut-off	No	≤ 30	II - IV	SR	Yes	6MWT +47m p=0.024	MLHFQ −8.1 p=0.004	Peak Vo$_2$ +2.5 p<0.001
MUSTIC-SR[18]	48	Crossover	3	> 150	174 ± 20	> 60	No	< 35	III	SR	No	6MWT +73m p<0.001	MLHFQ −13.6 p<0.001	Peak Vo$_2$ +1.2 p=0.029
MUSTIC-AF[97]	37	Crossover	3	> 200 paced	209 ± 18 paced	> 60	No	< 35	III	AF	No	6MWT +32m p=0.05	MLHFQ −4.3 p=0.11	Peak Vo$_2$ +1.7 p=0.04
MIRACLE[17]	453	Parallel	6	≥ 130	166 ± 20	≥ 55	No	≤ 35	III, IV	SR	No	6MWT +29m p=0.005	MLHFQ −9.0 p<0.001	NYHA p<0.001
MIRACLE -ICD[98]	369	Parallel	6	≥ 130	164 ± 22	≥ 55	No	≤ 35	III, IV	SR	Yes	6MWT +2m p=0.36	MLHFQ −6.5 p=0.02	NYHA p=0.007
MIRACLE - ICD II[99]	186	Parallel	6	≥ 130	165 ± 23	≥ 55	No	≤ 35	II	SR	Yes	6MWT +5m p=0.59	MLHFQ −2.6 p=0.49	Peak Vo$_2$ +0.3 p=0.87
CONTAK-CD[100]	490	Parallel	6	≥ 120	158 ± 26	No cut-off	No	≥ 35	II - IV	SR	Yes	6MWT+20m p=0.043	MLHFQ −2 p=0.39	Peak Vo$_2$ +0.8 p=0.03
COMPANION[21]	1520	Parallel	16.2 median	≥ 120	160 median	≥ 60	No	≤ 35	III, IV	SR	Yes	Death, Admission HR 0.81 p=0.015	Death HR 0.76 p=0.06	HF Death, Admission HR 0.66 p=0.002
CARE-HF[22]	813	Parallel	29.4 mean	≥ 150 ≥ 120 +echo	160 median	30 height indexed	Yes n=92	≤ 35	III, IV	SR	No	Death or MACE HR 0.63 p<0.001	Death HR 0.64 p=0.002	HF Admission HR 0.48 p<0.001

6MWT, 6-minute walk test
AF, atrial fibrillation
HF, heart failure
HR, hazard ratio
ICD, implantable cardioverter defibrillator
LVEDD, left ventricular end diastolic diameter
LVEF, left ventricular ejection fraction
MACE, major adverse cardiovascular event
MLHFQ, Minnesota Living with Heart Failure Questionnaire
NYHA, New York Heart Association
SR, sinus rhythm
Vo$_2$, oxygen consumption (ml/min/kg)

nonresponders in a number of studies.[23–26] This correlation between QRS narrowing and clinical efficacy suggests that after LV lead implantation, positioning the RV lead to produce maximal QRS shortening may improve resynchronization.[26] In 139 consecutive patients, ΔQRS was an independent predictor of response after multivariate adjustment. The RV lead was positioned for maximum reduction in QRS duration at the apex, septum, anterior wall, or RV outflow tract, guided by intra-operative biventricular pace mapping.[23]

MECHANICAL DYSSYNCHRONY

What Is Mechanical Dyssynchrony?

Mechanical dyssynchrony may be considered in terms of interventricular and intraventricular components. Interventricular dyssynchrony refers to delayed activation of the LV relative to the right ventricle. Intraventricular dyssynchrony refers to delayed activation of one left ventricular region relative to another. Correction of intraventricular delay frequently simultaneously improves interventricular delay through ventricular interdependence. CRT aims to correct both aspects of mechanical dyssynchrony.

Why Is Mechanical Dyssynchrony Important?

Baseline QRS duration consistently fails to predict response (Table 4.2). The ECG is unable to convey the presence and severity of electrical delay in all ventricular segments, and correlates particularly poorly with disturbance of distal conduction tissue. QRS morphology and duration are only influenced by significant myocardial masses. Regional changes represented by small vectors are inadequately displayed. In failing myocardium, heterogeneous interstitial fibrosis occurs with localized rearrangement of extracellular matrices and myocytes. Consequently, normal depolarization is replaced by a diffuse activation wave front travelling throughout the myocardial wall.[27] This disorganized depolarization generates abnormal regional loading conditions, inducing further localized fibrosis and hypertrophy with consequent mechanical dyssynchrony.

Although coupling of electrical activation and mechanical contraction remains incompletely defined, there is convincing evidence of electromechanical dissociation. QRS duration has no correlation with intraventricular dyssynchrony, and only a limited relationship with interventricular dyssynchrony. Regional delays in time to peak systolic velocity (Ts) occur in addition to delays in isovolumic contraction, suggesting further mechanical limitation occurs after electrical activation.[28] In myocardial ischemia, impaired regional contractility and wall motion abnormalities frequently produce mechanical dyssynchrony without disturbing electrical conduction. Hemodynamic studies indicate both BiV and LV pacing similarly augment systolic function regardless of different electrical activation.[8–9] In fact, cardiac output improves during LV pacing despite a significant increase in QRS duration.[29–30] This suggests benefit from CRT relates to improved mechanical rather than electrical coordination.

TABLE 4.2 Studies Defining Change in QRS Duration Following CRT

First Author (Ref. No.)	n	Inclusion QRS Duration (ms)	Follow-up (Months)	Response Criteria	Nonresponders (%)	QRS Responders vs. Nonresponders (ms) Baseline	ΔQRS
Lecoq.[23]	139	> 150	6	Survival, and HF hospitalization, and NYHA ≥ 1 class, or peak Vo$_2$ ≥ 10% or 6 min walk ≥ 10%	28	192 vs. 180 p=0.018	37 vs. 11 p<0.001
Pitzalis.[24]	60	> 130	14	Survival, and heart failure hospitalization	27	168 vs. 179 p=NS	45 vs. 31 p<0.05
Bax.[25]	85	≥ 120	6	NYHA ≥ 1 class, and 6 min walk ≥ 25%	26	174 vs. 171 p=NS	32 vs. 6 p<0.01
Molhoek.[101]	61	> 120	6	NYHA ≥ 1 class	26	179 vs. 171 p=NS	29 vs. 11 p=0.07
Alonso.[26]	26	> 120	6	Survival, and NYHA ≥ 1 class, and peak Vo$_2$ ≥ 10%	27	179 vs. 176 p=NS	23 vs. 4 p=0.04
Penicka.[56]	49	≥ 130	6	≥ 25% LVEF	45	190 vs. 171 p<0.01	38 vs. 17 -
Sassone[36]	48	≥ 120	6	≥ 15% LVESV	35	152 vs. 151 p=NS	10 vs. 3 p<0.001
Pitzalis.[37]	20	≥ 140	1	≥ 15% LVESV	40	173 vs. 164 p=NS	21 vs. 22 p=NS
Yu.[68]	30	> 140	3	≥ 15% LVESV	43	166 vs. 150 p=NS	24 vs. 19 p=NS

LVEF, left ventricular ejection fraction
LVESV, left ventricular end systolic volume
NYHA, New York Heart Association
Vo$_2$, oxygen consumption

How Do We Measure Mechanical Dyssynchrony Using Echocardiography?

Mechanical dyssynchrony may be assessed using conventional M-mode and Doppler echocardiography. Newer modalities include tissue Doppler imaging (TDI), tissue synchronization imaging (TSI), triplane tissue Doppler imaging, real-time three-dimensional echocardiography (RT3DE), strain rate imaging (SRI), and speckle tracking strain.

What Are the Limitations of Echocardiographic Parameters Using Conventional Measurements?

Left ventricular pre-ejection period (LVPEP), the time interval between QRS onset and beginning of the aortic Doppler flow velocity curve,[31] represents a complex interaction between ventricular contraction, preload, and afterload. A delay ≥ 140 ms is considered indicative of intraventricular dyssynchrony.[31–33]

Interventricular mechanical delay (IVMD) is the difference in left and right ventricular pre-ejection periods (LVPEP – RVPEP), measured from QRS onset to the beginning of aortic and pulmonary Doppler flow velocity curves respectively.[31] An IVMD ≥ 40 ms, 2SD above the mean of normal controls,[34] represents interventricular dyssynchrony.[31–32, 35] Multiple factors influence ventricular ejection, including changes in preload and afterload. In particular, prolonged RVPEP in pulmonary hypertension or right ventricular dysfunction reduces IVMD and accuracy of assessment.[35]

Left lateral wall diastolic contraction (LLWDC) describes delayed lateral wall contraction (using M-mode) after onset of diastolic filling (transmitral Doppler E wave onset).[22, 31, 32, 36] Coexistence of postsystolic contraction and diastolic relaxation signifies severe intraventricular dyssynchrony. Specificity is thus high, but sensitivity low.

Septal-to-posterior wall motion delay (SPWMD) measures time between maximal incursion of the septum and posterior wall on M-mode, with delay ≥ 130 ms considered significant intraventricular dyssynchrony.[24, 36–41] Many drawbacks exist. It is one dimensional, comparing only two basal segments and neglecting the more frequently delayed lateral wall. Septal motion reflects interventricular in addition to intraventricular dyssynchrony.[36] Feasibility is variably reported between 55% and 100%.[24, 36–41] Maximal septal or posterior wall motion is often diminished or absent in ischemic populations, causing inaccurate assessment.[36, 38–40] Parasternal acoustic windows may be inadequate.[40] Perpendicular M-mode sections of the proximal left ventricle are often not possible.[39] A calculated anatomical M-mode lowers temporal resolution, while a skewed M-mode produces artefactual dyssynchrony by comparing segments at different longitudinal positions.

TISSUE DOPPLER IMAGING

Temporal vs. Spatial Dyssynchrony

Tissue Doppler imaging evaluates longitudinal myocardial contraction in varying numbers of basal and mid-segments from apical four-, three-, and two- chamber views. Either time to peak systolic velocity (Ts) or time to onset of systolic velocity (To) is measured relative to QRS onset. LV dyssynchrony is quantified either by the standard deviation of 12 segments (Ts-SD-12 or "dyssynchrony index") or the maximal temporal difference between two (Ts-2, To-2) or more LV segments (e.g., Ts-6, Ts-12). Larger values indicate more severe dyssynchrony. The parameters neglect fundamental principles. Reduced cardiac ejection occurs through displacement of blood volume from early- to late-activated regions. More contractile force is accommodated when delayed segments are clustered together. The net impact is less when delays are dispersed throughout the ventricle.[42] Variance in timing alone cannot differentiate between spatial patterns of dyssynchrony.

Alignment

The limitations of TDI are similar to those of conventional Doppler. Excessive gain causes spectral broadening and velocity overestimation. Alignment of the insonating beam and direction of myocardial movement is crucial. Error is unavoidable given the limited number of acoustic windows through the human thorax. Deviation underestimates velocities and creates erroneous peaks through inclusion of nonlongitudinal motion. Alignment is particularly challenging in dilated, thinned, and spherically distorted ventricles.

Longitudinal Motion

Transducer orientation and insonation angle restricts TDI assessment to the longitudinal plane. However, ventricular contraction involves complex torsional deformation originating in oppositely wound myocardial fiber helices.[42,43] In systole the base rotates clockwise, and the apex rotates counterclockwise.[43] This wringing motion combines longitudinal, circumferential, and radial vectors. Of these, longitudinal indexes have several disadvantages, including low amplitude, greater variance, and limited contribution to systolic function.[42]

Pulsed Wave Analysis

Pulsed wave and color-coded TDI are compared in Table 4.3. Pulsed wave TDI is widely available and offers high temporal resolution. Sampling is restricted to a single position during each cardiac cycle, precluding post-hoc repositioning and analysis. Comparison of multiple segments requires separate acquisitions in different cycles, and is limited by differences in heart rate, loading conditions, and respiration. Atrial fibrillation is notably problematic.[44] By contrast, color-coded TDI stores time velocity data superimposed on 2-D cine loops, allowing offline analysis of multiple segments simultaneously during the same cardiac cycle.

Timing Velocities

Numerous issues confound timing of tissue Doppler velocities relative to the surface electrocardiogram. Errors may

TABLE 4.3 Differences Between Color-Coded and Pulsed Wave Tissue Doppler Imaging

Color-coded TDI	Pulsed Wave TDI
Limited availability	Wider availability
Myocardial velocities 10%-20% lower compared to pulsed wave TDI	Myocardial velocities 10%-20% higher compared to color-coded TDI.
Lower temporal resolution	Higher temporal resolution
Higher spatial resolution	Lower spatial resolution
Rapid acquisition	Slower acquisition
Offline analysis	Online analysis
Post-hoc sample volume repositioning possible	Post-hoc sample volume repositioning impossible
Simultaneous comparison of multiple segments	Simultaneous comparison of segments impossible

result from imprecise identification of QRS onset, depending on morphology and electrical trace clarity. Measurement from a uniform point on the electrocardiogram is recommended if the QRS onset is unclear.[45] The period during which to measure peak velocity is controversial. Although analysis is typically confined to the ejection interval, extension into diastole has been advocated.[46–48] However, inclusion of postsystolic shortening yielded inferior results in comparative studies.[49–50]

Inconsistencies in choosing peak velocity greatly impair reproducibility. Suboptimal image quality, misalignment, translational vectors, and signal noise all create artefacts. Multiphasic or ambiguous velocity curves hinder uniform interpretation. A recent study invited nine expert faculty members of an international echocardiography congress to analyze velocity traces from 18 consecutive patients.[51] Full agreement was achieved in just three cases, with an intraclass correlation coefficient of 0.42. For double peaks, selection of the highest was advised in the Cardiac Resynchronization Therapy in Patients with Heart Failure and Narrow QRS (RethinQ) trial.[52]

Measuring the time to onset of systolic velocity avoids errors in identifying peak velocity, and is considered a surrogate for regional electromechanical coupling.[34–35, 53–56] The rationale for measuring time to onset as opposed to peak velocity depends on the perceived purpose of CRT. The former aims to synchronize ventricular depolarization, the latter synchronize mechanical contraction. Few studies have compared strategies, some favoring time to onset,[54] others time to peak.[28]

Positioning Region of Interest (ROI)

Timing and velocities are neither homogeneous within segments, nor abruptly demarcated between segments. Delayed contraction occurs in all segments and all levels of the ventricle. Any given parameter will vary depending on the location interrogated. Moving the region of interest (ROI) within segments significantly alters timing. Mean septal-lateral delay (Ts-2) was 28 ms higher when comparing low-basal and mid-basal ROIs in 41 consecutive patients (p<0.01).[51] Bland-Altman limits of agreement were correspondingly wide (± 129 ms). Recent publications now advocate manually adjusting the ROI within the segment (up or down, left or right)

to produce the most "representative" peak velocity.[45–57] This contrasts starkly with the methods in earlier reports.

Feasibility

Remarkably few studies reported feasibility, given the aforementioned limitations (Table 4.4). Many enrolled nonconsecutive patients, or excluded patients with inadequate measurements from analysis.[41–44, 54–58] Whether such perfect data acquisition translates to real-world practice is highly questionable. Exponents of echocardiographic dyssynchrony ignore the realities of clinical practice. Who will arbitrate image quality? What is suboptimal? Which patients are suitable for a dyssynchrony study? Contrast this with QRS duration, readily measured in every patient by anyone with basic technical training.

TISSUE SYNCHRONIZATION IMAGING

The TSI algorithm automatically detects peak systolic velocity. Color coding superimposed on real-time images displays regional delays, ranging from green (earliest) to red (latest). A quantitative tool automatically calculates the median Ts within a manually positioned sample volume, enabling rapid comparison of segments.[49, 59] As with traditional TDI, moving the region of interest within segments alters the measured delay. The TSI algorithm detects velocity peaks within a specified time interval. Systole must be manually defined according to aortic valve opening and closure. Incorrect timing introduces error through inclusion of peaks outside the ejection phase.

TRIPLANE TISSUE DOPPLER IMAGING

Color-coded TDI only compares opposing walls within one plane. Interrogation of all segments requires three separate acquisitions in orthogonal planes, neglecting heart rate variability. A single 3-D triplane dataset allows simultaneous comparison of all 12 segments during the same cardiac cycle. The technique reduces acquisition time, eliminates heart rate

TABLE 4.4 Design of Studies Investigating Parameters Predicting Response to CRT

First Author (Ref. No.)	n	Follow-Up (Months)	Prospective	Consecutive Patients	Blinded Analysis	Dyssynchrony Parameter	Cut-off (ms)	Cut-off Derivation	Feasibility (%)	Variability Intra-	Variability Inter-
Conventional Parameters											
Pitzalis[37]	20	1	Yes	Yes	Yes	SPWMD	130	ROC curve	100	0.96	0.91
Pitzalis[24]	51	14	Yes	Yes	Yes	SPWMD	130	previous study	93	-	-
Marcus[38]	79	6	No	No	Yes	SPWMD	130	previous study	55	High	High
Diaz-Infante[39]	67	6	Yes	Yes	Yes	SPWMD	130	previous study	79	0.97	0.98
Sassone[36]	48	6	No	Yes	No	SPWMD	130	previous study	67	-	-
						LLWDC	present	present/absent	96	-	-
Da Costa[77]	67	12	Yes	No	Yes	IVMD	50	previous study	100	-	-
Achilli[53]	133	6	No	Yes	Yes	IVMD	44	ROC curve	100	-	-
Duncan[76]	39	6	No	No	Yes	t-IVT	-	-	100	-	-
Tissue Doppler Imaging											
Bleeker[40]	98	6	No	Yes	Yes	Ts-2	65	previous study	96	4%	10%
						SPWMD	130	previous study	59	8%	14%
Bax[70]	25	Acute	No	Yes	Yes	Ts-2	60	selected	100	-	-
Bleeker[71]	40	6	Yes	Yes	Yes	Ts-2	65	previous study	100	-	-
Soliman[44]	60	12	No	Yes	Yes	Ts-2 Pulsed	60	previous study	93	Low	Low
Bax[25]	80	6	No	Yes	Yes	Ts-4	65	ROC curve	100	-	-
Heist[58]	39	Acute	No	Yes	No	dP/dt	600 mmHg/s	previous study	-	-	-
					Ts-4	100	previous study				
Notabartolo[48]	49	3	No	Yes	No	Ts-6	110	EP study	100	-	-
Yuan[102]	18	3	Yes	Yes	Yes	Ts-6 Annular	105	ROC curve	100	-	-
Yu[68]	30	3	No	No	No	Ts-SD-12	32.6	2 SD controls	100	<5%	<5%
Yu[50]	54	3	No	No	No	Ts-SD-12	31.4	ROC curve	100	3%	5%
Yu[69]	55	3	No	No	No	Ts-SD-12	31.4	ROC curve	100	-	-
						Ts-12	98.5				
Yu.[57]	256	6	No	No	Yes	Ts-SD-12	33	ROC curve	100	5%	10%
						Ts-12	100	ROC curve			
						Ts-2	60	ROC curve			
De Boeck[51]	41	7	Yes	Yes	Yes	Ts-SD-12	32	previous study	100	13%	-
						Ts-2	60	previous study	100	11%	-
						IVMD	40	previous study	100	14%	-
						Strain-2	150	previous study	100	9%	-
Penicka[56]	49	6	Yes	Yes	Yes	To-3	60	ROC curve	100	7%	9%
						To LV-RV	56	ROC curve	100	6%	7%
						To Sum	102	ROC curve	100	-	-

(Continued)

TABLE 4.4   Design of Studies Investigating Parameters Predicting Response to CRT (Continued)

First Author (Ref. No.)	n	Follow-Up (Months)	Prospective	Consecutive Patients	Blinded Analysis	Dyssynchrony Parameter	Cut-off (ms)	Cut-off Derivation	Feasibility (%)	Intra-	Inter-
Jansen[54]	69	3	No	Yes	No	To-SD-6	20	ROC curve	100	3%	5%
						To-6	60	ROC curve	100		
Jansen[103]	53	3	No	Yes	Yes	Shuffle	present	present/absent	100	6%	11%
Cannesson[72]	23	8	Yes	Yes	No	Velocity Vector	75	ROC curve	92	3%	4%
Tissue Synchronization Imaging											
Tada[47]	22	27	No	No	No	TSI Ts Sep Lat	150	selected	100	–	–
Gorcsan[73]	29	Acute	Yes	Yes	No	TSI Ts-2	65	ROC curve	100	4%	6%
Van de Veire[59]	60	6	No	Yes	Yes	TSI Ts-2	65	previous study	100		
Yu[49]	56	3	No	No	No	TSI Ts-SD-12	34.4	ROC curve	100	4%	6%
						TSI Ts-12	105	ROC curve	100		
						TSI Ts-SD-6	34.5	ROC curve	100		
						TSI Ts-6	78	ROC curve	100		
Three-Dimensional											
Van de Veire[61]	49	Acute	No	Yes	No	3D Ts-SD-12	35.8	ROC curve	100	–	–
Van de Veire[60]	60	6	No	Yes	No	3D Ts-SD-12	33	ROC curve	100	–	–
Marsan[63]	56	Acute	No	Yes	Yes	3D SDI	5.6	ROC curve	93	Low	Low
Strain Rate Imaging											
Porciani[80]	59	6	Yes	No	No	oExcT	760	ROC curve	89	–	0.97
						Ts-SD-12	32	ROC curve		–	–
Mele[41]	37	6	Yes	Yes	Yes	Ts-SD-12	60	median	97	0.99	0.97
						Tε-2 Sep-Post	194	median	87	0.97	0.99
Dohi[74]	38	Acute	No	Yes	No	Tε-2 Sep-Post	130	selected	97	2%	4%
Capasso[104]	28	12	Yes	Yes	No	Tε-2	–	–	–	–	–
Speckle Tracking											
Kneble[83]	38	9	No	No	No	Tε-6	–	–	100	–	–
						Ts-6	105	ROC curve	100	–	–
Suffoletto[67]	50	8	Yes	Yes	No	Tε-2 Sep-Post	130	ROC curve	94	6%	8%
Gorcsan[45]	176	6	Yes	Yes	Yes	Tε-2 & Ts-2	130 / 60	ROC curve	93	–	–

variability, and more accurately defines LV volumes.[60–61] However, many inherent TDI failings remain, including angle dependency, timing of peak velocities, ROI positioning, and assessment of only longitudinal motion.

REAL-TIME THREE-DIMENSIONAL ECHOCARDIOGRAPHY

Dyssynchrony may be characterized without TDI using a three-dimensional model of the left ventricle.[62–64] Four consecutive cardiac cycles are combined to form a larger pyramidal volume.[62–63] Acquisition requires end-expiratory breath holding and a stable heart rate to minimize translation artefacts between the four subvolumes. Application in patients with atrial fibrillation or frequent ectopy is limited. Regional time-volume curves allow measurement of time to minimum systolic volume. The standard deviation of 12 or 16 segments creates a systolic dyssynchrony index, expressed as percentage of the cardiac cycle.[62–64] The parameter encompasses longitudinal, radial, and circumferential contraction. The problems are different, but no less significant, than those of TDI. Translational artefacts and suboptimal endocardial delineation often preclude analysis, confounding 23% of 100 patients with ischemic cardiomyopathy attending a high-volume center.[64] Image quality was deemed optimal in only 34% of cases. Lower frame rates and temporal resolution impede accurate timing. Time-volume curves are critically dependent on positioning of the center point, and ambiguous for akinetic segments.[64] Different software produces different values.[63]

STRAIN RATE IMAGING

TDI myocardial velocities are inherently inaccurate through incorporation of translational cardiac motion, rotation, and tethering by adjacent segments. Strain (ϵ) measures localized myocardial deformation, thus differentiating between passive displacement and active systolic contraction. Dyssynchrony is characterized by dispersion of time to peak strain ($T\epsilon$) between segments, analogous to TDI parameters (e.g., Te-SD-12). Strain rate is traditionally derived from tissue Doppler velocities. High signal noise, artefacts, angle dependence, respiratory drift, and complex data processing all overshadow the theoretical merits.[65] The resulting high intra- and interobserver variability ($> 16\%$)[50,66] limits reproducibility. Interpretation is difficult in ischemic populations as strain delays, particularly postsystolic shortening, may signify myocardial ischemia or viability rather than dyssynchrony.[65]

SPECKLE TRACKING

Speckle tracking is a novel method of quantifying regional strain from routine B-mode gray-scale images.[43–45,67] Tracking patterns of acoustic markers (speckles) quantifies tissue deformation without the directionality constraints of Doppler

techniques. Longitudinal and radial functions are measured from apical and parasternal views respectively. Several shortcomings exist. High quality, high frame rate, second harmonic images are required. Image degradation and through-plane motion both impair speckle tracking.[43] Temporal resolution is lower than TDI techniques. Defining the region of interest remains user dependent. The endocardial and epicardial borders are manually traced and fine-tuned to include all segments throughout the cardiac cycle.[45,67] Further adjustment is undertaken to optimize the tracking stability score.[45]

PREDICTING RESPONSE TO THERAPY

Numerous parameters of intraventricular dyssynchrony have been proposed as predictors of response to CRT (Table 4.4). These largely derive from retrospective, exploratory analyses of multiple measurements in small, single-center, nonrandomized studies. Interpretation is confounded by varying definitions of both dyssynchrony and response. The duration of CRT was frequently only six months or less, inadequate for assessing hard clinical end-points. The majority of evidence derives from three academic programs in Hong Kong,[49–50,57,68,69] Leiden,[25–40,59–61,63–70,71] and Pittsburgh.[45,67,72-74] Among these, it is unclear whether patients from earlier studies were included in subsequent ones. The manuscripts are often not specific regarding whether or not consecutive patients were recruited and whether or not observers performing analysis were blinded. Intra- and interobserver variability is frequently either not presented or quoted from previous studies. Cut-offs derived from one tissue Doppler parameter are inappropriately applied to another: 50 ms from 8 to 2 segment models;[35,53] 65 ms from 4 to 2 segment models,[25,40] 100 ms from 12 to 4 segment models.[58–75] Sensitivity and specificity are proportions for which confidence intervals guide interpretation. Only two studies present such intervals.[45,67] One hundred percent sensitivity and specificity are meaningless in small patient groups. In many studies, the lower confidence interval would equate to tossing a coin. Results are frequently over-interpreted, without statistical confidence that observations are not simply the play of chance.

Predicting Response Using Conventional Parameters

In two studies, SPWMD ≥ 130 ms predicted reverse remodeling in patients with predominantly nonischemic cardiomyopathy (n = 20 and n =60).[24,37] Predictive accuracy (84% and 85%) and correlation between SPWMD and volumetric change were remarkably consistent. In the larger study, SPWMD ≥ 130 ms independently predicted long-term clinical improvement following CRT (median follow-up 14 months).[24] Five subsequent studies unequivocally refuted the clinical applicability and predictive value of SPWMD.[36,38–41] Feasibility ranged from just 55% to 79%

(Table 4.4). Baseline SPWMD consistently failed to differentiate between responders and nonresponders, or correlate with LV remodeling. Sensitivity ranged from 24% to 66%, and specificity from 38% to 66%.

Echocardiographic inclusion criteria in the Cardiac Resynchronization in Heart Failure (CARE-HF) study were in addition to, rather than replacing, intermediate QRS prolongation (120-150 ms).[22] Ninety-two (11%) patients were enrolled, requiring two of three echocardiographic indicators of dyssynchrony: LVPEP > 140 ms; IVMD > 40 ms; or left lateral wall diastolic contraction (LLWDC). All three are relatively insensitive markers of dyssynchrony. Furthermore, by definition IVMD and LVPEP are highly interdependent, demonstrating co-linearity in multivariate models.[51]

A number of small, single-center studies observed no correlation between remodeling after CRT and IVMD, assessed using conventional or tissue Doppler.[25, 36, 50] However, in other reports IVMD predicted both clinical and volumetric response.[51, 76, 77] Two multicenter studies have confirmed the importance of IVMD. The Italian SCART (Selection of CAndidates to cardiac Resynchronization Therapy) trial retrospectively analyzed 6-month outcomes in 133 consecutive patients, defining response by clinical composite score combined with improved LVEF ≥ 5%.[53] Multivariate analysis identified longer IVMD as an independent predictor of positive response (OR = 1.017 [95% CI 1.005-1.029], p = 0.007). However, sensitivity and specificity were limited using the ROC derived cut-off of 44 ms (66% and 55%, respectively). In the CARE-HF trial, prolonged IVMD was an independent predictor of response to CRT (HR 0.99 [95% CI 0.98-1.00], p = 0.0084).[78] A degree of caution is warranted, as both analyses were exploratory, and the interactions between IVMD and response were limited.

Predicting Response Using Tissue Doppler Imaging

The simplest tissue Doppler assessment, septal to lateral delay (Ts-2), predicted short-term remodeling and symptomatic response in studies from three centers.[40,50,57,70,71] A retrospective analysis combined data from 256 patients attending these centers.[57] Septal-to-lateral delay predicted LV remodeling at 6 months with a sensitivity of 70% and specificity of 76%. Less favorable results were obtained elsewhere in 60 and 41 patients.[44,51] Sensitivity for identifying remodeling over similar time periods ranged from 33% to 62%, and specificity from 23% to 65%. Beyond the inherent limitations of TDI described previously, two segment models also neglect the majority of delayed segments. Interrogating more segments improved predictive accuracy in comparative studies.[50, 51, 54, 57]

The maximum time difference between peak systolic velocities in four basal segments (Ts-4) was examined in 85 patients.[25] Dyssynchrony ≥65 ms yielded a sensitivity and specificity of 80% to predict clinical improvement and of 92% to predict reverse remodeling. Patients with dyssynchrony (>65 ms) had improved prognosis compared to those without (6% vs. 50% one year mortality or HF hospitalization, p <0.001). Contrary evidence emerged from the Italian multicenter SCART trial.[53] Time to onset of systolic velocity was measured using pulsed wave Doppler in 133 consecutive patients. Septal to lateral delay (To-2) failed to predict the composite clinical and remodeling end-point in multivariate analysis. Subgroup analysis further discredited TDI techniques.[55] Despite employing a more complex 6-basal segment model, neither clinical nor volumetric response differed in patients with dyssynchrony.

Yu et al. have championed the 12-segment "dyssynchrony index" (Ts-SD-12).[49, 50, 57, 68, 69, 79] All but one report assessed remodeling at 3 months, defined as reduction in LVESV by 15%.[49, 50, 68, 69, 79] The original study included 30 patients.[68] The dyssynchrony index was the only independent predictor of reverse remodeling, with a pre-implant cut-off of 32.6 ms (two SD from the mean of 88 normal controls), remarkably separating responders from nonresponders completely. Four subsequent reports included 54, 55, 56, 58 patients, all with similar baseline characteristics.[49–50, 69, 79] Whether separate patient cohorts were involved is unclear. None of the publications report blinded analysis, prospective study design, or consecutive recruitment. For predicting remodeling, sensitivity ranged from 94% to 100%, and specificity from 78% to 100%.[50–68, 69, 79] Accuracy was similar in a combined analysis of 256 patients attending the universities of Hong Kong, Leiden, and Pittsburgh.[57] Whether comparable results are attainable beyond academic institutions is doubtful. Two other single-center studies have failed to reproduce such high predictive values.[51, 80] Ts-SD poorly predicted volumetric remodeling after 6 months in 41 and 59 patients, respectively. Sensitivity was reasonable (83% and 82%, respectively) but specificity poor (24% and 39%, respectively). As discussed in further detail later, the feasibility and accuracy of tissue Doppler parameters were critically flawed in the multicenter PROSPECT trial.[81]

Predicting Response Using Tissue Synchronization Imaging

The Hong Kong and Leiden groups compared automatic TSI and manual TDI parameters in 56 and 60 patients, respectively.[49, 59] High correlations validated the TSI software (r = 0.97 and r = 0.95 respectively, both p <0.001). Baseline TSI dyssynchrony was significantly greater in responders,[49, 59] and correlated with volumetric change after CRT (Table 4.5).[49] Predictive accuracy for remodeling was similar in 2-, 6-, and 12-segment parameters. Furthermore, the method of quantifying dispersion was only of minor importance. Measurement of standard deviation or range yielded similar overall accuracy and correlations in both the 6- and 12-segment models. No multicenter or randomized trial has employed TSI techniques.

TABLE 4.5 Parameters of Systolic Dyssynchrony Predicting Response to CRT

First Author (Ref. No.)	Responder Definition	% Non Respond	Dyssynchrony Parameter	Responders vs. Nonresponders Parameter (ms)	p	Correlation* r	Correlation* p	Accuracy Sn	Accuracy Sp
Conventional Parameters									
Pitzalis[37]	15% LVESV	40	SPWMD	246 vs. 110	<0.001	0.70	<0.001	100	63
Pitzalis[24]	5% LVEF	53	SPWMD	-	-	0.69	<0.0001	92	78
Marcus[38]	15% LVESV	-	SPWMD	77 vs. 59	0.63	0.10	0.41	24	66
Diaz-Infante[39]	Death, transplant, 6MW 10%	25	SPWMD	158 vs. 144	0.7	-	-	47	48
	15% LVESV	56	SPWMD	-	-	0.2	0.1	50	38
Sassone[36]	15% LVESV	35	SPWMD	96 vs. 108	0.555	-	-	-	-
			LLWDC	9 vs. -12	0.003	Independent predictor		-	-
			IVMD	46 vs. 52	0.308	Independent predictor		-	-
Da Costa[77]	HF death or admission, transplant	30	IVMD	64 vs. 57	0.09	-	-	-	-
Achilli[53]	5% LVEF, Clinical Score	32	IVMD	52 vs. 36	0.029	-	-	66	55
Duncan[76]	NYHA ≥ 1	26	t-IVT	16 vs. 9 (s/min)	<0.001	-	-	-	-
			IVMD	59 vs. 9	<0.001	-	-	-	-
Tissue Doppler Imaging									
Bleeker[40]	NYHA ≥ 1	23	Ts-2	103 vs. 41	<0.05	-	-	90	82
			SPWMD	188 vs. 155	NS	-	-	66	50
Bax[70]	5% LVEF	32	Ts-2	86 vs. 39	<0.01	0.47	0.017	76	88
Bleeker[71]	NYHA ≥ 1 and 6MW ≥ 25%	40	Ts-2	-	-	Independent predictor		-	-
Soliman[44]	NYHA ≥ 1 and 6MW ≥ 25%	17	Ts-2 Pulsed	-	-	-	-	62	20
	15% LVESV	22	Ts-2 Pulsed	81 vs. 78	NS	-	-	62	23
Bax[25]	NYHA ≥ 1 and 6MW ≥ 25%	26	Ts-4	87 vs. 35	<0.01	-	-	80	80
	15% LVESV	-	Ts-4	-	-	0.70	<0.001	92	92
Heist[58]	ΔdP/dt ≥ 25%	54	Ts-4	-	-	0.60	<0.0001	100	38
			dP/dt	-	-	0.47	0.002	89	76
Notabartolo[48]	15% LVESV	41	Ts-6	289 vs. 188	<0.01	-	-	97	55
	NYHA ≥ 1, 6MW 50m, QOL 15	24	Ts-6	264 vs. 198	-	-	-	78	33
Yuan[102]	5% LVEF	39	Ts-6 Annular	111 vs. 86	0.005	0.79	0.033	86	73
Yu[68]	15% LVESV	43	Ts-SD-12	45.0 vs. 24.8	<0.001	0.76	<0.001	100	100
Yu[50]	15% LVESV	43	Ts-SD-12	-	-	0.74	<0.001	96	78
Yu[69]	15% LVESV	47	Ts-SD-12	-	-	0.76	<0.001	96	78
			Ts-12	-	-	0.64	<0.001	90	76
Yu[57]	15% LVESV	45	Ts-SD-12	46 vs. 29	<0.001	-	-	93	73
			Ts-12	137 vs. 91	<0.001	-	-	92	68
			Ts-2	90 vs. 42	<0.001	-	-	70	76
De Boeck[51]	15% LVESV	41	Ts-SD-12	47 vs. 42	NS	0.27	0.086	83	24
			Ts-2	29 vs. 32	NS	0.12	0.453	33	65
			IVMD	67 vs. 41	<0.01	0.46	0.003	91	47
			Strain-2	330 vs. 182	<0.01	0.45	0.003	96	47

(Continued)

"response" criteria is not necessarily "nonresponsive." Without CRT a patient may have undergone further adverse remodeling, been unable to achieve his or her current walking distance, or indeed be dead. A crucial weakness of echocardiographic studies is the absence of "hard" end-points—all cause mortality, cardiovascular death, and hospitalizations.

Reasons for Nonresponders

Lack of response has been attributed to absence of sufficient baseline dyssynchrony to allow improvement with therapy. However, no echocardiographic indicator of dyssynchrony will completely predict a successful response, given the numerous other potential reasons for nonresponse: suboptimal lead placement; nonviable ischemic or infarcted myocardium;[86,87,90] poor threshold or inadequate device optimization; severe LV dilatation;[86] irreversible mitral annular dilatation and severe regurgitation;[86] and development of atrial fibrillation after implantation. Most importantly of all, perhaps, is the duration of CRT. It is highly unlikely, for example, that beta-blockers would have shown clear-cut clinical or volumetric benefits in similarly small-scale and short-duration studies with the end-points used.

THE PROSPECT STUDY

Predictors of Response to Cardiac Resynchronization Therapy

PROSPECT was an observational trial that was expected to inform the cardiologic community of the best echocardiographic indicator to select patients for CRT.[81] The trial proved to be more informative than expected. As part of the trial design, the investigators aimed to ensure that the 12 selected echocardiographic parameters were reproducible when used in multiple international centers (n = 53). Three core laboratories were used. The striking lack of reproducibility of the measures proved to be the principal finding of the study. The echocardiographic indicators also poorly predicted response to CRT, whether defined clinically or echocardiographically.

ECHOCARDIOGRAPHIC DYSSYNCHRONY IN PATIENTS WITH NARROW QRS COMPLEXES

What Is Narrow QRS?

The 120 ms QRS threshold adopted by international guidelines is based on the enrollment criteria of landmark clinical trials. However, the true meaning of "narrow" QRS duration is controversial. The median QRS duration in both COMPANION and CARE-HF was 160 ms, while the mean QRS duration ranged from 155 to 175 ms in the remaining trials (Table 4.1). This has prompted many to question the benefit of CRT in patients with an "intermediate" QRSd between 120 and 150 ms.[91] In the CARE-HF and COMPANION trials,

only those patients with QRS ≥ 160 ms and 169 ms, respectively, experienced a significant risk reduction.[21–22] Such dichotomies are misleading. Efficacy and dyssynchrony are likely to correlate. This does not justify extrapolating arbitrary, nonprespecified cut-offs to patient care. QRS duration is a continuous variable whose threshold must reflect the entry criteria of landmark clinical trials. In these trials the number and outcomes of patients with an intermediate QRS duration is unknown. Withholding CRT in this group is both unfounded and unethical.

Echocardiographic Selection in Narrow QRS Patients

Three nonrandomized, single-center studies have compared CRT in patients with broad and narrow QRS durations (120 ms cut-off), the latter selected using tissue Doppler or conventional parameters (Table 4.6).[92–94] All three studies were small, including between 14 and 51 patients. All three reported no significant difference in clinical and remodeling end-points, including NYHA class and LV ejection fraction. However, the largest narrow QRS study to date yielded similar results without echocardiographic selection. In 331 and 45 patients, respectively, with a wide and narrow QRS, respectively, increases in NYHA class, LVESV, and 6-minute walk distance were similar over a mean 28-month follow-up.[95] The echocardiographic studies are critically flawed. None included a narrow QRS control group without echocardiographic dyssynchrony, or without CRT activated. No hard clinical end-point was evaluated. Most importantly, failure to detect a difference does not imply equivalence.

The only randomized trial in patients with a narrow QRS confirms these misgivings. Following device implantation, the RethinQ trial randomly assigned 172 patients with echocardiographic dyssynchrony to CRT or no CRT.[52] Most patients (96%) were selected using one tissue Doppler criterion (Ts-4 ≥ 65 ms). After 6 months, neither the primary end-point of peak VO2 nor other indicators such as reverse remodeling or 6-minute walk distance improved. In summary, no robust evidence supports echocardiographic selection in patients with a narrow QRS. An appropriate trial would require a reproducible measurement of dyssynchrony tested prospectively with hard clinical end-points.

CONCLUSION

Improving clinical outcomes is clearly desirable. However, proposals that would deny patients an effective treatment with a Class IA guideline recommendation are misguided, unique to devices (as opposed to drugs), and in part driven by limited health care budgets. Landmark trials have demonstrated unequivocal morbidity and mortality benefits in over 4,000 patients enrolled on the basis of their electrocardiogram. Echocardiographic parameters of dyssynchrony are not robust enough to withhold CRT from patients. Extending

TABLE 4.6   CRT in Patients with Narrow QRS Duration

Study	n	n with narrow QRSd	Randomized	Prospective	Blinded	Control Group QRSd	Follow-Up (Months)	Echo Parameter	Main end-points
RethinQ[52]	172	172 <130ms	Yes	Yes	Yes	CRT Off Narrow	6	Ts-4 SPWMD	Peak Vo$_2$ ≥1.0 46% vs. 41%, p=0.63
Yu[92]	102	51 <120ms	No	Yes	No	Wide ≥120ms	3	Ts-SD-12 ≥32.6ms	No significant difference: 6MWT, NYHA, LVEF, LVESV
Bleeker[93]	66	33 <120ms	No	Yes	Yes	Wide ≥120ms	6	Ts-4 ≥65ms	No significant difference: 6MWT, NYHA, LVEF, LVESD, MR
Achilli[94]	52	14 ≤120ms	No	Yes	Yes	Wide >120ms	18 mean	IVMD LLWDC	No significant difference: NYHA, LVEF, LVESD, MR
Gasparini[95]	376	45 ≤120ms	No	Yes	No	Wide >120ms	28 mean	None	No significant difference: mortality, 6MWT, NYHA, LVESV
Gasparini[105]	158	30 <150ms	No	Yes	No	Wide ≥150ms	11 mean	None	No significant difference: 6MWT, QOL, LVEF, LVESV

6MWT, 6-minute walk test; AV, atrioventricular; CRT, cardiac resynchronization therapy; HF, heart failure; IVMD, interventricular mechanical delay; LLWDC, left lateral wall diastolic contraction; LVEDD, left ventricular end diastolic diameter; LVESV, left ventricular end systolic volume; LVEF, left ventricular ejection fraction; LVPEP, left ventricular pre-ejection period; MR, mitral regurgitation; NYHA, New York Heart Association; QOL, quality of life; SPWMD, septal-to-posterior wall motion delay; Vo$_2$, oxygen consumption (ml/min/kg)

CRT to patients with narrow QRS complexes based on echocardiographic parameters has yet to be shown to benefit patients. Echocardiographic assessment will only become credible and applicable to clinical practice once used to select patients for large prospective randomized trials which show an improvement in clinical outcome. From existing evidence, we believe it neither mandatory to alter current guidelines for patient selection (to either restrict or expand the indication for CRT), nor essential to include echocardiographic assessment. For now, the cornerstone of dyssynchrony assessment remains the parameter prospectively validated in landmark clinical trials—the ECG-documented QRS duration.

PRACTICAL POINTS

1. CRT should be implanted in patients with NYHA III or IV symptoms of heart failure, QRS duration > 120ms-1, EF<35%, and SR.
2. CRT selection should not be guided by echocardiographic parameters of dyssynchrony.
3. CRT should not be implanted in patients with a narrow QRS complex.

REFERENCES

1. Swedberg K, Cleland J, Dargie H, et al. Guidelines for the diagnosis and treatment of chronic heart failure: executive summary (update 2005): The Task Force for the Diagnosis and Treatment of Chronic Heart Failure of the European Society of Cardiology. *Eur Heart J.* 2005; 26(11): 1115–1140.
2. Bax JJ, Abraham T, Barold SS, et al. Cardiac resynchronization therapy part 1—issues before device implantation. *J Am Coll Cardiol.* 2005; 46(12):2153–2167.
3. Shenkman HJ, Pampati V, Khandelwal AK, et al. Congestive heart failure and QRS duration: establishing prognosis study. *Chest.* 2002; 122(2):528–534.
4. McCullough PA, Hassan SA, Pallekonda V, et al. Bundle branch block patterns, age, renal dysfunction, and heart failure mortality. *Int J Cardiol.* 2005; 102(2):303–308.
5. Silvet H, Amin J, Padmanabhan S, et al. Prognostic implications of increased QRS duration in patients with moderate and severe left ventricular systolic dysfunction. *Am J Cardiol.* 2001; 88(2):182-5, A6.
6. Baldasseroni S, Opasich C, Gorini M, et al. Left bundle-branch block is associated with increased 1-year sudden and total mortality rate in 5517 outpatients with congestive heart failure: a report from the Italian network on congestive heart failure. *Am Heart J.* 2002; 143(3):398–405.
7. Gottipaty VK, Krelis SP, Lu F, et al. The resting electrocardiogram provides a sensitive and inexpensive marker of prognosis in patients with chronic congestive heart failure. *J Am Coll Cardiol.* 1999; 33(A): 145A.
8. Blanc JJ, Etienne Y, Gilard M, et al. Evaluation of different ventricular pacing sites in patients with severe heart failure: results of an acute hemodynamic study. *Circulation.* 1997; 96(10):3273–3277.
9. Kass DA, Chen CH, Curry C, et al. Improved left ventricular mechanics from acute VDD pacing in patients with dilated cardiomyopathy and ventricular conduction delay. *Circulation.* 1999; 99(12):1567–1573.
10. Auricchio A, Stellbrink C, Block M, et al. Effect of pacing chamber and atrioventricular delay on acute systolic function of paced patients with congestive heart failure. The Pacing Therapies for Congestive Heart Failure Study Group. The Guidant Congestive Heart Failure Research Group. *Circulation.* 1999; 99(23):2993–3001.
11. Leclercq C, Cazeau S, Le Breton H, et al. Acute hemodynamic effects of biventricular DDD pacing in patients with end-stage heart failure. *J Am Coll Cardiol.* 1998; 32(7):1825–1831.
12. Breithardt OA, Sinha AM, Schwammenthal E, et al. Acute effects of cardiac resynchronization therapy on functional mitral regurgitation in advanced systolic heart failure. *J Am Coll Cardiol.* 2003; 41(5):765–770.
13. Stellbrink C, Breithardt OA, Franke A, et al. Impact of cardiac resynchronization therapy using hemodynamically optimized pacing on left ventricular remodeling in patients with congestive heart failure and ventricular conduction disturbances. *J Am Coll Cardiol.* 2001; 38(7):1957–1965.
14. St. John Sutton MG, Plappert T, Abraham WT, et al. Effect of cardiac resynchronization therapy on left ventricular size and function in chronic heart failure. *Circulation.* 2003; 107(15):1985–1990.
15. Saxon LA, De Marco T, Schafer J, et al. Effects of long-term biventricular stimulation for resynchronization on echocardiographic measures of remodeling. *Circulation.* 2002; 105(11):1304–1310.
16. Lau CP, Yu CM, Chau E, et al. Reversal of left ventricular remodeling by synchronous biventricular pacing in heart failure. *Pacing Clin Electrophysiol.* 2000; 23(11 Pt 2):1722–1725.
17. Abraham WT, Fisher WG, Smith AL, et al. Cardiac resynchronization in chronic heart failure. *N Engl J Med.* 2002; 346(24):1845–1853.
18. Cazeau S, Leclercq C, Lavergne T, et al. Effects of multisite biventricular pacing in patients with heart failure and intraventricular conduction delay. *N Engl J Med.* 2001; 344(12):873–880.
19. Auricchio A, Kloss M, Trautmann SI, et al. Exercise performance following cardiac resynchronization therapy in patients with heart failure and ventricular conduction delay. *Am J Cardiol.* 2002; 89(2): 198–203.
20. Auricchio A, Stellbrink C, Sack S, et al. Long-term clinical effect of hemodynamically optimized cardiac resynchronization therapy in patients with heart failure and ventricular conduction delay. *J Am Coll Cardiol.* 2002; 39(12):2026–2033.
21. Bristow MR, Saxon LA, Boehmer J, et al. Cardiac-resynchronization therapy with or without an implantable defibrillator in advanced chronic heart failure. *N Engl J Med.* 2004; 350(21):2140–2150.
22. Cleland JG, Daubert JC, Erdmann E, et al. The effect of cardiac resynchronization on morbidity and mortality in heart failure. *N Engl J Med.* 2005; 352(15):1539–1549.
23. Lecoq G, Leclercq C, Leray E, et al. Clinical and electrocardiographic predictors of a positive response to cardiac resynchronization therapy in advanced heart failure. *Eur Heart J.* 2005; 26(11):1094–1100.
24. Pitzalis MV, Iacoviello M, Romito R, et al. Ventricular asynchrony predicts a better outcome in patients with chronic heart failure receiving cardiac resynchronization therapy. *J Am Coll Cardiol.* 2005; 45(1):65–69.
25. Bax JJ, Bleeker GB, Marwick TH, et al. Left ventricular dyssynchrony predicts response and prognosis after cardiac resynchronization therapy. *J Am Coll Cardiol.* 2004; 44(9):1834–1840.
26. Alonso C, Leclercq C, Victor F, et al. Electrocardiographic predictive factors of long-term clinical improvement with multisite biventricular pacing in advanced heart failure. *Am J Cardiol.* 1999; 84(12):1417–1421.
27. Auricchio A, Yu CM. Beyond the measurement of QRS complex to ward mechanical dyssynchrony: cardiac resynchronisation therapy in heart failure patients with a normal QRS duration. *Heart.* 2004; 90(5): 479–481.
28. Yu CM, Yang H, Lau CP, et al. Regional left ventricle mechanical asynchrony in patients with heart disease and normal QRS duration: implication for biventricular pacing therapy. *Pacing Clin Electrophysiol.* 2003; 26(2 Pt 1):562–570.
29. Turner MS, Bleasdale RA, Mumford CE, et al. Left ventricular pacing improves haemodynamic variables in patients with heart failure with a normal QRS duration. *Heart.* 2004; 90(5):502–505.
30. Leclercq C, Faris O, Tunin R, et al. Systolic improvement and mechanical resynchronization does not require electrical synchrony in the dilated failing heart with left bundle-branch block. *Circulation.* 2002; 106(14): 1760–1763.
31. Cazeau S, Bordachar P, Jauvert G, et al. Echocardiographic modeling of cardiac dyssynchrony before and during multisite stimulation: a prospective study. *Pacing Clin Electrophysiol.* 2003; 26(1 Pt 2):137–143.
32. Cleland JG, Daubert JC, Erdmann E, et al. The CARE-HF study (CArdiac REsynchronisation in Heart Failure study): rationale, design and endpoints. *Eur J Heart Fail* 2001; 3(4):481–489.
33. Yu CM, Abraham WT, Bax J, et al. Predictors of response to cardiac resynchronization therapy (PROSPECT)—study design. *Am Heart J.* 2005; 149(4):600–605.
34. Bader H, Garrigue S, Lafitte S, et al. Intra-left ventricular electromechanical asynchrony. A new independent predictor of severe cardiac events in heart failure patients. *J Am Coll Cardiol.* 2004; 43(2):248–256.

35. Ghio S, Constantin C, Klersy C, et al. Interventricular and intraventricular dyssynchrony are common in heart failure patients, regardless of QRS duration. *Eur Heart J.* 2004; 25(7):571–578.

36. Sassone B, Capecchi A, Boggian G, et al. Value of baseline left lateral wall postsystolic displacement assessed by M-mode to predict reverse remodeling by cardiac resynchronization therapy. *Am J Cardiol.* 2007; 100(3):470–475.

37. Pitzalis MV, Iacoviello M, Romito R, et al. Cardiac resynchronization therapy tailored by echocardiographic evaluation of ventricular asynchrony. *J Am Coll Cardiol.* 2002; 40(9):1615–1622.

38. Marcus GM, Rose E, Viloria EM, et al. Septal to posterior wall motion delay fails to predict reverse remodeling or clinical improvement in patients undergoing cardiac resynchronization therapy. *J Am Coll Cardiol.* 2005; 46(12):2208–2214.

39. Diaz-Infante E, Sitges M, Vidal B, et al. Usefulness of ventricular dyssynchrony measured using M-mode echocardiography to predict response to resynchronization therapy. *Am J Cardiol.* 2007; 100(1):84–89.

40. Bleeker GB, Schalij MJ, Boersma E, et al. Relative merits of M-mode echocardiography and tissue Doppler imaging for prediction of response to cardiac resynchronization therapy in patients with heart failure secondary to ischemic or idiopathic dilated cardiomyopathy. *Am J Cardiol* 2007; 99(1):68–74.

41. Mele D, Pasanisi G, Capasso F, et al. Left intraventricular myocardial deformation dyssynchrony identifies responders to cardiac resynchronization therapy in patients with heart failure. *Eur Heart J.* 2006; 27(9):1070–1078.

42. Helm RH, Leclercq C, Faris OP, et al. Cardiac dyssynchrony analysis using circumferential versus longitudinal strain: implications for assessing cardiac resynchronization. *Circulation.* 2005; 111(21):2760–2767.

43. Notomi Y, Lysyansky P, Setser RM, et al. Measurement of ventricular torsion by two-dimensional ultrasound speckle tracking imaging. *J Am Coll Cardiol.* 2005; 45(12):2034–2041.

44. Soliman OI, Theuns DA, Geleijnse ML, et al. Spectral pulsed-wave tissue Doppler imaging lateral-to-septal delay fails to predict clinical or echocardiographic outcome after cardiac resynchronization therapy. *Europace* 2007; 9(2):113–118.

45. Gorcsan J III, Tanabe M, Bleeker GB, et al. Combined longitudinal and radial dyssynchrony predicts ventricular response after resynchronization therapy. *J Am Coll Cardiol.* 2007; 50(15):1476–1483.

46. Sogaard P, Egeblad H, Kim WY, et al. Tissue Doppler imaging predicts improved systolic performance and reversed left ventricular remodeling during long-term cardiac resynchronization therapy. *J Am Coll Cardiol.* 2002; 40(4):723–730.

47. Tada H, Toide H, Okaniwa H, et al. Maximum Ventricular Dyssynchrony Predicts Clinical Improvement and Reverse Remodeling during Cardiac Resynchronization Therapy. *Pacing Clin Electrophysiol.* 2007; 30 Suppl 1:S13–S18.

48. Notabartolo D, Merlino JD, Smith AL, et al. Usefulness of the peak velocity difference by tissue Doppler imaging technique as an effective predictor of response to cardiac resynchronization therapy. *Am J Cardiol.* 2004; 94(6):817–820.

49. Yu CM, Zhang Q, Fung JW, et al. A novel tool to assess systolic asynchrony and identify responders of cardiac resynchronization therapy by tissue synchronization imaging. *J Am Coll Cardiol* 2005; 45(5):677–684.

50. Yu CM, Fung JW, Zhang Q, et al. Tissue Doppler imaging is superior to strain rate imaging and postsystolic shortening on the prediction of reverse remodeling in both ischemic and nonischemic heart failure after cardiac resynchronization therapy. *Circulation.* 2004; 110(1):66–73.

51. De Boeck BW, Meine M, Leenders GE, et al. Practical and conceptual limitations of tissue Doppler imaging to predict reverse remodeling in cardiac resynchronisation therapy. *Eur J Heart Fail* 2008; 10(3):281–290.

52. Beshai JF, Grimm RA, Nagueh SF, et al. Cardiac-Resynchronization Therapy in Heart Failure with Narrow QRS Complexes. *N Engl J Med.* 2007; 357(24):2461–2471.

53. Achilli A, Peraldo C, Sassara M, et al. Prediction of response to cardiac resynchronization therapy: the selection of candidates for CRT (SCART) study. *Pacing Clin Electrophysiol.* 2006; 29 Suppl 2:S11–S19.

54. Jansen AH, Bracke F, van Dantzig JM, et al. Optimization of pulsed wave tissue Doppler to predict left ventricular reverse remodeling after cardiac resynchronization therapy. *J Am Soc Echocardiogr.* 2006; 19(2):185–191.

55. Peraldo C, Achilli A, Orazi S, et al. Results of the SCART study: selection of candidates for cardiac resynchronisation therapy. *J Cardiovasc Med* (Hagerstown). 2007; 8(11):889–895.

56. Penicka M, Bartunek J, De Bruyne B, et al. Improvement of left ventricular function after cardiac resynchronization therapy is predicted by tissue Doppler imaging echocardiography. *Circulation.* 2004; 109(8):978–983.

57. Yu CM, Gorcsan J III, Bleeker GB, et al. Usefulness of tissue Doppler velocity and strain dyssynchrony for predicting left ventricular reverse remodeling response after cardiac resynchronization therapy. *Am J Cardiol.* 2007; 100(8):1263–1270.

58. Heist EK, Taub C, Fan D, et al. Usefulness of a novel "response score" to predict hemodynamic and clinical outcome from cardiac resynchronization therapy. *Am J Cardiol.* 2006; 97(12):1732–1736.

59. Van de Veire NR, Bleeker G, De Sutter J, et al. Tissue synchronization imaging accurately measures left ventricular dyssynchrony and predicts response to cardiac resynchronization therapy. *Heart.* 2007; 93(9):1034–1039.

60. Van de Veire NR, Yu CM, Ajmone-Marsan N, et al. Triplane tissue Doppler imaging: a novel three-dimensional imaging modality that predicts reverse left ventricular remodelling after cardiac resynchronisation therapy. *Heart.* 2008; 94(3):e9.

61. Van de Veire NR, Bleeker GB, Ypenburg C, et al. Usefulness of triplane tissue Doppler imaging to predict acute response to cardiac resynchronization therapy. *Am J Cardiol.* 2007; 100(3):476–482.

62. Kapetanakis S, Kearney MT, Siva A, et al. Real-time three-dimensional echocardiography: a novel technique to quantify global left ventricular mechanical dyssynchrony. *Circulation.* 2005; 112(7):992–1000.

63. Marsan NA, Bleeker GB, Ypenburg C, et al. Real-time three-dimensional echocardiography permits quantification of left ventricular mechanical dyssynchrony and predicts acute response to cardiac resynchronization therapy. *J Cardiovasc Electrophysiol.* 2008; 19(4):392–399.

64. Burgess MI, Jenkins C, Chan J, et al. Measurement of left ventricular dyssynchrony in patients with ischaemic cardiomyopathy: A comparison of real-time three-dimensional and tissue doppler echocardiography. *Heart.* 2007; 93(10):1191–1196.

65. Marwick TH. Measurement of strain and strain rate by echocardiography: ready for prime time? *J Am Coll Cardiol.* 2006; 47(7):1313–1327.

66. Popovic ZB, Grimm RA, Perlic G, et al. Noninvasive assessment of cardiac resynchronization therapy for congestive heart failure using myocardial strain and left ventricular peak power as parameters of myocardial synchrony and function. *J Cardiovasc Electrophysiol.* 2002; 13(12):1203–1208.

67. Suffoletto MS, Dohi K, Cannesson M, et al. Novel speckle-tracking radial strain from routine black-and-white echocardiographic images to quantify dyssynchrony and predict response to cardiac resynchronization therapy. *Circulation.* 2006; 113(7):960–968.

68. Yu CM, Fung WH, Lin H, et al. Predictors of left ventricular reverse remodeling after cardiac resynchronization therapy for heart failure secondary to idiopathic dilated or ischemic cardiomyopathy. *Am J Cardiol.* 2003; 91(6):684–688.

69. Yu CM, Zhang Q, Chan YS, et al. Tissue Doppler velocity is superior to displacement and strain mapping in predicting left ventricular reverse remodelling response after cardiac resynchronisation therapy. *Heart.* 2006; 92(10):1452–1456.

70. Bax JJ, Marwick TH, Molhoek SG, et al. Left ventricular dyssynchrony predicts benefit of cardiac resynchronization therapy in patients with end-stage heart failure before pacemaker implantation. *Am J Cardiol.* 2003; 92(10):1238–1240.

71. Bleeker GB, Kaandorp TA, Lamb HJ, et al. Effect of posterolateral scar tissue on clinical and echocardiographic improvement after cardiac resynchronization therapy. *Circulation.* 2006; 113(7):969–976.

72. Cannesson M, Tanabe M, Suffoletto MS, et al. Velocity vector imaging to quantify ventricular dyssynchrony and predict response to cardiac resynchronization therapy. *Am J Cardiol.* 2006; 98(7):949–953.

73. Gorcsan J III, Kanzaki H, Bazaz R, et al. Usefulness of echocardiographic tissue synchronization imaging to predict acute response to cardiac resynchronization therapy. *Am J Cardiol.* 2004; 93(9):1178–1181.

74. Dohi K, Suffoletto MS, Schwartzman D, et al. Utility of echocardiographic radial strain imaging to quantify left ventricular dyssynchrony and predict acute response to cardiac resynchronization therapy. *Am J Cardiol.* 2005; 96(1):112–116.

75. Yu CM, Lin H, Zhang Q, et al. High prevalence of left ventricular systolic and diastolic asynchrony in patients with congestive heart failure and normal QRS duration. *Heart.* 2003; 89(1):54–60.

76. Duncan AM, Lim E, Clague J, et al. Comparison of segmental and global markers of dyssynchrony in predicting clinical response to cardiac resynchronization. *Eur Heart J.* 2006; 27(20):2426–2432.

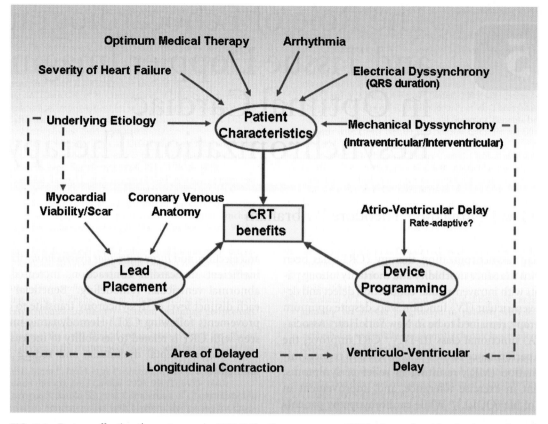

FIG. 5.1. Factors affecting the outcome in CRT. Patient's response to CRT is determined by the interaction of one's individual clinical characteristics with intraprocedural outcome and the device programming. The determinants of these three factors are in turn multifactorial, and interplay (broken red line) among these determinants will impact the net benefit from pacing therapy.

ventricular systole to follow atrial contraction. Ventriculo-atrial gradient resulting from atrial relaxation and initiation of ventricular contraction may result in a "diastolic" MR, which further reduces preload and therefore stroke volume (SV).[17–18] Short AV delay, on the other hand, modifies late diastolic filling dynamics. Interruption of the active atrial transport by the premature closure of the MV resulting from the onset of the ventricular contraction compromises SV.[19] As such, defining the optimal AV delay for each individual patient is deemed important to create an impact on the hemodynamic improvement and clinical benefits from CRT. Echocardiography can provide information on the timing of LV filling and atrial transport critical to maximizing preload and SV.

Echocardiographic Interrogation of Optimal AV Delay

Optimization of AV delay following device implantation has been more commonly achieved by performing Doppler echocardiography and analyzing flow velocity profiles at the level of mitral, aortic, and left ventricular outflow tract

(LVOT), as well as the MR flow profile.[20–22] Optimal AV delay can be calculated from the LV filling times during long and short AV delays or determined by dynamic AV delay programming with measures of acute hemodynamic benefit as surrogates.

Assessment of Transmitral Flow Pattern

Pulsed-wave (PW) Doppler analysis of the mitral inflow pattern provides insight into the role of left atrial (LA) contribution to LV filling. Proper timing of ventricular contraction relative to atrial contraction and relaxation is characterized by an increase in the LV filling time and complete separation of the mitral E and A waves without causing truncation on the latter.

Doppler interrogation of the mitral inflow is best performed on the apical four-chamber view, where flow is usually parallel to the ultrasound beam. PW sample volume, 1-2 mm in size, is placed either on the tip of the ventricular side of the open mitral leaflets or at the level of mitral annulus, depending on which parameter is being assessed. Parameters of diastolic function that relate to the transmitral gradient are best obtained at the tips of the valve leaflets while those reflecting changes in flow should be measured from recordings of the inflow velocity at the mitral annulus, where the cross-sectional area (CSA) is more stable.[23] Spectral display of mitral A wave is also more defined when sample volume is placed in the mitral annulus.[24]

Technical Considerations

Pitfalls in recording mitral E and A wave velocities are related to misalignment of the ultrasound beam, misplacement of sample volume, and suboptimal machine settings.

Poorly defined signals arising from improper alignment of the beam with the direction of the blood flow may also render measurements unreliable. Hence, optimizing ultrasound beam alignment and proper adjustment of the machine settings should be done. Overestimation of mitral velocity time integral (VTI) may result from incorrect placement of sample volume too far into the left ventricle. Respiration as well as changes in the position of intracardiac structures during contraction and relaxation may relatively vary the location of the sample volume during the entire cardiac cycle. Attention to consistency of sample volume location is important in serial or comparative studies. Technically this error can be minimized by performing the assessment on a breath-hold and by placing the sample volume in midway between the level of the mitral annulus and the mitral leaflets.[24] Alternately, in patients for whom breath-holding is a problem, turning the respirometer signals may aid in identifying VTI spectral display recorded at expiration.

Error may also arise from improper tracking of the Doppler trace. Failure to trace the modal velocity or the brightest line may result in inconsistent measurements. When tracing the velocity to derive a VTI, it is best to trace the outer edge of the most dense (or brightest) portion of the spectral tracing and ignore the dispersion that occurs near peak velocity.[23]

Iterative Method Using Diastolic Filling Time (DFT) or Mitral Inflow VTI (E-A VTI)

The iterative method using transmitral PW Doppler optimizes AV delay by allowing maximal separation of the early passive filling "E" wave and the active atrial transport "A" wave without being extremely short as to produce early closure of the mitral valve. It is performed by programming a long AV delay that is shorter than the intrinsic PR interval, but long enough to preserve biventricular capture. Alternately some authors programmed long AV delay 30 ms short of the intrinsic PR interval. The AV delay is gradually shortened at decrements of 20 ms until truncation of the A wave is observed (Fig. 5.2A and Fig. 5.2B). Gradual prolongation of AV delay at increments of 10 ms is performed until truncation is eliminated (Fig. 5.2C).[20, 22, 25] DFT, the interval from the onset of E wave to A wave terminus, is measured for each programmed AV delay. Alternately, one can measure EA VTI, a surrogate of diastolic filling volume for a given length of AV delay.[26] Measurement of E wave or A wave VTI alone is

not encouraged because at long AV delay, fusion of E and A waves (Fig. 5.2A) resulting from near simultaneous occurrence of early filling and the atrial kick may interfere with the accuracy and consistency in the measurements. Optimal AV delay is set at the setting corresponding to the E and A wave separation with the greatest VTI. Iterative method using DFT and/or EA VTI is performed at both atrial-sensed (AS) and atrial-paced (AP) biventricular pacing.

Ritter Method

Ritter's formula aims to maximize LV diastolic filling time without interruption of the "atrial kick." This method was originally developed for patients with high-grade AV block requiring a dual-chamber pacemaker. In a small study by Melzer et al. Ritter's formula was found to have good correlation with radionuclide ventriculography when used in optimizing AV interval among patients with reduced LV function.[27] According to Ritter, pacing in DDD with a long AV delay results in the abbreviation of the DFT as a result of premature MV closure before the onset of ventricular contraction. Conversely, when AV delay is shortened inappropriately, end-diastolic filling flow is abruptly interrupted by the ventricular contraction when LA pressure is still high.[28] The Ritter method requires PW Doppler imaging of the mitral inflow during a long and an inappropriately short AV delay. At each AV delay setting, the time interval from the termination of mitral A wave to the onset of the paced QRS is measured and designated as QA long and QA short, respectively (Fig. 5.3A and Fig. 5.3B). Optimal AV delay is derived using the following formula: Optimal AV delay = SAV short + ([SAV long + QA long] − [SAV short + QA short]) where SAV long and SAV short are long and short sensed AV delay, respectively.[26]

Ishikawa Method (Ishikawa and Inoue)

A modification of Ritter's formula was devised by Ishikawa et al. who theorized that the AV delay at which the end of the mitral A wave coincides with complete MV closure may be optimal. This method is carried out by simultaneous recording of phonocardiogram and the PW Doppler of transmitral flow at a slightly long AV delay. The time interval from the termination of A wave to the complete MV closure (mitral component of S1) is measured. Alternately this interval can also be derived from the termination of mitral A wave to the end of diastolic MR. Using this method, optimal AV delay is predicted by decreasing the long AV delay by the measured time interval. The optimal AV delay predicted by this formula correlated positively with optimal AV delay determined by an increase in invasively measured cardiac output (CO) and a decrease in pulmonary capillary wedge pressure (PCWP).[29–30]

Meluzin Method

Further modification of the Ritter and Ishikawa methods was proposed by Meluzin et al. Instead of using the onset of paced QRS (Ritter method), the mitral component of S1 on phonocardiogram or the duration of low velocity diastolic MR (Ishikawa method), Meluzin used the

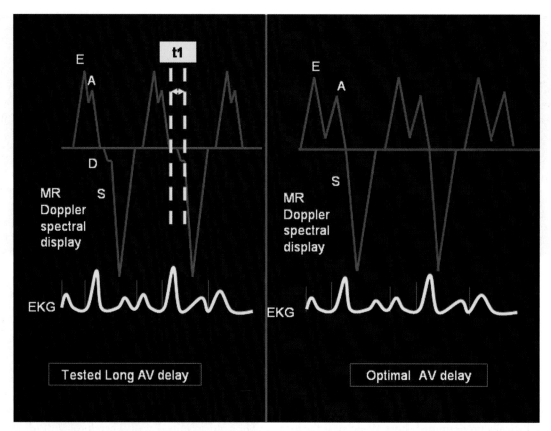

FIG. 5.4. Meluzin Method: Precise determination of the end of atrial and onset of ventricular contractions is of utmost importance in the identification of optimal AV delay. The high velocity systolic (S) component of mitral regurgitation (MR) used to identify the onset of ventricular contraction in this technique should be easily differentiated from the diastolic component of the MR jet. With long AV delay diastolic MR (D) occurs as a result of the reversal of left atrio-ventricular pressure gradient during atrial relaxation before the onset of ventricular contraction and is therefore characterized by low velocity signals. Using this method, the programmed long AV delay should be shortened by t1 which is the time interval between the termination of the A wave and the onset of systolic MR (S) to time the onset of ventricular contraction immediately after the end of atrial contraction. Thus, optimal AV delay = tested long AV delay − t1

the summation of isovolumic contraction time, LV ejection time, and isovolumic relaxation time (Fig. 5.7A). The LV ejection time (b) is measured from the interval between the onset and cessation of LVOT velocity curve (Fig. 5.7B). The sum of isovolumic times was obtained by subtracting the ejection time from the A-E interval. The index is the sum of isovolumic times divided by ejection time. Thus, MPI = (a−b)/b.[36,40] The optimal AV delay is that AV interval that yields the lowest MPI. Setting of various AV interval during interrogation proceeds in a dynamic sequential pattern of iterative method.[40]

Assessment of Left Ventricular Outflow Tract or Aortic Flow Velocity Profile

LVOT or Aortic VTI Method Compared with diastolic AV delay optimization whose rationale rests primarily on

improving preload through achieving maximal atrial contribution to LV filling, systolic AV delay optimization aims at improving SV and CO. Serial evaluation of SV and CO is a primary application of PW or CW Doppler interrogations of the LVOT and aortic flow respectively. Given that the LVOT or aortic annulus cross-sectional area (CSA) is relatively stable in the same patient, the VTI can accurately track beat to beat changes in SV resulting from dynamic manipulation of the AV interval. Hence, optimal AV delay is defined as the setting which produced greatest LVOT/ aortic VTI.

Spectral Doppler interrogation of blood flow within the LVOT is best performed using the apical five-chamber or apical long axis view. PW sample volume of 3-5 mm gate is positioned just proximal to the aortic valve. Wall filter should be adjusted to allow delineation of the commencement and cessation of flow. Gain, velocity scale,

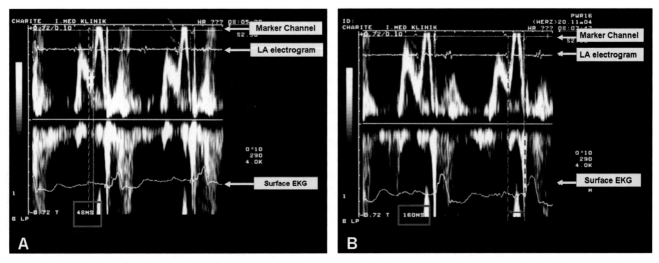

FIG. 5.5. **A:** Measurement of the interatrial conduction time (IACT) in the VDD Mode: IACT is the time interval from the right atrial sensing marker (red arrow, Marker Channel) to the left atrial deflection (red arrow, LA electrogram). In this particular patient, the IACT is 48 ms. **B:** Assessment of the left-atrial electromechanical action, (LA-EAC long.). During an uphysiologically long AV interval, LA-EAC long is defined as the time interval between the left atrial deflection (red arrow, LA electrogram) and the end of mitral A wave. In this particular patient, the LA-EAC long is 160 ms. (A, B Modified from Melzer et al. Influence of the atrio-ventricular delay optimization on the intra left ventricular delay in cardiac resynchronization therapy. *Cardiovascul Ultrasound* 2006 4:5 doi:10.1186/1476-7120-4-5)

and baseline should be adjusted accordingly to optimally display the entire Doppler spectrum without excessive background noise. Blood flow detected within LVOT is displayed in a V-shaped configuration, depicting steep acceleration and deceleration slopes, with the aortic valve closing click following immediately after end-ejection. The LVOT VTI is measured by tracing the outer edge of the brightest signal.[23]

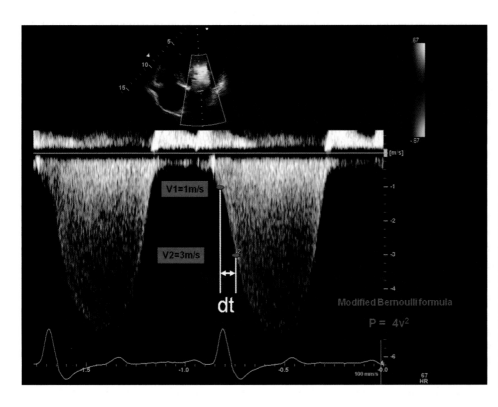

FIG. 5.6. Doppler-derived dP/dt. The rate of pressure rise (RPR) is calculated using the MR jet CW Doppler profile. Two velocity time points, 1m/s and 3m/s, in the MR jet are used as reference, and the respective pressures are derived from these velocities using the modified Bernoulli formula. The time that it takes for the velocity to change from 1m/s to 3m/s (dt) is measured. The velocity derived pressure difference is corrected for dt.

escape detection during guided lead placement. In addition, variability in the coronary venous anatomy and the complexity of the technique of LV lead implantation may render lead placement suboptimal thereby causing persistent abnormal LV activation and depolarization when pacing was applied. Tailoring the timing of ventricular pre-excitation may address the varying patterns of ventricular activation and overcome conduction abnormalities across regions of infarcted myocardium in the setting of a suboptimal lead placement.

Optimal Interventricular Interval (V-V delay)

The goal of V-V optimization is to determine an optimal V-V delay that further reduces inter- and intra-ventricular *mechanical* dyssynchrony promoting cardiac mechanical efficiency and resultant improvement in SV. In HF patients, slow conduction of activation within the LV resulting from fibrosis, ischemia, and myocardial scarring may necessitate earlier activation of the affected site to restore balanced electrical activation and effect synchronized contraction. Studies have demonstrated that sequential biventricular pacing results in an improved systolic and diastolic performance with reduction in the extent of myocardium displaying DLC and intraventricular dyssynchrony with corresponding improvement in LVEF and LV dP/dt, and reduction in MR volume[53, 55–56] when compared with simultaneous pacing. Long-term benefit associated with tailored optimal interventricular interval translated to hemodynamic and clinical improvements and significant reduction in the percentage of nonresponders to CRT.[57] In the In-Synch III study, incremental benefit of tailored sequential biventricular pacing, with an earlier LV pre-excitation, over nominal V-V setting was evident with significant improvement in the echocardiographically determined SV among patients with history of myocardial infarction (MI). Hemodynamic improvement with sequential biventricular pacing translated to a greater exercise capacity but did not improve NYHA functional class or QOL.[58] Bordachar et al. reported otherwise. In their study on 41 CRT recipients, not only did NYHA functional class and QOL improve but echocardiographic evidence of LV reverse remodeling was observed after 3 months of tailored sequential bi-ventricular pacing.[56] On the contrary, the Resynchronization for Hemodynamic Treatment for Heart Failure Management II Implantable Cardioverter Defibrillator (RHYTHM II ICD) found no significant incremental benefits with optimized V-V delay. The magnitude of clinical improvement achieved after 6 months of CRT in terms of symptom alleviation, functional capacity, and QOL were comparable between those whose V-V delays were nominally and optimally programmed.[59]

Echocardiographic Methods of Optimizing V-V Delay

Interventricular mechanical delay (IMD) can be determined by measuring the difference between the pulmonic and aortic pre-ejection intervals using PW Doppler technique. Optimal V-V delay can be defined simply as that interventricular interval that yields the least V-V mechanical delay. However, it has been previously shown that reduced V-V dyssynchrony is not correlated with improved left ventricular systolic function.[56] Thus V-V echocardiographic V-V delay optimization is best performed by using hemodynamic surrogates of improved LV systolic function or assessing the magnitude of achieved reduction in intraventricular dyssynchrony.

Assessment of Doppler-Derived Hemodynamic Surrogates of Improved Systolic Function

Interrogation of optimal V-V delay is commonly performed at the pre-determined optimal AV delay setting.[55, 57] Depending on the design of the implanted device, dynamic sequential programming of the V-V delay at varying ranges and increments (up 80 ms difference at increments of 20-40 ms)[40, 55–57] may be performed by an earlier stimulation of one ventricle over the other. Optimal V-V delay is set at that sequence and interval that produces the maximum improvement in the Doppler aortic VTI[57, 59–60] or, less commonly, MPI.[40]

Assessment of the Magnitude of Achieved Reduction in Intraventricular Dyssynchrony

Tissue Doppler Imaging   TDI provides information on regional myocardial peak systolic velocities and displacement and their timing relative to the initiation of the electrical stimulation represented by the QRS complex in the EKG tracing. It provides insight to the electromechanical coupling alterations and therefore can reflect the degree of dyssynchrony and the magnitude of its reduction as a consequence of CRT. Sogaard et al. utilized TT, a color-coded display of regional myocardial shortening calculated as the integral of tissue velocity, in assessing the extent of myocardium displaying DLC (Fig. 5.8A-C). Strain rate (SR) analysis was performed on myocardial segments showing motion toward the apex (Fig. 5.8D). Display of motion toward the apex after closure of the aortic valve was only registered as DLC if negative SR documented that the motion reflected true shortening.[15] For all the interrogated V-V intervals, TT was performed using the 16-segment model of LV[61] and global systolic contraction amplitude (GCSA) was derived from the average systolic shortening amplitude of all the segments. The optimum interventricular delay was defined by the maximum GCSA. TDI-guided optimization of V-V delay translated to improvement in the LV systolic performance and dimensions with a resultant NYHA functional class improvement and increase in the 6-minute hall walk during a short-term pacing.[53]

As with any Doppler studies, effects of angle of insonation, stationary artifacts, and noise are to be considered in the interpretation of any TDI-derived curves. Presence of multiple peaks is a common source of error (Fig. 5.8A). Necessary caution is warranted in utilizing this technique. TDI analysis re-

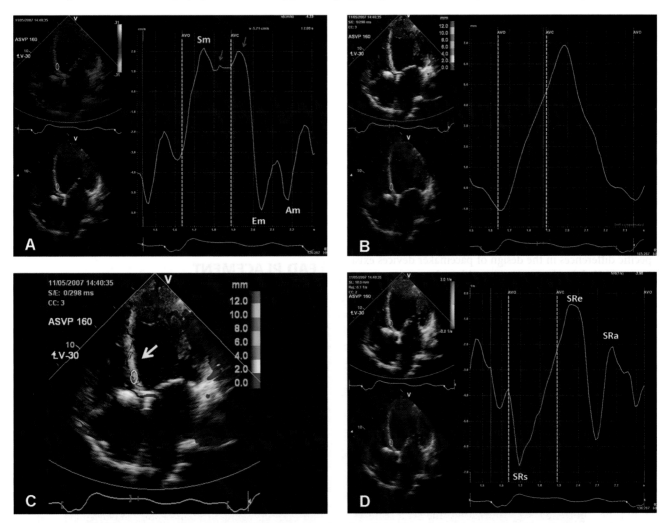

FIG. 5.8. A: Tissue Doppler image in the apical 4-chamber view of a patient with dilated cardiomyopathy paced at an AV delay of 160 ms with LV paced 30 ms earlier than RV (upper left panel) and the corresponding velocity profile at the base of the inter-ventricular septum (right panel). Green broken lines mark the systolic ejection period measured at 250 ms. Peak systolic velocity (Sm) is 2.10 cm/s occurring at 120 ms after aortic valve opening (AVO). Note the presence of a second lower peak (red arrow) occurring at 200 ms after AVO followed by another distinct peak (red arrow) after aortic valve closure (AVC) These two peaks can influence the resultant amplitude of myocardial displacement on Tissue Tracking. **B:** Corresponding Tissue Tracking (TT) image (upper left panel) and profile (right panel). The peak amplitude of systolic shortening is 6.9 occurring at 100 ms after aortic valve closure (AVC), suggestive of delayed longitudinal contraction (DLC). **C:** Tissue Tracking display in color-coded format from figure B. The regional myocardial displacement in each segment is calculated automatically as the integral of the digitally stored velocity tracing during systole for each segment. Note that part of the basal to mid-segment of the interventricular septum where the sample volume (yellow oblong) was placed is gray (yellow arrow), signifying absence of motion towards the apex/transducer, or myocardial relaxation. **D:** Corresponding Strain Rate (SR) image (upper left panel) and SR profile (right panel). To confirm if the measured amplitude in TT is a true DLC, SR imaging must be performed. Peak systolic strain rate (SRs) is −6.79 1/s occurring early in systole (50 ms after AVO). Occurrence of peak Srs during early systole does not support the DLC found in TT (figure B). *Sm, myocradial peak systolic velocity; Em, myocardial peak early diastolic velocity; Am, myocardial peak late diastolic velocity; SRe, peak early diastolic strain rate, Sra, peak late diastolic strain rate.*

Cardiac Magnetic Resonance Assessment of Ventricular Dyssynchrony

Subha V. Raman • Michael Donnally

urrent patient selection for cardiac resynchronization therapy (CRT) relies on global measures of electrical conduction delay (the electrocardiographic QRS duration) and overall systolic function (the left ventricular ejection fraction) combined with clinical assessment of functional status (New York Heart Association class). Approximately one-third of patients diagnosed with heart failure demonstrate electrical conduction abnormalities [1–3] by surface electrocardiography, usually in the form of a complete left bundle branch block (LBBB) or nonspecific intraventricular conduction delay (IVCD).[4] Such electrical conduction abnormalities have been shown to be associated with structural changes resulting in impaired left ventricular function[5] as well as increased morbidity and mortality.[4] In large multicenter trials, responders to CRT have experienced improvements in exercise tolerance, heart failure symptoms, heart failure hospitalizations,[6–7] and mortality.[8–9] These benefits of CRT have been accompanied by reductions in LV chamber size, improvements in ejection fraction, and decreases in the severity of mitral regurgitation.[10–11]

If dyssynchrony is a measurable condition that identifies patients who should benefit from resynchronization, it may have different facets depending on the technique used for measurement. For instance, QRS duration and tissue-Doppler indices (TDI) of dyssynchrony bear only modest overlap. In a study of heart failure patients with LVEF <35%, up to 40%, of patients with QRS duration >120 ms did not exhibit left ventricular dyssynchrony by TDI, and 27% of patients with TDI >60 ms between the septum and lateral wall had normal QRS duration.[12] Some studies have shown a better response to CRT in patients with wider QRS,[13, 14] while others have shown baseline QRS duration to be a poor predictor of long-term response.[6, 15–17] Achilli et al., for example, found a favorable response to CRT seen in patients with dyssynchrony as assessed by echocardiography and QRS <120 ms.[16]

Thus, a potential role for cardiac magnetic resonance (CMR) in patient assessment for CRT emerges from two observations. First, approximately one-third of patients undergoing CRT device implantation do not respond to therapy.[6, 18] Second, the currently used electrocardiographic and echocardiographic measures of electrical and mechanical dyssynchrony perform poorly in discriminating responders from nonresponders. However, postdevice CMR remains relatively contraindicated pending uniform use of MR-compatible lead systems, limiting the use of CMR in CRT to evaluating patients prior to device placement. Here, too, a further limitation becomes apparent when recognizing that many patients referred for CRT already have implanted pacemakers or defibrillators that currently preclude elective magnetic resonance examination. Despite these limitations, CMR identifies important myocardial characteristics not feasible with other approaches that, when feasible, should be performed to improve patient selection for CRT. In addition to the assessment of dyssynchrony, CMR allows for the determination of the size, shape, and function of the LV as well as the presence and transmurality of scar tissue in the location where the LV lead should be positioned.[19–20] Better patient selection should improve outcomes twofold for patients with heart failure as it 1) reduces the cost and complications associated with invasive device implantation in patients who are unlikely to respond and 2) identifies patients who may benefit from CRT yet are deemed ineligible according to conventional ECG and echo parameters. In this chapter we will discuss CMR-based assessment of myocardial strain and their applications to dyssynchrony measurement for CRT. Specific CMR techniques including myocardial tagging, velocity-encoded cine, and late postgadolinium enhancement (LGE) will be examined. We have also included details of a novel approach developed in our laboratory that uses frequency domain-based segmentation of routinely acquired cine CMR images that may overcome some of the variability seen in time domain-based dyssynchrony evaluation. Finally, the safety of CMR in patients with implanted devices will also briefly be discussed.

TAGGED CINE CMR

Tagged cine CMR involves application of saturation bands applied noninvasively during the imaging process by a spatial modulation of magnetization technique (SPAMM). These tags deform in moving tissues and yield quantifiable regional myocardial function through measurement of tag line and grid deformation through the cardiac cycle. Regional myocardial deformation can be analyzed to provide information about three-dimensional strain, including the magnitude of the strain of the LV during the cardiac cycle.[21–22] This method has been used in several studies to track and quantify regional myocardial mechanical dyssynchrony via the assessment of tagged cine CMR.[23]

Initial methods to quantify strain from tagged CMR images focused on tracking the position of tag lines. However, acquiring the tagged images is only clinically useful if strain calculations can be made without time-consuming post-processing.[24]

Using tagged CMR imaging assessment of longitudinal and circumferential dyssynchrony from both temporal and regional strain variance analysis, dyssynchrony assessed by longitudinal motion is less sensitive, follows different time courses than those from circumferential motion, and may manifest CRT benefit during specific cardiac phases depending on pacing mode.[25] These findings concur with those of Zwanenburg et al., who demonstrated that circumferential delays are more sensitive than their longitudinal counterparts.[26] These results highlight potential limitations to longitudinal-based analyses and support further efforts to develop noninvasive synchrony measures based on circumferential deformation.

Two techniques, displacement encoding of stimulated echoes (DENSE)[27] and the harmonic phase (HARP) method, have been described, which allow for a full automatic assessment of principal strain values.[28] DENSE arose from the framework of stimulated echo and displacement encoding using bipolar gradients for high-resolution myocardial systolic strain mapping. Data processing requires minimal user intervention and provides rapid quantitative feedback. Aletras et al. demonstrated successful application of this method to quantify myocardial strain.[29]

HARP uses isolated spectral peaks in SPAMM-tagged magnetic resonance images, which contain information about cardiac motion. This approach permits rapid and accurate analysis and visualization of myocardial strain within 5 to 10 min after the scan is complete, thus shortening the postprocessing analysis time. Its performance has been demonstrated on MR image sequences reflecting both normal and abnormal cardiac motion, including patients with coronary artery disease and wall motion abnormalities.[30] Results from this method compare very well with a previously validated tracking algorithm,[28] and inter- and intra-observer reproducibility have been demonstrated in assessing both circumferential and radial principal strain.[31] Both techniques have evolved since their introduction, thereby becoming more similar over time and losing their distinct features.[24]

Although faster, HARP analysis still requires significant postprocessing. A more automatic alternative is strain-encoded (SENC) MRI, a method for direct imaging of regional strain.[32] SENC imaging is derived from a standard myocardial tagging sequence that tags the tissue at end-diastole with a sinusoidal tag pattern designed to modulate the longitudinal magnetization orthogonal to the imaging plane. Deformations of tissue during systole change the local frequency of the pattern in proportion to the through-plane strain component. The distribution of regional contraction (circumferential shortening in long-axis views or longitudinal compression in short-axis views) is then displayed as contrast in the images. The SENC technique has several features that make it especially well suited for assessing dyssynchronous heart failure and CRT, in that it provides: 1) instantaneous real-time quantitative strain measurements without the need for user intervention; 2) higher spatial resolution over standard tagging as a result of reduced tag spacing; 3) acquisition of both circumferential and longitudinal myocardial strain information; and 4) application to assessment of regional function of the right as well as the left ventricle.[33]

Indices of Dyssynchrony

Once the strain data has been obtained, an index of myocardial dyssynchrony needs to be defined. Regional temporal variance of strain is similar to many commonly used indexes based on tissue Doppler functional imaging with echocardiography. The limitation to this method is that one obtains the same results with clustered myocardial dyssynchrony as one does with diffuse dyssynchrony. To compensate for this limitation, regional variance strain vector of the principal strain has been implemented.[25, 34] Temporal and spatial elements of dyssynchrony are included in the latter method which allows for more accurate quantification of LV dyssynchrony.[34] Temporal uniformity of strain has been used by Leclercq et al.[35] and has been described in more detail by Helm et al.,[25] who also reported that the temporal uniformity of strain/circumferential uniformity ratio estimates compare favorably with vector sum methods used in regional variance vector of principal strain.

Segmental radial wall motion data has been used to derive a global dyssynchrony measure, the tissue synchronization index (CMR-TSI). Increasing LV dyssynchrony, quantified using the CMR-TSI, predicts survival and morbidity. At a cutoff of 110 ms, CMR-TSI predicted cardiovascular death with a sensitivity of 93% and a specificity of 67%. CMR-TSI, however, is comparatively crude, insofar as it is based solely on radial motion. Notwithstanding, this relatively simple measure may provide prognostic information in patients undergoing CRT.[36]

T(Onset) versus T(Max)

Timing parameters of myocardial contraction used to evaluate dyssynchrony include time of onset or T(onset) of circumferential shortening and time to peak or T(peak) of circumferential shortening. The peak time to circumferential shortening is often used to select patients for cardiac resynchronization therapy, whereas pacing directly influences only the onset times. These parameters of myocardial contraction have been studied in healthy individuals as well as in patients with ischemic and nonischemic cardiomyopathies. In healthy volunteers, a distinct spatial pattern for T(onset) was found, with earliest onset in the lateral wall, and latest onset in the septum. Compared with T(onset), T(peak) had a larger width and an opposite spatial pattern, with peak shortening occurring earlier in the septum than in the lateral wall. Shortening in these segments continued after aortic valve closure, during which circumferential shortening increased. Maps of the timing of contraction in normal subjects may serve as a reference in detecting mechanical asynchrony due to intraventricular conduction defects or ischemia.[37]

Both onset and peak shortening are earlier in the septum and later in the lateral wall, indicating a discoordinate contraction in patients with LBBB.[23, 38] Several other studies have shown that ischemic regions continue shortening after aortic valve closure. Furthermore, it is unclear whether there is a consistent direction of propagation delay and whether this depends on the etiology of the heart failure. The relationship between T(peak) and T(onset) has been demonstrated to be stronger in nonischemic patients than in the ischemic patients. In addition, nonischemic patients had a propagation of T(onset) consistently from septum to lateral wall; however, in the ischemic patients no consistent direction of propagation was found. The relation between peak time and onset time of shortening was strongest in nonischemic patients and is most consistent when time to first peak is used instead of time to maximum peak.[26]

VE-CMR

Velocity-encoded (VE) cine CMR potentially allows direct myocardial wall motion measurements similar to echocardiography using tissue Doppler imaging (TDI). In this technique, signal intensity represents magnitude and direction of velocity, which may be encoded in both in-plane as well as through-plane directions. Patients with nonischemic cardiomyopathy are categorized similarly with regards to the degree of dyssynchrony, with 95% of patients being classified as similar. Both VE-CMR and TDI provide reproducible results for LV dyssynchrony assessment, with low intraobserver and interobserver variation.[12] In the current study, only patients with nonischemic cardiomyopathy were included; additional studies in patients with ischemic cardiomyopathy are needed. Velocity-encoded (VE) CMR quantification of LV intraventricular dyssynchrony correlates well with that found by TDI.[39]

Velocity-encoded (VE) MRI, when applied for myocardial wall motion measurement, potentially allows direct myocardial wall motion measurement similar to echocardiography.[39]

Contrast-CMR

As noted earlier, a moderate proportion of individuals do not respond to treatment with CRT. As the search for improved selection has proceeded, it has become clear that the presence of LV dyssynchrony is likely central to realizing a benefit from CRT.[40–41] However, this may not be the final determinate of CRT success because not all patients with documented dyssynchrony on imaging respond to CRT. This may be explained by the presence of scar tissue in the posterolateral left ventricular segment over which percutaneously-deployed LV leads are typically placed, which may result in ineffective LV pacing and inadequate LV resynchronization.[12, 42] The impact of pacing lead placement in the scar as detected by LGE-CMR has been demonstrated to be a strong independent predictor of the composite end-point of cardiovascular death or hospitalization for worsening heart failure, particularly if the scar is transmural.[43]

Late gadolinium-enhanced (LGE) CMR provides an assessment of the presence of posterolateral scar[12, 42] and total scar burden prior to CRT.[44–45] It is not surprising that attempting to influence myocardial contraction by pacing scar does not produce significant therapeutic impact.

Not only might it be beneficial to determine the presence of posterolateral scar prior to CRT, one may be able to predict response to CRT based on total scar burden as assessed by LGE-CMR. Total scar burden and the transmurality of the scar have been shown to predict the response to CRT.[44–45] However, Jansen et al. recently suggested that LV dyssynchrony, even in the presence of posterolateral scar, may predict response to CRT if there is optimization of atrioventricular and interventricular pacing intervals.[46]

Prediction of Pacing Site

CMR wall motion models have been used to characterize mechanical dyssynchrony and predict optimal pacing sites for CRT. Wall motion series (a time series of radial length or wall motion change) has been demonstrated, by using a hierarchical agglomerative clustering technique, to perform better than radial motion series in identifying the areas of maximal conduction delay in the LV and elucidating the optimal pacing site to obtain maximal benefit from CRT.[47]

Tagged-CMR has been used to elucidate the 3-D location of optimal LV pacing site via assessment of maximally delayed activation by strain analysis. Optimal CRT was achieved from LV lateral wall sites, slightly more anterior than posterior and more apical than basal. LV sites yielding > or = 70% of the maximal dP/dtmax increase covered approximately 43% of the LV free wall.[48]

Fourier Shape Descriptor-Based LV Characterization

Our laboratory has developed a novel computer vision-based approach to characterizing LV myocardial deformation from routinely acquired cine CMR images, and this approach has shown promise in detecting intraventricular dyssynchrony.[49] Beginning from recognition that endocardial and epicardial borders of the myocardium deform in a periodic fashion, we can classify motion of these borders based on the frequency-domain coefficients generated using the Fourier transform in 2-dimensions for each imaging plane under consideration. We found that, in comparison to electrocardiographic QRS duration and LV ejection fraction, the main current determinants of CRT eligibility in addition to clinical status, our Fourier shape descriptor-based approach using only a single midventricular short axis cine CMR correctly classified 90.9% of cases, including those with abnormal cardiac function but without dyssynchrony, compared to 62.5% based on QRS duration and EF alone. Ongoing work incorporates open contour segmentation of the right ventricle as well as long axis deformation, recognizing the contribution of apical twisting and base-to-apex fiber shortening.

Safety

Implanted devices, such as pacemakers and cardioverter/defibrillators (ICDs), have historically been considered absolute contraindications to MRI. However, gradually accruing data in patients undergoing MRI with such devices suggest that clinically significant device dysfunction may not occur. Furthermore, image quality may be sufficient despite susceptibility artifact with distortion dependent on the scan sequence and plane. These data raise the possibility of performing CMR post-device placement.[50–51] Ideally, device manufacturers will increase their incorporation of lead systems that have been specifically designed to be MR-compatible so that patients with cardiovascular disease requiring implantable devices may still benefit from the unique diagnostic and prognostic data afforded by CMR.

PRACTICAL POINTS

1. The presence of transmural inferolateral scarring on late postgadolinium enhancement imaging of the myocardium reliably predicts lack of response to cardiac resynchronization therapy (CRT) using standard lateral cardiac vein-directed LV lead placement.
2. Cardiac magnetic resonance (CMR) affords measurement of velocities, displacement, and strain over the entire heart with high spatial and temporal resolution.
3. CMR-based approaches to global inter- and intra-ventricular dyssynchrony measurement may guide the development of novel multiple lead CRT approaches.

REFERENCES

1. Shamim W, Francis DP, Yousufuddin M. Intraventricular conduction delay: a prognostic marker in chronic heart failure. *Int J Cardiol.* 1999;70:171–178.
2. Aaronson KD, Schwartz JS, Chen TM. Development and prospective validation of a clinical index to predict survival in ambulatory patients referred for cardiac transplant evaluation. *Circulation.* 1997;95:2660–2667.
3. Farwell D, Patel NR, Hall A. How many people with heart failure are appropriate for biventricular resynchronization? *Eur Heart J.* 2000;21:1246–1250.
4. Wilensky RL, Yudelman P, Cohen AI. Serial electrocardiographic changes in idiopathic dilated cardiomyopathy confirmed at necropsy. *Am J Cardiol.* 1988;62:276–283.
5. Grines CL, Bashore TM, Boudoulas H. Functional abnormalities in isolated left bundle branch block: The effect of interventricular asynchrony. *Circulation.* 1989;79:845–853.
6. Abraham WT, Fisher WG, Smith AL. Cardiac resynchronization in chronic heart failure. *N Engl J Med.* 2002;346:1845–1853.
7. Cazeau S, Leclercq C, Lavergne T. Effects of multisite biventricular pacing in patients with heart failure and intraventricular conduction delay. *N Engl J Med.* 2001;344:873–880.
8. Bristow MR, Feldman AM, Saxon LA. Heart failure management using implantable devices for ventricular resynchronization: Comparison of Medical Therapy, Pacing, and Defibrillation in Chronic Heart Failure (COMPANION) trial. COMPANION Steering Committee and COMPANION Clinical Investigators. *J Card Fail.* 2000;6:276–285.
9. Cleland JG, Daubert JC, Erdmann E. The effect of cardiac resynchronization on morbidity and mortality in heart failure. *N Engl J Med.* 2005;352:1539–1549.
10. Breithardt OA, Sinha AM, Schwammenthal E. Acute effects of cardiac resynchronization therapy on functional mitral regurgitation in advanced systolic heart failure. *J Am Coll Cardiol.* 2003;41:765–770.
11. Yu CM, Fung JW, Zhang Q. Tissue Doppler imaging is superior to strain rate imaging and postsystolic shortening on the prediction of reverse remodeling in both ischemic and nonischemic heart failure after cardiac resynchronization therapy. *Circulation.* 2004;110:66–73.
12. Bleeker GB, Schalij MJ, Molhoek SG. Relationship between QRS duration and left ventricular dyssynchrony in patients with end-stage heart failure. *J Cardiovasc Electrophysiol.* 2004;15:544–549.
13. Auricchio A, Stellbrink C, Butter C. Clinical efficacy of cardiac resynchronization therapy using left ventricular pacing in heart failure patients stratified by severity of ventricular conduction delay. *J Am Coll Cardiol.* 2003;42:2109–116.
14. Bristow MR, Saxon LA, Boehmer J. Cardiac-resynchronization therapy with or without an implantable defibrillator in advanced chronic heart failure. *N Engl J Med.* 2004;350:2140–2150.
15. Penicka M, Bartunek J, De Bruyne B. Improvement of left ventricular function after cardiac resynchronization therapy is predicted by tissue Doppler imaging echocardiography. *Circulation.* 2004;109:978–983.
16. Achilli A, Sassara M, Ficili S. Long-term effectiveness of cardiac resynchronization therapy in patients with refractory heart failure and "narrow" QRS. *J Am Coll Cardiol.* 2003;42:2117–1124.
17. Mollema SA, Bleeker GB, van der Wall EE. Usefulness of QRS duration to predict response to cardiac resynchronization therapy in patients with end-stage heart failure. *Am J Cardiol.* 2007;100:1665–1670.
18. Kass DA, Chen CH, Curry C. Improved left ventricular mechanics from acute VDD pacing in patients with dilated cardiomyopathy and ventricular conduction delay. *Circulation.* 1999;99:1567–1573.
19. Isbell DC, Kramer CM. Cardiovascular magnetic resonance: structure, function, perfusion, and viability. *J Nucl Cardiol.* 2005;12:324–336.
20. Schuijf JD, Kaandorp TA, Lamb HJ. Quantification of myocardial infarct size and transmurality by contrast-enhanced magnetic resonance imaging in men. *Am J Cardiol.* 2004;94:284–288.
21. Moore CC, Lugo-Olivieri CH, McVeigh ER. Three-dimensional systolic strain patterns in the normal human left ventricle: characterization with tagged MR imaging. *Radiology.* 2000;214:453–466.
22. Rosen BD, Berger RD. Resynchronization therapy upgrades: turning coach into first class. *J Cardiovasc Electrophysiol.* 2004;15:1290–1292.
23. Curry CW, Nelson GS, Wyman BT. Mechanical dyssynchrony in dilated cardiomyopathy with intraventricular conduction delay as depicted by 3D tagged magnetic resonance imaging. *Circulation.* 2000;101:E2.
24. Kuijer JP, Hofman MB, Zwanenburg JJ. DENSE and HARP: two views on the same technique of phase-based strain imaging. *J Magn Reson Imaging.* 2006;24:1432–1438.
25. Helm RH, Leclercq C, Faris OP. Cardiac dyssynchrony analysis using circumferential versus longitudinal strain: implications for assessing cardiac resynchronization. *Circulation.* 2005;111:2760–2767.
26. Zwanenburg JJ, Gotte MJ, Marcus JT. Propagation of onset and peak time of myocardial shortening in time of myocardial shortening in ischemic versus nonischemic cardiomyopathy: assessment by magnetic resonance imaging myocardial tagging. *J Am Coll Cardiol.* 2005;46: 2215–2222.
27. Aletras AH, Ding S, Balaban RS. DENSE: displacement encoding with stimulated echoes in cardiac functional MRI. *J Magn Reson Imaging.* 1999;137:247–252.
28. Osman NF, Kerwin WS, McVeigh ER. Cardiac motion tracking using CINE harmonic phase (HARP) magnetic resonance imaging. *Magn Reson Med.* 1999;42:1048–1060.

29. Aletras AH, Balaban RS, Wen H. High-resolution strain analysis of the human heart with fast-DENSE. *J Magn Reson.* 1999;140:41–57.

30. Garot J, Bluemke DA, Osman NF. Fast determination of regional myocardial strain fields from tagged cardiac images using harmonic phase MRI. *Circulation.* 2000;101:981–988.

31. Castillo E, Osman NF, Rosen BD. Quantitative assessment of regional myocardial function with MR-tagging in a multi-center study: interobserver and intraobserver agreement of fast strain analysis with Harmonic Phase (HARP) MRI. *J Cardiovasc Magn Reson.* 2005;7:783–791.

32. Osman NF, Sampath S, Atalar E. Imaging longitudinal cardiac strain on short-axis images using strain-encoded MRI. *Magn Reson Med.* 2001;46:324–334.

33. Lardo AC, Abraham TP, Kass DA. Magnetic resonance imaging assessment of ventricular dyssynchrony: current and emerging concepts. *J Am Coll Cardiol.* 2005;46:2223-8.

34. Wyman BT, Hunter WC, Prinzen FW. Effects of single- and biventricular pacing on temporal and spatial dynamics of ventricular contraction. *Am J Physiol Heart Circ Physiol.* 2002;282:H372–H379.

35. Leclercq C, Faris O, Tunin R. Systolic improvement and mechanical resynchronization does not require electrical synchrony in the dilated failing heart with left bundle-branch block. *Circulation.* 2002;106:1760–1763.

36. Chalil S, Stegemann B, Muhyaldeen S. Intraventricular dyssynchrony predicts mortality and morbidity after cardiac resynchronization therapy: a study using cardiovascular magnetic resonance tissue synchronization imaging. *J Am Coll Cardiol.* 2007;50:243–252.

37. Zwanenburg JJ, Gotte MJ, Kuijer JP. Timing of cardiac contraction in humans mapped by high-temporal-resolution MRI tagging: early onset and late peak of shortening in lateral wall. *Am J Physiol Heart Circ Physiol.* 2004;286:H1872–H1880.

38. Nelson GS, Curry CW, Wyman BT. Predictors of systolic augmentation from left ventricular preexcitation in patients with dilated cardiomyopathy and intraventricular conduction delay. *Circulation.* 2000;101:2703–2079.

39. Westenberg JJ, Lamb HJ, van der Geest RJ. Assessment of left ventricular dyssynchrony in patients with conduction delay and idiopathic dilated cardiomyopathy: head-to-head comparison between tissue doppler imaging and velocity-encoded magnetic resonance imaging. *J Am Coll Cardiol.* 2006;47:2042–2048.

40. Bax JJ, Bleeker GB, Marwick TH. Left ventricular dyssynchrony predicts response and prognosis after cardiac resynchronization therapy. *J Am Coll Cardiol.* 2004;44:1834–1840.

41. Yu CM, Chau E, Sanderson JE. Tissue Doppler echocardiographic evidence of reverse remodeling and improved synchronicity by simultaneously delaying regional contraction after biventricular pacing therapy in heart failure. *Circulation.* 2002;105:438–445.

42. Bleeker GB, Kaandorp TA, Lamb HJ. Effect of posterolateral scar tissue on clinical and echocardiographic improvement after cardiac resynchronization therapy. *Circulation.* 2006;113:969–976.

43. Chalil S, Stegemann B, Muhyaldeen SA. Effect of posterolateral left ventricular scar on mortality and morbidity following cardiac resynchronization therapy. *Pacing Clin Electrophysiol.* 2007;30:1201–1209.

44. Chalil S, Foley PW, Muyhaldeen SA. Late gadolinium enhancement-cardiovascular magnetic resonance as a predictor of response to cardiac resynchronization therapy in patients with ischaemic cardiomyopathy. *Europace.* 2007;9:1031–1037.

45. Ypenburg C, Roes SD, Bleeker GB. Effect of total scar burden on contrast-enhanced magnetic resonance imaging on response to cardiac resynchronization therapy. *Am J Cardiol.* 2007;99:657–660.

46. Jansen AH, Bracke F, Dantzig JM. The influence of myocardial scar and dyssynchrony on reverse remodeling in cardiac resynchronization therapy. *Eur J Echocardiogr.* 2007.

47. Huang H, Shen L, Zhang R. Cardiac motion analysis to improve pacing site selection in CRT. *Acad Radiol.* 2006;13:1124–1134.

48. Helm RH, Byrne M, Helm PA. Three-dimensional mapping of optimal left ventricular pacing site for cardiac resynchronization. *Circulation.* 2007;115:953–961.

49. Gotardo PFU, Boyer KL, Saltz J. A new deformable model for boundary tracking in cardiac MRI and its application to the detection of intraventricular dyssynchrony. In: *Proc IEEE Conf Computer Vision and Pattern Recognition.* 2006:736–743.

50. Martin ET, Coman JA, Shellock FG. Magnetic resonance imaging and cardiac pacemaker safety at 1.5-Tesla. *J Am Coll Cardiol.* 2004;43:1315–1324.

51. Roguin A, Zviman MM, Meininger GR. Modern pacemaker and implantable cardioverter/defibrillator systems can be magnetic resonance imaging safe: in vitro and in vivo assessment of safety and function at 1.5 T. *Circulation.* 2004;110:475–482.

Reverse Remodeling in Heart Failure with Cardiac Resynchronization Therapy

Hind W. Rahmouni • Martin G. St. John Sutton

Cardiac resynchronization therapy (CRT) is an effective therapy for patients with all NYHA symptom classes of systolic heart failure, left ventricular dilatation, prolonged QRS duration, and low ejection fraction. In contrast to pharmaceutical agents that usually only attenuate remodeling, CRT reverses the remodeling process in both ischemic and nonischemic heart failure. The effects of CRT on remodeling are immediate and sustained up to at least 2 years. A reduction in LVESV of ≥10% has a high sensitivity and specificity for prediction of long-term all-cause and cardiovascular mortality. This review discusses remodeling, focusing on the evidence base for CRT-induced reverse remodeling

Left ventricular mechanical dyssynchrony is associated with increased morbidity and mortality in patients with congestive heart failure.[1-4] Dyssynchrony exacerbates heart failure, not only by retardation of regional contraction, but also by facilitating remodeling at the macroscopic and molecular levels. Indices of ventricular remodeling include increasing LV size, degree of hypertrophy, and extent of interstitial fibrosis, which are all associated with adverse clinical outcome, including death from pump failure. In addition, interstitial myocardial fibrosis and scar formation following myocardial repair form an ideal substrate for slow impulse conduction that increases the propensity for life-threatening ventricular dysrhythmias and sudden death.[5-6] Reversing remodeling is now an established objective of heart failure therapy. Cardiac resynchronization therapy (CRT) has been shown to reverse this remodeling process in the majority of heart failure with prolonged QRS duration on the surface electrocardiogram primarily by reducing left ventricular size, and secondarily by restoring near-normal LV chamber architecture and reducing the severity of mitral regurgitation.

Remodeling

Ventricular remodeling is the process by which heart size, shape, and function are regulated by the interaction of biomechanical, neurohormonal, local trophic, and genetic factors. It is a dynamic interaction of molecular, cellular, and organ-level processes. Ventricular remodeling may be physiological during normal growth and pregnancy, or patho-

logical as in chronic pressure or volume overload from hypertension, valvular, and congenital heart disease—especially in transposition with ventricular inversion, from genetically programmed primary cardiomyopathies and most commonly following acute ischemic cardiac injury. If unchecked, remodeling can result in molecular maladaptations, cellular dysfunction, reorganization of the extracellular matrix, and vascular changes that culminate in progressive dilatation, interstitial fibrosis, increased myocardial stiffness, chamber distortion, and heart failure. The initial biological trigger for ventricular dilatation varies but most frequently it is acute infarction following which the injured myocardium stops contracting with concomitant stretching and thinning of the infarct zone. This combination increases wall stress, which is the patho-etiological mechanism that drives the remodeling process and triggers the stretch-induced changes in the extracellular matrix that begin the process of infarct repair. As the heart remodels, LV geometry changes from a prolate ellipse to a more spherical shape.[7-8] These changes in chamber shape are accompanied by increase in ventricular volume and mass, and alteration in the equilibrium between collagen deposition and degradation. Increasing the myocardial collagen content during repair changes the material properties of the myocardium, resulting in increased chamber stiffness. Alteration in left ventricular composition, architecture, and stiffness affect LV filling dynamics, rate of cross-bridge formation, and sarcoplasmic sequestration of cytosolic calcium that impact upon systolic as well as diastolic function. Progressive increase in LV volume is associated with deterioration in LV performance and a poor clinical outcome.[9] Functional mitral regurgitation (MR) is ubiquitous during LV remodeling because of an imbalance between tethering forces—annular dilatation, disruption of the mitral valve and subvalve apparatus, increased LV sphericity and LV dilatation—versus closing forces—reduction of LV contractility, global and regional LV dyssynchrony, papillary muscle asynchrony, and altered mitral systolic annular contraction.[10] Functional MR is typically dynamic and exacerbated during exercise. Increase in MR during exercise identifies a subgroup of patients at particularly high risk for adverse cardiovascular events.[11] Development of MR is important because it results in an additional volume overload to an already severely dysfunctional LV that often escalates the deterioration of LV function and the early onset of failure.

Remodeling in the Dyssynchronous Heart

In the normal heart the electrical pacemaker impulse is initiated by the sinus node and conducted rapidly via specialized Purkinje network in such a temporal and spatial distribution as to activate synchronous mechanical ventricular contraction within 40 ms. Mechanical contraction begins earlier at the apex and then a wavefront of electrical depolarization spreads to the base of the heart, resulting in concentric inward wall motion during ventricular emptying and similar temporally coordinated outward wall motion during relaxation and diastolic filling. Left ventricular dyssynchrony in the broadest terms is when there is heterogeneity of systolic contraction, that is, when some regions of the myocardium are contracting early and some are contracting late, typically resulting from a delay in activation of the lateral LV free wall resulting in prolongation of the QRS duration >120 ms on the surface electrocardiogram. Dyssynchrony compromises mechanical efficiency, with transmission of the ventricular blood pool between two intracavitary sinks (the stretched lateral wall in early systole and the anteroseptal region in late systole). Functional MR may further aggravate this "intracavity" volume overload. Dyssynchrony also causes changes in regional hypertrophy, blood flow, and oxygen consumption, resulting in local alterations in myocardial protein expression.[12] (Table 7.1)

Reverse Remodeling

Pharmacologic therapies for chronic, advanced heart failure include β-adrenergic receptor blocking agents, angiotensin converting enzyme inhibitors/angiotensin receptor blockers that attenuate LV remodeling but with rare exception do not reverse LV remodeling. However, their use is the accepted standard of care and is associated with improved survival, enhanced exercise capacity, decreased adverse cardiovascular events, and symptomatic relief. Traditional surgical therapies including myocardial revascularization, correction of mitral regurgitation by valve repair or replacement, ventricular volume reduction, and epicardial restraint devices have all aimed at reducing LV loading conditions but have not achieved LV reverse remodeling long term. Occasionally obligate use of a left ventricular assist device (LVAD) has resulted in reverse remodeling such that the LVAD has been removed with sustained recovery of LV function.

The current goal of heart failure therapy is not simply to attenuate, but to reverse the remodeling process. Reverse remodeling involves reduction in LV size, near-normalization of LV architecture, increase in contractile function, and accompanying symptomatic benefit. Reduction of volumes is often but not always accompanied by a reversal of the deranged molecular processes. Clinical and experimental data are still limited regarding the correlation between macroscopic and molecular remodeling.[13] Reverse remodeling is accompanied by improved survival, exercise capacity, and quality of life.

ASSESSMENT OF REMODELING AND REVERSE REMODELING

LV remodeling and reverse remodeling have been assessed echocardiographically in the randomized CRT trials either as changes in linear LV cavity dimensions, wall thickness, end diastolic and systolic LV volumes, ejection fraction, sphericity index,[14] LV mass, and severity of mitral regurgitation. Assessment of LV volumes and ejection fraction are important because they are powerful predictors of long-term mortality and adverse cardiovascular events.[15–16] More recently tissue Doppler imaging (TDI) has been used prior to CRT to detect dyssynchrony in patients likely to benefit from CRT and also post CRT to demonstrate improvement in the synchrony of regional LV contraction from baseline values. A few studies have attempted to characterize remodeling associated with CRT using 3-dimensional (3D) echocardiographic imaging.[17] Three-dimensional echocardiographic techniques currently available enable comprehensive characterization of right ventricular size, shape, function, degree of dyssynchrony, and extent of RV remodeling in heart failure at baseline and after CRT. Thus, structural RV remodeling can be correlated with improvement in symptoms following CRT.

TABLE 7.1 Myocardial Changes in the Dyssynchronous Heart

	Early-activated Wall	Late-activated Wall
Cardiac mass	Reduction in wall thickness	Hypertrophy
Perfusion	Low	High
Conduction velocity	Epicardium slower than endocardium	Endocardium slower than epicardium
The gap protein connexin 43	Usual distribution: intercalated disk	Lateral sarcolemma
Mitogen activated kinase ERK42/44		Highly phosphorylated
Calcium handling proteins (SERCA2a; phospholamban)		Down regulated

Effect of CRT on Remodeling

LV Size, Mass, and Shape

The change in LV size over time with CRT can be assessed by linear M-Mode echocardiographic measurements of cavity dimensions. However, with the certain knowledge that >50% of any heart failure population have an ischemic etiology and wall motion abnormalities, LV volume computations using transthoracic echocardiography are preferable using modified Simpson's method of discs as recommended by the American Society of Echocardiography.[8,19] This methodology is not confounded by the presence of segmental wall motion abnormalities.

The extent of reduction of LV volume was measured in five major CRT trials as a part of the remodeling assessment (Table 7.2). In these randomized studies involving approximately 4,000 patients, echocardiographic images of the left ventricle were obtained as part of the study protocol.

Changes in LV morphology are observed within a single beat upon activating CRT. CRT abruptly enhances LV systolic function by increasing stroke volume by between 10% to 30%, reducing LV end-systolic volume without any change in LV mass, thus reducing LV end-systolic stress. These changes become statistically significant at one week compared to control patients.[20]

Longer-term studies have shown that ≥10% decline in LV end-systolic and end-diastolic volumes is associated with an increase in LVEF. In the majority of patients (65% to 75%) with advanced (NYHA symptom class III/IV) heart failure, CRT results in progressive reduction in end-diastolic and end-systolic LV diameters and LV volumes at 3, 6, and 12 months (Figs. 7.1 and 7.2) compared to baseline values or

compared to the control group. A similar degree of structural and functional LV reverse remodeling was recently demonstrated in minimally symptomatic patients with NYHA symptom class I/II heart failure, LVEF <40%, and QRS duration >120ms in the REVERSE trial unveiled at the late-breaking trials at the American College of Cardiology scientific sessions in Chicago in 2008.

The MIRACLE trial provided a unique opportunity to quantify the magnitude and frequency of reverse remodeling after one year, specifically, LV volumes and ejection fraction in more than 200 patients who were initially randomized to the active CRT arm and followed for a minimum of one year of continuous CRT.

LV end-diastolic (EDV) and end-systolic (ESV) volumes both decreased as compared to baseline values at 12 months. However, the mean difference for both EDV and ESV between baseline and 6 months and baseline and one year were greater at 6 months, consistent with a trend for LV volumes to return to baseline by one year in spite of continuous biventricular pacing. The proportion of patients who experienced a decrease in LVEDV and LVESV at 6 months was 71% and 74%, respectively, and at one year 58% and 60%, respectively. By contrast LV ejection fraction increased progressively from a mean of 24% at baseline to 29% at 6 months (Fig. 7.3) and to 31% at 12 months.

Examination of the baseline demographics that correlated with structural remodeling (change in LVEDV) at 6 months were age ≥65 years, female sex, QRS duration ≥170 ms, and a LVEF ≤25%; at 12 months the only correlations were QRS duration ≥170 ms and an LVEF ≤ 25%

Concomitant with the reduction in LV cavity size, LV mass decreased progressively with CRT at 3 and 6 months but at a

TABLE 7.2   **CRT Randomized Clinical Trials with Remodeling Parameters**

Trials	Design	QRS (ms)	NYHA	Patients (n)	Primary End-points	Remodeling Parameters
CARE-HF	Open label	≥120	III, IV	814	All cause mortality	LVEF LV end-systolic volume index Degree of MR (area of the MR jet)
CONTAK-CD	Crossover, Parallel controlled	≥120	II-IV	490	6MWT NYHA class QOL	LVEF LV volumes
MIRACLE	Parallel arms	≥130	III, IV	453	6MWT NYHA class QOL	LVEF Internal diastolic dimensions Degree of MR (area of the MR jet)
MIRACLE-ICD	Parallel arms	≥130	III, IV	555	6MWT NYHA class QOL	LVEF LV systolic and diastolic volumes LV size
MUSTIC-SR	Crossover	>150	III	58	6MWT	LVEF LV systolic and diastolic volumes Degree of MR (area of the MR jet)

CARE-HF, Cardiac Resynchronization-Heart Failure; CONTAK, CD, CONTAK-Cardiac Defibrillator; MIRACLE, Multicenter InSync Randomized Clinical Evaluation; MIRACLE-ICD, MIRACLE implantable Cardioverter Defibrillator trial; MUSTIC, Multisite Simulation in Cardiomyopathy; LV, left ventricle; LVEF, left ventricular ejection fraction; MR, mitral regurgitation; 6MWT, 6-minute walk test; QOL, quality of life; NYHA, New York Heart Association

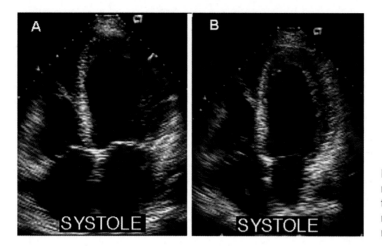

FIG. 7.1. Transthoracic apical four-chamber view before resynchronization **(A)**, and after cardiac resynchronization therapy **(B)**. At 6 months, the end systolic volume is reduced compared to baseline, and the left ventricle has a more elliptical shape reflecting the reverse remodeling.

slower rate than the decrease in LV volumes. LV cavity shape assessed as a sphericity index changed from a globular to a more normal ellipsoidal configuration in the treatment group while neither LV volumes, LV mass, nor cavity shape improved in the control group over time.[21]

Mitral Regurgitation

Mitral regurgitation occurs in more than 70% of all patients with chronic severe systolic heart failure. Ypenburg et al.[22] showed that the severity of mitral regurgitation decreases almost instantaneously after initiation of CRT using the vena contracta measurement and mitral deformation indexes. These authors also reported a decrease in dyssynchrony between the papillary muscles assessed by speckle tracking strain analysis. There was progressive reduction in MR severity at 3 and at 6 months (Figs. 7.4 and 7.5). These beneficial effects were maintained at 12 months' follow-up unless CRT was acutely interrupted, at which time there was immediate recurrence of MR and worsening in mitral deformation indexes.

There are several potential mechanisms by which CRT decreases the severity of MR. CRT recoordinates the timing and duration of contraction of the two papillary muscles that synchronizes initiation and completion of LV filling and ejection.[23] The structural and functional reverse remodeling that reduces the diameter of the LV short axis also plays a role

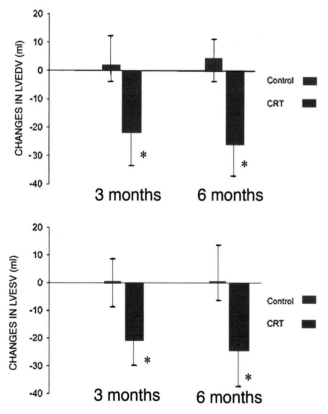

FIG. 7.2. Median change (with 95% confidence intervals) in LVEDV (top), LVESV (bottom), at 3 and 6 months after randomization in the control group and the CRT group (LVEDV, left ventricular end-diastolic volume; LVESV, left ventricular end-systolic volume) in the MIRACLE trial. (* = p <0.001)

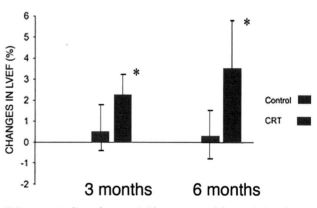

FIG. 7.3. Median change (with 95% confidence intervals) in ejection fraction (EF), at 3 and 6 months after randomization in the control group and the CRT group in the MIRACLE trial. (* = p <0.001)

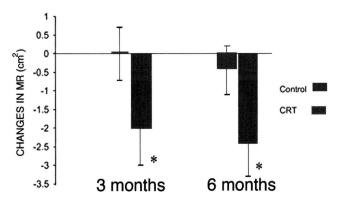

FIG. 7.4. Median change (with 95% confidence intervals) in mitral regurgitation (MR) volume, at 3 and 6 months after randomization in the control group and the CRT group in the MIRACLE trial. (* = p <0.001)

in restoring the mitral annular area and subvalve geometry to near-normal, and it approximates the papillary muscles to facilitate appropriate coaptation of the anterior and posterior mitral valve leaflets (Fig. 7.6).

Diastolic Dysfunction

The true importance of diastolic function has really emerged over the last decade because currently between one-third and one-half of all patients presenting with clinical heart failure have severe diastolic dysfunction and preserved systolic function.[24–25] In addition, severe LV diastolic dysfunction and especially restrictive LV filling defined by transmitral blood flow velocities is a powerful predictor of death independent of LV size or ejection fraction. However, no CRT trials have been conducted on primary diastolic LV heart failure, and most major CRT trials have not evaluated diastolic function post-resynchronization.

The data that is available[21] shows that optimization of atrioventricular delay and synchronous biventricular pacing resulted in significant prolongation of LV filling time at 6 months, which by Starling's law of the heart augments diastolic resting myofiber length and, in turn, increases LV stroke volume. Normalized LV filling time calculated by dividing filling time by RR interval was also prolonged. The LV dyssynchrony was also reduced as reflected by the reduction in the interventricular mechanical delay (IVMD) and reduction of isovolumic contraction time. Although the variables that are commonly used to evaluate LV diastolic function—transmitral peak velocities during passive filling (E wave), atrial contraction (A wave), and E/A ratio—do not change, the E wave deceleration slope significantly decreased and the deceleration time was significantly prolonged in the CRT group compared with no change in the control group.

Noninvasive Doppler-derived myocardial performance (Tei) index reflects combined systolic and diastolic cardiac function.[26–27] This novel index is defined as the sum of the isovolumetric relaxation time (IVRT) and isovolumetric contraction (IVCT) time divided by ejection time (LVET).

$$\text{Tei index} = (\text{IVRT} + \text{IVCT}) / \text{LVET}$$

The Tei index does not depend on geometric assumptions and can be easily measured noninvasively. The Tei index improved significantly in the CRT patients by 6 months but did not change from baseline in the control group.

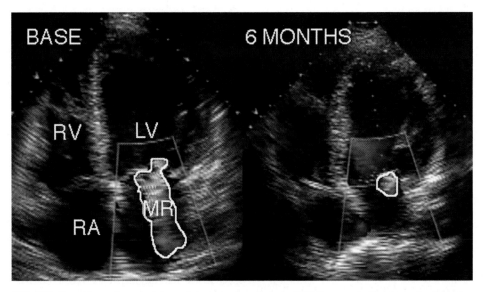

FIG. 7.5. Transthoracic apical four-chamber view before CRT demonstrating by color-Doppler regurgitant flow in the left atrium during systole indicating a severe mitral regurgitation (Base) and 6 months after CRT with a significant reduction in the severity of the mitral regurgitation (6 months).

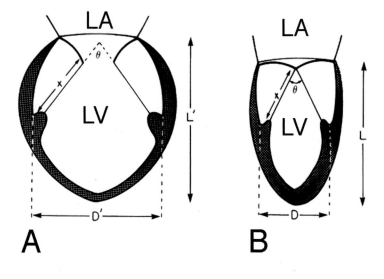

FIG. 7.6. Schematic demonstrating the possible mechanism of mitral regurgitation. Left ventricular dilatation due to volume overload results in the left ventricle becoming more spherical (A, B). The mitral valve ring circumference increases. The angle subtended by the papillary muscles to the mitral annulus increases, but there is no elongation of the mitral valve leaflets or chordae, which results in incomplete cusp coaptation and mitral regurgitation. (From St John Sutton M, Oldershaw PJ, Kotler MN. *Textbook of Echocardiography and Doppler in Adults and Children.* 2nd ed, Cambridge, Mass: Blackwell Science; 1996:164.

Right Ventricle

There are very few data on the effects of CRT on RV size or function. Donal et al.[28] reported acute improvement in tricuspid annular velocities with biventricular pacing but long-term effects were not studied. Bleeker et al.[29] showed improvement in RV dimension in patients with heart failure after 6 months of CRT with significant improvement in pulmonary artery pressures. Rajagopalan et al.[30] also showed an improvement in RV function using color tissue Doppler imaging. This improvement was seen in both ischemic and nonischemic patients and was independent of left ventricular ejection fraction and baseline left ventricular dyssynchrony. The precise mechanism by which CRT may lead to improved RV function is not clear. The ubiquitous improvement in mitral regurgitation can lead to lower pulmonary artery pressures, thereby decreasing RV afterload and improving RV systolic function. Another possible mechanism is the beneficial effects of CRT on left ventricular remodeling and dilation. A decrease in left ventricular dilation can improve RV diastolic filling and thereby improve systolic function.[31] Additional research is still needed to determine the impact of CRT on the right ventricle in patients with advanced heart failure in whom pulmonary hypertension is common.

Atrial Remodeling

Yu et al.[32] assessed atrial remodeling and atrial function at 3 months in heart failure patients who received CRT using conventional and new echocardiographic imaging tools consisting of tissue Doppler and myocardial strain analysis. Active contractile function was observed to improve significantly in both atria, particularly in the LA. Atrial remodeling was also demonstrated by the reduction of atrial area and volume before and after atrial systole. These findings were concordant with the improvement of atrial function, including the increase of atrial emptying fraction, peak atrial contraction velocity by tissue Doppler velocity, and atrial strain. These changes were observed mainly in responders to CRT in whom LV reverse remodeling was clearly evident.

Molecular Remodeling after CRT

In a recent study by Vanderheyden et al.[33] the LV messenger ribonucleic acid (mRNA) levels of contractile and calcium regulatory genes were measured before and after CRT. Before CRT, the HF patients showed lower LV mRNA levels of alpha-myosin heavy chain (alpha-MHC), beta-myosin heavy chain (beta-MHC), sarcoplasmic reticulum calcium ATPase 2 alpha (SERCA), phospholamban (PLN), and higher brain natriuretic peptide (BNP) mRNA levels as compared with control subjects. In addition to an increase in LVEF, a decrease in left ventricular end-diastolic diameter and NYHA class, responders to CRT showed a reduction in N-terminal proBNP levels associated with an increase in mRNA levels of alpha-MHC, SERCA, a decrease in BNP mRNA levels, and an increase in the ratio of alpha-/beta-MHC and SERCA/PLN. No significant changes in molecular profile were observed in nonresponders to CRT.

Over the long term, collagen type I turnover influences response to CRT. The ability of CRT to restore the balance between collagen type I synthesis and degradation is associated with a beneficial response.[34]

Factors Influencing Ventricular Remodeling

HF Etiology (Ischemic vs. Nonischemic)

All eight large randomized CRT trials enrolled mostly NYHA symptom class III/IV heart failure patients with diverse patho-etiologies. The major causes of heart failure in the approximately 5,000 patients enrolled in these CRT trials were ischemic cardiomyopathy and idiopathic primary dilated cardiomyopathies. Most trials in accordance with optimal clinical practice guidelines do not require that every patient with heart failure undergo coronary arteriography to assign an ischemic versus nonischemic patho-etiology. The diagnostic assignment to ischemic dilated cardiomyopathy is made by the referring physician on the basis of clinical history of chest pain, prior myocardial infarction, or evidence of coronary artery disease by electrocardiography, echocardiography, or by radionuclide myocardial perfusion scan and often but not always supported by cardiac catheterization. Therefore, there is potential for ambiguity or misclassification and subsequent incorrect patho-etiologic assignment.

The MIRACLE trial provided an opportunity to compare and contrast the timeframe and extent of LV remodeling in ischemic versus nonischemic patients. NYHA symptom class, quality of life, and 6-minute walk test were not different in patients with ischemic versus nonischemic pathoetiologies for heart failure at 6, 12, 18, or 24 months.

Reverse LV remodeling and increase in ejection fraction occurred in patients with heart failure of ischemic and nonischemic etiologies.[21] However, the magnitude of reduction in LV end-diastolic volume and the increase in ejection fraction after 6 months of CRT was significantly greater by two- to threefold in the heart failure patients with a nonischemic pathoetiology as compared to those with an ischemic pathoetiology (Fig. 7.7). The greater degree of LV remodeling occurred in those nonischemic patients in spite of the fact that the nonischemic patients had significantly larger LV end-systolic and end-diastolic volumes and lower ejection fractions at baseline. These discrepancies in reverse remodeling profiles between ischemic and nonischemic heart failure patients cannot be attributed either to differences in clinical demographics at baseline between the two patho-etiologies or to the disparate use of β-adrenergic receptor blocking

agents. Examination of changes in LV volumes between 6 and 12 months of continuous CRT showed that CRT had a persistent and consistently different effect on reverse remodeling in ischemic heart failure as compared to those with nonischemic heart failure. When the time-dependent changes in LV volumes were assessed by cause of heart failure at 6 and 12 months using a statistical model adjusted for age, sex, and baseline heart rate, QRS duration, ejection fraction, and LV volumes, because of differences between ischemic and nonischemic patients, the difference in changes in LV end-diastolic volume by etiology of heart failure remained significant.[21] In the ischemic heart failure patients, the beneficial reduction in LV volumes achieved at 6 months had almost completely regressed by 12 months. By contrast, the reduction in LV volumes in the nonischemic heart failure patients at 6 months was more than threefold greater than in the ischemic patients, and this difference was sustained at 12 months.

The late recurrence of LV dilatation in ischemic heart failure with CRT beyond 6 months may be associated with the decline in LV function due to repetitive episodes of ischemia and the inevitable progressive loss of viable myocardium that characterizes ischemic cardiomyopathy, rather than loss of efficacy of cardiac resynchronization therapy.

Pacing Mode

Three major CRT modalities have emerged: simultaneous BiV pacing, sequential BiV pacing, and LV pacing. In the DECREASE-HF trial, Rao et al.[35] compared the effect of these different modes of pacing on left ventricular remodeling, systolic and diastolic function at baseline, 3 months, and 6 months. Simultaneous BiV pacing was associated with a trend toward a greater reduction in ventricular size. In contrast, LV pacing showed much weaker benefit on LV size and function, and may exacerbate MR in a small subset of patients.

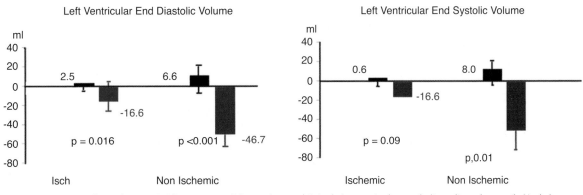

FIG. 7.7. Median change (with 95% confidence intervals) in left ventricular end diastolic volume (left), left ventricular end-systolic volume (right), at baseline and 6 months after biventricular pacing in the control group and the CRT group in ischemic vs. nonischemic patients in the MIRACLE trial. (LVEDV, left ventricular end-diastolic volume; LVESV, left ventricular end-systolic volume).

Concomitant Medical Therapy

CRT results in LV reverse remodeling, regardless of β-blocker treatment status. Control patients who receive β-blocker show no evidence for change in LV size or function at 6 months, while CRT patients taking β-blockers exhibit a significant improvement in LV remodeling.[21]

All randomized CRT trials have compared optimal medical therapy with optimal medical therapy plus CRT.

Left Ventricular Resynchronization

LV resynchronization in patients with echocardiographic evidence of LV dyssynchrony at baseline occurs almost immediately after initiation of CRT and predicts response to CRT at 6-month follow-up as demonstrated by color-coded tissue Doppler imaging per Bleeker et al.[36] The majority of CRT trials have used QRS duration >130ms as an enrollment criterion as evidence for LV dyssynchrony.

The influence of a number of factors on remodeling after CRT has been studied. The effect of QRS duration has recently been studied in the RethinQ trial[37] and showed that patients with heart failure, LV dyssynchrony, and narrow QRS intervals do not exhibit structural or functional reverse remodeling with CRT. In a group of patients with QRS of more than 120 seconds, Mollema et al.[38] showed that there was no significant difference in QRS duration at baseline between echocardiographic responders, defined as a decrease >10% in LV end-systolic volume, and nonresponders after 6 months follow-up. No significant relation was demonstrated between baseline QRS duration and improvement in clinical or echocardiographic variables at 6-month follow-up. Thus, baseline QRS duration is not predictive for clinical and echocardiographic responses to CRT at 6-month follow-up.

Persistence of Reverse Remodeling

The symptomatic benefits and reverse remodeling of CRT are dependent on the continuation of the biventricular pacing stimulus. Cessation of CRT results in recurrent LV dilatation, acute deterioration in ejection fraction, and return of the mitral regurgitation to the level of severity at baseline.[39] Worsening of clinical status and loss of reverse remodeling has also been reported in individual patients in whom either the right or left ventricular (coronary sinus) lead has become dislodged or fractured with loss of synchronous bi-ventricular pacing corroborating the need for continuous CRT.

How long the symptomatic benefit and the structural and functional remodeling are sustained is not known. In the MIRACLE program NYHA symptom class, quality of life and 6-minute walking distance all improved in the population as a whole, and these changes for the better were maintained to two years from device deployment in the those patients with continuous CRT. In CARE-HF benefits continued at least for 18 months, with further data analysis pending at 29 months. The extent of reverse remodeling achieved at 18 months in CARE-HF was an increase in LVEF of 6.9 units and a decrease in LV end-systolic volume index of 26 ml/m^2.

Correlation Between Clinical Outcome and Remodeling in CRT Patients

At first glance there appears to be no direct correlation between clinical outcome and the extent of LV structural remodeling with CRT. This is partially explained by the 20% to 30% "placebo effect" that describes the subjective improvement in symptoms and well-being in the absence of any objective accompanying reverse remodeling. However, when patients were divided into quartiles by increasing severity of LV remodeling, the preponderance of patients with greatest symptom benefit were in quartile 3 and 4, in which the greatest remodeling occurred.

CRT in Special Categories of Patients

Patients with Narrow QRS

The RethinQ (Cardiac Resynchronization Therapy in Patients with Heart Failure and Narrow QRS) study explored the effects of CRT in 172 patients with heart failure (EF ≤35%), and a narrow QRS complex, but with mechanical dyssynchrony assessed by the opposite wall delay method by color tissue Doppler imaging. In this randomized double-blind study, CRT did not result in a significant change in the primary end-point, which was the peak oxygen consumption. The Minnesota Living with Heart Failure score, 6-minute walk test, LV volumes, and EF at 6 months were not different. Until additional studies are done in this population, caution is warranted before considering CRT in this population.

Patients with NYHA Class I and II: REVERSE Trial

In a randomized, double-blind, parallel-controlled clinical trial (REVERSE) the effects of CRT on disease progression over 12 months in 610 patients with asymptomatic and mildly symptomatic (NYHA class II and I) heart failure and ventricular dyssynchrony was assessed. All patients had a QRS ≥120ms, a left ventricular ejection fraction (LVEF) <40% and left ventricular end diastolic dimensions >55mm. A composite primary end-point was used that included all cause mortality, HF hospitalizations, NYHA class, and the patient global assessment. A change in left ventricular end-systolic volume index (LVESVi) of greater than 15% was a secondary end-point. After 12 months, the group with CRT on had a significantly greater reduction in LVESVi and improvement in LVEF than the control group.

Elderly Patients

The prevalence of heart failure increases with age. HF is the leading medical cause of hospitalization among people aged ≥65 years and they represent an important proportion of patients with heart failure encountered in daily practice. However, the mean age in major CRT trials was <67 years. A recent study by Delnoy et al.[40] examined the clinical and echocardiographic response to CRT in a large group of 107 elderly (age >75 years) patients and compared them to a group of 159 younger patients (age ≤75 years). During follow-up, there was a comparable and sustained improvement in both groups according to New York Heart Association (NYHA) class and quality of life score. Reverse LV remodeling defined as LV end-systolic volume reduction ≥10% was seen in 79% and 87% (group aged ≤75 years), respectively, versus 71% and 79% (group aged >75 years), respectively, after 3 months and 1 year, respectively. A subgroup analysis of 39 octogenarians (>80 years) also showed a significant improvement in NYHA class and LV ejection fraction in this subgroup. LV reverse remodeling occurred in a similar extent (75% and 84%, respectively) after 3 months and 1 year, respectively.

Nonresponders to CRT

In all CRT trials, there are consistently 30% of patients who do not respond favorably to resynchronization despite rigorous selection criteria. The following are a few of many hypotheses that have been raised:

1. Lead placement: Left ventricular (LV) lead placement at an optimal anatomic pacing site is a critical determinant of outcome of cardiac resynchronization therapy (CRT). Selecting the "right" patient for CRT but stimulating the "wrong" site remains an important cause for the high incidence of nonresponders to CRT. The optimal left ventricular pacing location for cardiac resynchronization therapy should be individualized according to the site of maximal mechanical delay. In addition, optimal LV lead placement may not be possible due to unfavorable coronary sinus (CS) anatomy.
2. Scar burden: Total scar burden, assessed using contrast-enhanced magnetic resonance imaging, is an important factor influencing response to CRT and may be included in the selection process for CRT.[41] There is a linear relation between scar size and ejection fraction, and LV volumes. This relation is independent of scar location and transmurality.[42]
3. The need for a more accurate and clinically applicable direct measurement of mechanical dyssynchrony that is amenable to improvement and correction by CRT: The QRS duration is currently used as a surrogate for electromechanical dyssynchrony. However selection of patients using other parameters may lead to better selection of patients who will respond to CRT. PROSPECT "Predictors of response to cardiac resynchronization therapy," a prospective, multicenter, nonrandomized study, aimed to identify echocardiographic measures of dyssynchrony and evaluate their ability to predict response to CRT. A variety of conventional echocardiographic and tissue Doppler imaging parameters were tested against measures of clinical response. The primary response criteria were improvement in the heart failure Clinical Composite Score and left ventricular reverse remodeling. PROSPECT showed that, despite promising preliminary data from prior single-center studies, the various echocardiographic measures of ventricular dyssynchrony are unable to distinguish responders from nonresponders to a degree that would affect clinical decision making.

CONCLUSION

Cardiac resynchronization therapy (CRT) is an effective therapy for patients who are already refractory to optimal medical treatment with all NYHA symptom classes of systolic heart failure, LV dilatation, prolonged QRS duration, and low ejection fraction. In contrast to pharmaceutical agents that usually only attenuate remodeling, CRT reverses the remodeling process in both ischemic and nonischemic heart failure and in doing so reduces morbidity and mortality and alleviates symptoms in the majority of patients with heart failure. The effects of CRT on remodeling are immediate and sustained up to at least 2 years, which is as long as patients have been followed thus far.

Several issues regarding CRT and remodeling need clarification. These include elucidation of the mechanism via which the symptomatic benefit from CRT is transduced to reverse structural and functional remodeling; why up to 30% of patients who meet the enrollment criteria for clinical CRT trials do not respond to CRT; and the fact that there are currently no reliable noninvasive tools that predict response to CRT before CRT implantation.

PRACTICAL POINTS

1. The current goal of heart failure therapy is not simply to attenuate, but to reverse, the remodeling process. Reverse remodeling involves reduction in LV size, near-normalization of LV architecture, increase in contractile function, and accompanying symptomatic benefit. Reduction of volumes is often but not always accompanied by a reversal of the deranged molecular processes. Clinical and experimental data are still limited regarding the correlation between macroscopic and molecular remodeling. Reverse remodeling is accompanied by improved survival, exercise capacity, and quality of life.
2. Quantitative echocardiographic assessment of LV volumes and ejection fraction are important because

induces heterogeneity in electrical activation of the my-ocardium. Using endocardial mapping of the LV in 40 patients, Vassallo et al. demonstrated that the electrical acti-vation pattern during RV apical pacing is very similar to left bundle branch block.[17] A single breakthrough was located in the interventricular septum in the majority of the patients. In addition, the site of latest activation was predominantly located at the inferoposterior base of the LV, with a total endocardial activation time similar to left bundle branch block.[17]

Similar to the changes in electrical activation of the ven-tricles, the mechanical activation pattern of the LV is changed during RV apical pacing. Importantly, not only the onset of mechanical contraction is changed, but also the pattern of mechanical contraction.[16] In several studies using animal models, it has been demonstrated that the early-activated re-gions near the pacing site exhibit rapid early systolic shorten-ing, resulting in pre-stretch of the late activated regions.[18–19] As a consequence, these regions exhibit an increase in (de-layed) systolic shortening, imposing systolic stretch to the early activated regions exhibiting premature relaxation. This abnormal contraction pattern of the various regions of the LV may result in a redistribution of myocardial strain and work and subsequent less effective contraction.[19]

Both the abnormal electrical and mechanical activation patterns of the ventricles negatively affect cardiac function. An overview of the effects of RV apical pacing on cardiac function is provided in Figure 9.3. The most important effects are related to cardiac metabolism and perfusion, remodeling, hemodynamics, and mechanical function. The effects on cardiac metabolism and perfusion have been clearly demonstrated in an animal model of cardiac pacing, where it was noted that the abnormal activation pattern with paradoxical stretching of the different regions within the LV resulted in significant changes in regional myocar-dial perfusion.[20] Similarly, it has been demonstrated that RV apical pacing may negatively influence LV perfusion. Even in the absence of coronary artery disease, myocardial perfusion defects may be present in up to 65% of the patients after long-term RV pacing.[21–22] It has been noted that the perfusion defects are mainly located near the pacing site (inferior and apical segments) and tend to increase with time.[22]

In addition, cardiac pacing may result in regional and global LV remodeling. Changes in cardiac structure ranging from the cellular to macroscopic level have been noted after long-term cardiac pacing. Karpawich et al.[23] demonstrated histological changes in 14 patients with congenital complete

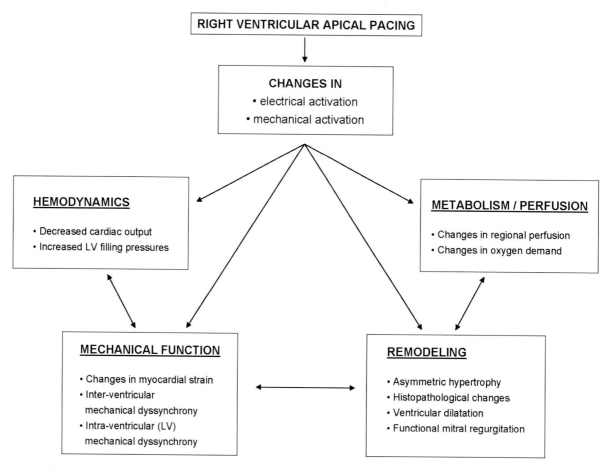

FIG. 9.3. By changing the electrical and mechanical activation pattern, RV apical pacing may negatively affect cardiac hemodynamics and mechanical function. In addition, RV apical pacing may result in ventricular remodeling and changes in cardiac metabolism.

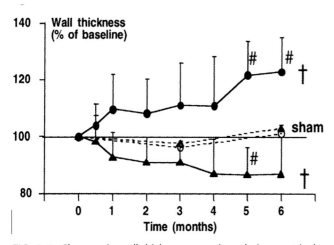

FIG. 9.4. Changes in wall thickness over time during ventricular pacing at physiological heart rate for 6 months at the base of the LV free wall in eight dogs and five controls (sham). After 6-month follow-up, wall thickness had decreased 17 ± 17% in the early-activated LV free wall (▲) and had increased 23 ± 12% in the late-activated septum (●). In the controls, no significant changes in wall thickness were observed. † Significant change over time by ANOVA; # p <0.05 compared with baseline. (Reprinted with permission from van Oosterhout MF, Prinzen FW, Arts T, et al. Asynchronous electrical activation induces asymmetrical hypertrophy of the left ventricular wall. *Circ.* 1998;98:588–595.)

atrioventricular block, requiring RV pacing. Endomyocardial biopsies were acquired after long-term (median 5.5 years) permanent RV pacing. In these patients, cellular and intracellular alterations were noted, including mitochondrial variations and degenerative fibrosis.[23]

Furthermore, RV pacing may result in asymmetrical remodeling of the LV. In an animal model of cardiac pacing, it was demonstrated that LV wall thickness may decrease in early-activated regions, whereas it may increase in late-activated regions (Fig. 9.4), accompanied by a change in myocyte thickness.[24] Finally, global remodeling resulting in an increase in LV volumes may occur after long-term pacing. Both in animal[24] and in human[25] studies, changes in LV size have been reported. Importantly, severe LV remodeling may subsequently lead to functional mitral regurgitation and left atrial remodeling.

In addition, the abnormal electrical and mechanical activation of the LV may result in changes in hemodynamic properties and global mechanical function. Pacing at the RV apex may result in a decrease in cardiac output and may change LV filling properties.[26] Finally, changes in myocardial strain and timing of regional strain may occur during RV apical pacing. Using magnetic resonance imaging in an animal model of cardiac pacing, Prinzen et al. demonstrated that regional myocardial strain is changed during pacing.[19] A significant decrease in strain was observed in the regions close to the pacing site, whereas an increase in myocardial strain was observed in remote regions. Importantly, timing of peak regional strain is also changed during pacing.

This is often referred to as "mechanical dyssynchrony."[27] The presence of LV dyssynchrony after long-term RV apical pacing has been related to a decrease in LV systolic function and deterioration in functional capacity.[28] However, not all patients will develop significant mechanical dyssynchrony after long-term RV apical pacing. In the following paragraphs, the assessment of ventricular dyssynchrony with echocardiography and the relation with RV apical pacing will be discussed.

MECHANICAL DYSSYNCHRONY IN RIGHT VENTRICULAR APICAL PACING

Transthoracic echocardiography is the most widely used technique to assess the extent of ventricular dyssynchrony. Right ventricular apical pacing may induce both interventricular dyssynchrony (between the RV and the LV), as well as intraventricular dyssynchrony (within the LV) in some patients. Various echocardiographic techniques are available for the assessment of cardiac mechanical dyssynchrony. These include conventional Doppler techniques, tissue Doppler imaging, strain analysis, and novel three-dimensional echocardiography. The majority of the techniques have been used to quantify inter- and intraventricular dyssynchrony in heart failure patients referred for CRT. Using echocardiography, the prediction of a favorable response to CRT may be improved, rather than using the conventional selection criteria (severe heart failure, LV ejection fraction <35%, QRS >120 ms) alone.[29] Similarly, these techniques can be used to detect the presence of ventricular mechanical dyssynchrony during acute and long-term RV apical pacing.

Interventricular Dyssynchrony

For the assessment of interventricular dyssynchrony (mechanical dyssynchrony between the RV and the LV), conventional Doppler techniques are typically used. For both ventricles, the electromechanical delay is calculated as the time from QRS to the onset of pulmonary systolic flow (RV electromechanical delay) or aortic systolic flow (LV electromechanical delay). The time difference between the RV and LV electromechanical delay represents interventricular dyssynchrony (Fig. 9.5). Previously, a difference of ≥40 ms in electromechanical delay between the RV and the LV has been used to indicate the presence of interventricular dyssynchrony.[30–31]

It has been demonstrated that RV apical pacing is associated with an increase in interventricular dyssynchrony. In 33 patients with a DDDR pacemaker for atrioventricular block or sinus node dysfunction, the effect of RV apical pacing on interventricular dyssynchrony was investigated.[32] After long-term RV apical pacing, an echocardiogram was performed during intrinsic rhythm and during RV pacing. An increase in interventricular dyssynchrony was observed, most prominent in patients with an LV ejection fraction <35% (mean interventricular delay increased from 22 ± 17 to 58 ± 14, p <0.001). During RV apical pacing, 15 of the 33 patients (45%) exhibited significant interventricular dyssynchrony.[32]

TABLE 9.2 **Completed and Ongoing Randomized Clinical Trials Comparing Right Ventricular *Versus* Biventricular Pacing (*Continued*)**

Trial (reference)	Number of Patients	Design	Inclusion Criteria	Primary End-point	Secondary End-point	Comment
BLOCK HF[73]	1200*	Parallel arms	- AV block - LV systolic dysfunction - Mild to moderate heart failure	Time to: - all-cause mortality - heart failure-related urgent care - increase in LVESVI	- (NT-pro) BNP, ANP - Heart failure hospitalization - Atrial tachyarrhythmia - NYHA class - QOL - Echocardiographic measures - All-cause mortality	Ongoing

*For the ongoing trials: number of patients to be randomized

AF, atrial fibrillation; AV, atrioventricular; AVN, atrioventricular node; BiV, biventricular; CRT, cardiac resynchronization therapy; LA, left atrial; LV, left ventricular; LVEF, left ventricular ejection fraction; LVEDD, left ventricular end-diastolic diameter; LVEDV, left ventricular end-diastolic volume; LVESD, left ventricular end-systolic diameter; LVESV, left ventricular end-systolic volume; LVESVI, left ventricular end-systolic volume index; MR, mitral regurgitation; NYHA, New York Heart Association; PM, pacemaker; QOL, quality of life; RV, right ventricular; 6MWT, 6-minute walking test

modest benefit[65,67] or no benefit at all.[66] Similarly, conflicting results on the effect of the different pacing modes on the quality of life have been reported (Table 9.2). Finally, no data is yet available on the outcome after long-term RV pacing versus biventricular pacing. The Biventricular Pacing for Atrioventricular Block to Prevent Cardiac Desynchronization (BioPace) trial[68] has included mortality as one of the primary end-points. This trial will randomize 1,200 patients with a conventional pacemaker indication and any LV systolic function, and will follow them systematically for up to 30 months after randomization. This trial and other prospective randomized trials will demonstrate if the benefits

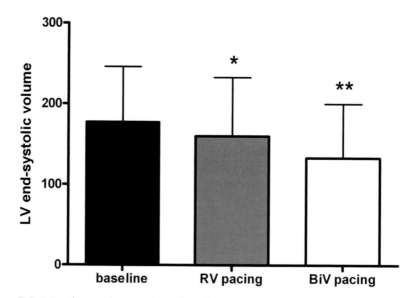

FIG. 9.9. Changes in LV end-systolic volume during 3 months of RV pacing and 3 months of biventricular pacing in 30 patients with a standard indication for permanent pacing and LV dysfunction (LV end-diastolic diameter ≥60 mm and LV ejection fraction ≤40%). The LV end-systolic volume was 177.3 ± 68.7 ml at baseline, and decreased modestly with RV pacing (160.2 ± 73.4 ml, p<0.05). When compared with RV pacing, BiV pacing significantly reduced LV end-systolic volume by 17% (133.1 ± 66.5 ml, p <0.001). *p <0.05 baseline vs. RV pacing; **p <0.001 baseline vs. BiV pacing and RV pacing vs. BiV pacing

of biventricular pacing, as demonstrated in the smaller acute and mid-term follow-up studies will actually provide benefit in outcome over conventional RV apical pacing.

SUMMARY AND CONCLUSIONS

Although the RV apex has been used for several decades as the preferred location of endocardial pacing leads, recent studies have demonstrated detrimental effects of conventional RV apical pacing. From large randomized clinical trials, it has become apparent that there is an association between RV apical pacing and cardiac morbidity (heart failure hospitalization and atrial fibrillation) and mortality. However, not all patients will experience clinical adverse effects from long-term RV apical pacing. New pacing algorithms that minimize RV apical pacing are promising, but data on outcome is scarce.

The underlying mechanism of these negative effects may be related to the changes in electrical and mechanical activation of the myocardium. As a result, cardiac metabolism, perfusion, and hemodynamics may be altered, and structural remodeling and changes in mechanical function may occur. In addition, in some patients, RV apical pacing may induce severe inter- and intraventricular dyssynchrony. Importantly, it has been demonstrated that the induction of mechanical inter- and intraventricular dyssynchrony by RV apical pacing is associated with a poor outcome, and therefore should be closely monitored. Upgrade from RV apical pacing to biventricular pacing may partially reverse the detrimental effects of RV apical pacing. A number of studies have demonstrated favorable effects of "upgrading" previously paced patients, both in the acute phase and during long-term follow-up. Finally, to avoid the detrimental effects of RV apical pacing, biventricular pacing may be considered even in patients with conventional pacemaker indications. Some studies have reported positive results of "de novo" biventricular pacing in these patients, but more data from ongoing trials is needed.

PRACTICAL POINTS

1. Cardiac pacing is the only effective treatment for patients with symptomatic sick sinus syndrome and atrioventricular conduction disorders. Indications for cardiac pacing are clearly defined in the current ACC/AHA/HRS and ESC guidelines.
2. Large clinical trials have demonstrated an association between RV apical pacing and cardiac morbidity and mortality.
3. Detrimental effects of RV apical pacing are mainly related to metabolism and perfusion, hemodynamics, structural remodeling, and changes in mechanical function.

4. RV apical pacing can induce mechanical inter- and intraventricular dyssynchrony. The deterioration of LV function during long-term RV apical pacing may be related to the induction of ventricular dyssynchrony by cardiac pacing.
5. Upgrading from RV apical pacing to biventricular pacing may partially reverse the detrimental effects of RV apical pacing.
6. If patients with permanent RV pacing develop ventricular dyssynchrony and heart failure during follow-up, an upgrade to biventricular pacing may result in an improvement in LV function and heart failure symptoms.

REFERENCES

1. Gregoratos G, Abrams J, Epstein AE, et al. ACC/AHA/NASPE 2002 guideline update for implantation of cardiac pacemakers and antiarrhythmia devices: summary article: a report of the American College of Cardiology/American Heart Association Task Force on Practice Guidelines (ACC/AHA/NASPE Committee to Update the 1998 Pacemaker Guidelines). *Circulation.* 2002;106:2145–2161.
2. Vardas PE, Auricchio A, Blanc JJ, et al. Guidelines for cardiac pacing and cardiac resynchronization therapy: the task force for cardiac pacing and cardiac resynchronization therapy of the European Society of Cardiology. Developed in collaboration with the European Heart Rhythm Association. *Eur Heart J.* 2007;28:2256–2295.
3. Mond HG, Irwin M, Morillo C, et al. The world survey of cardiac pacing and cardioverter defibrillators: calendar year 2001. *Pacing Clin Electrophysiol.* 2004;27:955–964.
4. Manolis AS. The deleterious consequences of right ventricular apical pacing: time to seek alternate site pacing. *Pacing Clin Electrophysiol.* 2006;29:298–315.
5. Sweeney MO, Prinzen FW. A new paradigm for physiologic ventricular pacing. *J Am Coll Cardiol.* 2006;47:282–288.
6. Nielsen JC, Kristensen L, Andersen HR, et al. A randomized comparison of atrial and dual-chamber pacing in 177 consecutive patients with sick sinus syndrome: echocardiographic and clinical outcome. *J Am Coll Cardiol.* 2003;42:614–623.
7. Hayes DL, Furman S. Cardiac pacing: how it started, where we are, where we are going. *J Cardiovasc Electrophysiol.* 2004;15:619–627.
8. Gillis AM. Redefining physiologic pacing: lessons learned from recent clinical trials. *Heart Rhythm.* 2006;3:1367–1372.
9. Lamas GA, Lee KL, Sweeney MO, et al. Ventricular pacing or dual-chamber pacing for sinus-node dysfunction. *N Engl J Med.* 2002;346: 1854–1862.
10. Sweeney MO, Hellkamp AS, Ellenbogen KA, et al. Adverse effect of ventricular pacing on heart failure and atrial fibrillation among patients with normal baseline QRS duration in a clinical trial of pacemaker therapy for sinus node dysfunction. *Circulation.* 2003;107:2932–2937.
11. Wilkoff BL, Cook JR, Epstein AE, et al. Dual-chamber pacing or ventricular backup pacing in patients with an implantable defibrillator: the Dual Chamber and VVI Implantable Defibrillator (DAVID) Trial. *JAMA.* 2002;288:3115–2123.
12. Healey JS, Toff WD, Lamas GA, et al. Cardiovascular outcomes with atrial-based pacing compared with ventricular pacing: meta-analysis of randomized trials, using individual patient data. *Circulation.* 2006;114:11–17.
13. Olshansky B, Day JD, Moore S, et al. Is dual-chamber programming inferior to single-chamber programming in an implantable cardioverter-defibrillator? Results of the INTRINSIC RV (Inhibition of Unnecessary RV Pacing With AVSH in ICDs) study. *Circulation.* 2007;115:9–16.
14. Sweeney MO, Bank AJ, Nsah E, et al. Minimizing ventricular pacing to reduce atrial fibrillation in sinus-node disease. *N Engl J Med.* 2007;357: 1000–1008.
15. Wiggers CJ. The muscular reactions of the mammalian ventricles to artificial surface stimuli. *Am J Physiol.* 1925;73:346–378.

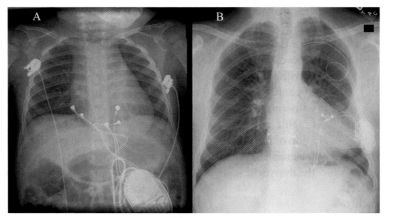

FIG. 10.6. Chest X-rays demonstrating multisite pacing techniques in (A) a child with an epicardial system, and (B) an adult with congenital heart disease with a mixed (epicardial and endocardial) system.

anatomic, hemodynamic, and electrical characteristics in these patients, it is very likely that the subset that may benefit from CRT differs substantially from those defined by the adult criteria.

Limited studies have evaluated chronic pacing in order to resynchronize the failing systemic right ventricle. Janousek et al evaluated eight patients with a systemic right ventricle and wide QRS who underwent resynchronization, with a follow-up of 18 months.[57] They noted an improvement in acute changes in echocardiographic measurements of systolic and diastolic function, dyssynchrony index, RV dP/dt and fractional area of change, and NYHA functional class.

CHRONIC RESYNCHRONIZATION PACING IN PATIENTS WITH A PULMONIC RIGHT VENTRICLE AND RIGHT BUNDLE BRANCH BLOCK

There have been no chronic pacing studies in patients with congenital heart disease with a right bundle branch block and pulmonic right ventricular failure, evaluating for improved hemodynamic parameters, decreased arrhythmia burden, improved symptomatology, or decreased mortality. Preliminary data on acute hemodynamic response to right ventricular pacing in patients with congenital heart disease, right ventricular dysfunction, and a right bundle branch block have been encouraging;[48,57] however, there has been a suggestion that right ventricular lead placement needs to be individualized in order to maximize acute hemodynamic response.[48]

A study by Stephenson et al. evaluated atrial synchronous right ventricular pacing in patients who had undergone repair of Tetralogy of Fallot and in whom an ICD had been placed.[58] They noted that attempts to shorten the QRS with adjusting the AV interval were successful in only 6 of 11 patients. Their study did not evaluate hemodynamic or echocardiographic parameters to further measure the effects of right ventricular apical pacing in this setting. A concept they raised was whether shortening the QRS would decrease the arrhythmia burden and potentially decrease mortality, as it has been noted that there is a higher incidence of sudden

cardiac death in patients with a QRS greater than 180 milliseconds following repair of Tetralogy of Fallot.[59]

In Dubin's evaluation of patients with right bundle branch block it was noted that the location of pacing in which the QRS morphology was narrowed was not consistent among the seven patients studies.[48] The site that produced the narrowest QRS correlated well with the largest improvement in cardiac index (six of seven patients), but not with right ventricular Dp/Dt. It seems clear that in order to affect acute improvement in hemodynamics and produce a narrower QRS, the lead would need to be placed in various locations within the right ventricle, on an individual basis. What parameter(s) would be most predictive of a long-term benefit remains unclear.

TECHNICAL ISSUES

Pediatric patients more frequently require epicardial pacing due to small patient size, the presence of intracardiac shunts, or limited access to cardiac chambers due to surgical palliation. While this may require a more invasive approach, it does facilitate access to areas of the heart that may be more difficult to approach from the endocardial surface. In the largest series of pediatric patients with multisite pacing, 44% had a transvenous system, 47% epicardial, and 10% a combination.[4] In children in whom a transvenous system is an option, one still needs to consider the issue of future growth and the stability of the left ventricular lead, as well as the presence of three leads traversing a small venous system and the likelihood of obstruction. The potential for decades needed for pacing makes decisions about venous access especially relevant in this population.

SUMMARY

Multisite pacing offers a promising therapeutic option in various groups within the pediatric and congenital heart disease populations. This patient population differs greatly from the typical adult heart failure population, and there is limited prospective data to guide patient selection for resynchronization therapy.

(7% vs. 15%, $p = 0.004$). Alth
was found in heart failure mor
of a major cardiac event (deatl
tion), this study was not powere
Results of the MIRACLE trial
CRT trials with hemodynamic
ment, but earlier studies were s
ther uncontrolled or not doubl

Following MIRACLE, the
investigate the safety and clir
CRT with an ICD, or the MIRA(
emerging data revealed the s
primary prevention of sudden
function.[21] The goal of combini
with defibrillator therapy was tc
toms in addition to the mortali
tricular tachyarrhythmias. The
was proarrhythmic or compror
Enrollment criteria was similar
ception of an ICD indication,
due to ventricular tachycardia
without a transient, reversible c
tolerated, and sustained ventr
spontaneous or inducible.

Patients were randomized to
active defibrillator ($n = 182$) an(
tive biventricular pacing and defi
MIRACLE-ICD found signific
NYHA functional class at 6 mor
group compared to the control
CRT patients also had a longer (
peak VO$_2$ compared to controls
Although there was no differer
with or without CRT (the study
such a difference and follow-up
supported the safety and efficac)
ICD. The InSync device used in
proved by the U.S. Food and Dr
August 2001 and the combined C

The MIRACLE-ICD II trial v
assess CRT in mild heart failt
whether it limited disease progre
capacity in patients with an EF
and similar ICD indication to M
pacity was not significantly impr
not moderately-to-severely imp
CRT was associated with reverse
end-diastolic and systolic volum
fraction, suggesting that CRT cou
ease progression. CRT in mild he
current trials, which will be discu

COMPANION TRIAL

The Comparison of Medical The
tion in Heart Failure (COMPAN

How To

- Resynchronization in pediatric and patients with congenital heart disease may require epicardial lead placement due to small patient size, the presence of right to left shunting, lack of a coronary sinus following surgery, or complex anatomy with limited venous access.
- Epicardial lead placement is routinely performed in pediatric patients less than approximately 13 years of age (about 40 kg) because of small venous anatomy, concerns for future growth and potential for lead dislodgement, and small coronary sinus anatomy.
- Epicardial lead placement offers the opportunity to choose the site of ventricular placement. In patients in whom site placement is not limited by scar tissue from previous surgical procedures, attempts have been made to utilize echocardiography to look for sites of late mechanical contraction and/or perform activation mapping to look for latest sites of electrical activation at the time of implant.

Troubleshooting

- Concerns over device failure are troublesome in children, with a higher percentage of epicardial leads which are more susceptible to fracture, especially in patients who tend to have a less sedentary lifestyle. Growth-related device malfunction is another potential concern. Transvenous pacing systems often cannot keep up with patient growth and lead advancement or replacement is not uncommon, especially during adolescence.

PRACTICAL POINTS

1. Pediatric and congenital heart disease patients differ significantly from the typical adult resynchronization candidate, without clearly defined indications for implantation.
2. Patients will more frequently require epicardial or mixed (epicardial and transvenous) systems because of small patient size, cardiac anatomy, or limited access to various cardiac chambers.
3. Due to a more active lifestyle, epicardial placement, and significant somatic growth, a high suspicion for lead fracture should be maintained.

REFERENCES

1. Cleland JG, Daubert JC, Erdmann E, et al. Cardiac Resynchronization-Heart Failure Study I. The effect of cardiac resynchronization on morbidity and mortality in heart failure. *N Engl J Med.* 2005;352(15):1539–1549.
2. Strickberger SA, Conti J, Daoud EG, et al. Council on Clinical Cardiology Subcommittee on Electrocardiography and Arrhythmias and the Quality of Care and Outcomes Research Interdisciplinary Working G, Heart Rhythm S. Patient selection for cardiac resynchronization therapy: from the Council on Clinical Cardiology Subcommittee on Electrocardiography and Arrhythmias and the Quality of Care and

Outcomes Research Interdisciplinary Working Group, in collaboration with the *Heart Rhythm Society. Circulation.* 2005;111(16):2146–2150.
3. Alexander ME, Berul CI, Fortescue EB, et al. Who is eligible for cardiac resynchronization therapy in pediatric cardiology? (Abstract). *Heart Rhythm.* 2004;1 (suppl 1):S122.
4. Dubin AM, Janousek J, Rhee E, et al. Resynchronization therapy in pediatric and congenital heart disease patients: an international multicenter study. *J Am Coll Cardiol.* 2005;46(12):2277–2283.
5. Thambo JB, Bordachar P, Garrigue S, et al. Detrimental ventricularremodeling in patients with congenital complete heart block and chronic right ventricular apical pacing. *Circulation.* 2004; 110(25):3766–3772.
6. Vanagt WY, Verbeek XA, Delhaas T, et al. The left ventricular apex is the optimal site for pediatric pacing: correlation with animal experience. *Pacing Clin Electrophysiol.* 2004;27(6 Pt 2):837–843.
7. Tantengco MV, Thomas RL, Karpawich PP. Left ventricular dysfunction after long-term right ventricular apical pacing in the young. *J Am Coll Cardiol.* 2001;37(8):2093–2100.
8. Karpawich PP. Chronic right ventricular pacing and cardiac performance: the pediatric perspective. *Pacing Clin Electrophysiol.* 2004;27 (6 Pt 2):844–849.
9. Janousek J, Tomek V, Chaloupecky V, et al. Dilated cardiomyopathy associated with dual-chamber pacing in infants: improvement through either left ventricular cardiac resynchronization or programming the pacemaker off allowing intrinsic normal conduction. *J Cardiovasc Electrophysiol.* 2004;15(4):470–474.
10. Deshmukh P, Casavant DA, Romanyshyn M, et al. Permanent, direct His-bundle pacing: a novel approach to cardiac pacing in patients with normal His-Purkinje activation. *Circulation.* 2000;101(8):869–877.
11. Scheinman MM, Saxon LA. Long-term His-bundle pacing and cardiac function. *Circulation.* 2000;101(8):836–837.
12. Deshmukh PM, Romanyshyn M. Direct His-bundle pacing: present and future. *Pacing Clin Electrophysiol.* 2004;27(6 Pt 2):862–870.
13. Blanc JJ, Etienne Y, Gilard M, et al. Evaluation of different ventricular pacing sites in patients with severe heart failure: results of an acute hemodynamic study. *Circulation.* 1997;96(10):3273–3277.
14. de Cock CC, Giudici MC, Twisk JW. Comparison of the haemodynamic effects of right ventricular outflow-tract pacing with right ventricular apex pacing: a quantitative review. *Europace.* 2003;5(3):275–278.
15. Tse HF, Yu C, Wong KK. Functional abnormalities in patients with permanent right ventricular pacing: the effect of sites of electrical stimulation. *J Am Coll Cardiol.* 2002;40(8):1451–1458.
16. Karpawich PP, Mital S. Comparative left ventricular function following atrial, septal, and apical single chamber heart pacing in the young. *Pacing Clin Electrophysiol.* 1997;20(8 Pt 1):1983–1988.
17. Prinzen FW, Peschar M. Relation between the pacing induced sequence of activation and left ventricular pump function in animals. *Pacing Clin Electrophysiol.* 2002;25(4 Pt 1):484–498.
18. Vanagt WY, Verbeek XA, Delhaas T, et al. Acute hemodynamic benefit of left ventricular apex pacing in children. *Ann Thorac Surg.* 2005; 79(3):932–936.
19. Cojoc A, Reeves JG, Schmarkey L, et al. Effects of single-site versus biventricular epicardial pacing on myocardial performance in an immature animal model of atrioventricular block. *J Cardiovasc Electrophysiol.* 2006;17(8):884–889.
20. Boucek MM, Aurora P, Edwards LB, et al. Registry of the International Society for Heart and Lung Transplantation: tenth official pediatric heart transplantation report—2007. *J Heart Lung Transplant.* 2007; 26(8):796–807.
21. Khoury GH, Dushane JW, Ongley PA. The Preoperative and Postoperative Vectorcardiogram in Tetralogy of Fallot. *Circulation.* 1965;31:85–94.
22. Horowitz LN, Simson MB, Spear JF, et al. The mechanism of apparent right bundle branch block after transatrial repair of tetralogy of Fallot. *Circulation.* 1979;59(6):1241–1252.
23. Thambo JB, Bordachar P, Garrigue S, et al. Magnitude of ventricular dyssynchrony in adults with surgical repair of tetralogy of Fallot and prolonged right ventricular conduction [Abstract]. *Europace Supplements.* 2005;7:229–230.
24. Dos L, Teruel L, Ferreira I J, et al. Late outcome of Senning and Mustard procedures for correction of transposition of the great arteries. *Heart.* 2005;91(5):652–656.
25. Graham TP Jr, Atwood GF, Boucek R J, Jr, et al. Abnormalities of right ventricular function following Mustard's operation for transposition of the great arteries. *Circulation.* 1975;52(4):678–684.

TABLE 11.1 Major (chroni:

Study (*n randomized*)
MIRACLE*(524)*[21†]
MUSTIC SR *(58)*[12]
MUSTIC AF *(43)*[18]
PATH CHF *(42)*[16]
CONTAK CD*(581)*[45]
MIRACLE ICD *(362)*[20]
PATH CHF II *(89)*[48]
COMPANION *(1520)*[1]
MIRACLE ICD II *(186)*[22]
CARE HF *(800)*[2]

*All trials required an ejection fra
†Literature cited for major clinica

produced significant imme
when compared to right v
also found further hemody
optimal AV delay. This was
epicardial LV leads; later t
ward intermediate and lon

MUSTIC STUDY

The Multisite Stimulation
study was a randomized, c
study in the 1990s designed
efficacy of transvenous biv
failure patients without a
maker.[12,17–18] Patients ha

TABLE 11.2 Primary
the Maj
in Cardi

Study (*n random.*)	Pri en
MIRACLE*(524)*	NYI €
MUSTIC SR *(58)*	6M
MUSTIC AF *(43)*	6M
PATH CHF *(42)*	pea € L
CONTAK CD*(581)*	cor
MIRACLE ICD*(362)*	NYI €
COMPANION *(1520)*	mo h
MIRACLE ICD II *(186)*	pea
CARE HF *(800)*	mo h

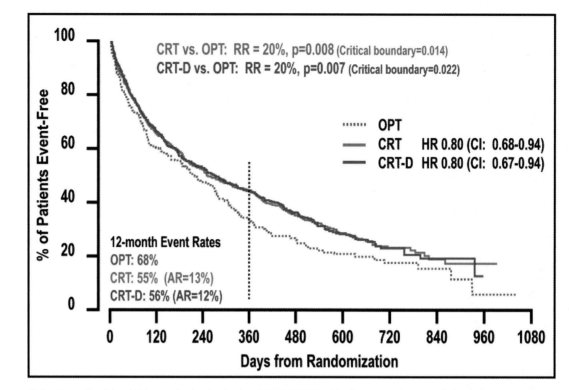

FIG. 11.1. Combined Primary End-point in the COMPANION trial of 12 month rates of death from any cause or hospitalization from any cause. Both treatment groups had a 20% reduction compared to the control of optimal pharmacologic therapy. CRT, Cardiac resynchronization therapy; CRT-D, Cardiac resynchronization therapy combined with defibrillator; OPT, Optimal pharmacologic therapy.

CRT versus CRT-ICD. Patients with advanced heart failure, NYHA Class III and IV, with an EF ≤35% were randomized to CRT without a defibrillator (n = 409) versus optimal pharmacologic therapy (n = 404) and was designed as a morbidity and mortality trial to investigate the effects of CRT on the risk of complications and death in this patient population.[2,25] Control patients did not receive a device in order to assess all effects of CRT, including implant-related complications. The primary end-point was a composite of death from any cause or unplanned hospitalization for a major cardiovascular event; the principal secondary end-point was death from any cause. Follow-up was an average of 29.4 months. Inclusion criteria for evidence of dyssynchrony was different compared to previous CRT trials. Patients were enrolled if QRS duration was ≥150 msec based on QRS duration only, or if QRS duration was between 120 msec and 150 msec, an additional two of three echocardiographic parameters were required. These parameters were an interventricular mechanical delay >40 msec, aortic pre-ejection delay >140 msec, or delayed posterolateral activation. CARE-HF was the first CRT trial to incorporate echocardiographic evidence of ventricular dysynchrony into inclusion criteria.

CARE-HF revealed a significant reduction in both the primary and secondary end-points from CRT. Compared to the control of optimal pharmacologic therapy, CRT significantly reduced the combined end-point of death from any cause or unplanned hospitalization for a major cardiac event by 37% (hazard ratio = 0.63, p <0.001). All-cause mortality was also significantly reduced by 36% with CRT (hazard ratio = 0.64, p <0.002), which is similar to the all-cause mortality benefit from CRT plus ICD in the COMPANION trial (hazard ratio = 0.64 p = 0.003). CRT benefits were similar in both ischemic and nonischemic etiology of heart failure, and significantly reduced heart failure hospitalizations by 52% (p <0.001). Echocardiographic evidence of reverse remodeling was also evident with improved LVEF, mitral regurgitation, and LV end-systolic volumes at 18 months. Device-related adverse events included lead displacement (n = 24), coronary sinus dissection (n = 10), pocket erosion (n = 8), pneumothorax (n = 6), and device-related infection (n = 3).

The mortality benefit from CRT alone likely reflects an improvement in cardiac function, as this trial also demonstrated a significant reduction in death from worsening heart failure. Addition of a defibrillator would then further improve survival by reducing the risk of sudden death from ventricular tachyarrhythmias. This trial confirmed the clinical benefits of CRT but also a survival and morbidity benefit, advocating the routine use of CRT in this patient population.

RECENTLY PUBLISHED CRT TRIALS

RethinQ Trial

Cardiac resynchronization therapy has been shown to improve survival, clinical symptoms, and exercise capacity, and also promote reverse remodeling in patients with moderate to severe heart failure and prolonged QRS, who were refractory to pharmacologic therapy. A wide QRS on surface ECG is considered to be evidence of prolonged ventricular conduction and regional ventricular delay in contraction, which is reduced with biventricular pacing. Current guidelines are based on QRS duration, but echocardiographic parameters, such as tissue Doppler imaging, have shown inter- and intraventricular dyssynchrony can predict cardiac events in heart failure independent of QRS duration.[5, 26] In fact, these measurements have revealed more than a third of narrow QRS heart failure patients display some degree of mechanical dyssynchrony. The Cardiac Resynchronization Therapy in Patients with Heart Failure and Narrow QRS trial was designed to further investigate the clinical efficacy of CRT in narrow QRS heart failure.[27–28] It was the first randomized controlled, multicenter double-blind trial in narrow QRS patients; previous studies suggesting a benefit were smaller in enrollment and single centers.[29–30] It was completed in early 2007 and results were published by the end of the year.

Patients had a standard indication for CRT and ICD (NYHA Class III heart failure, EF ≤35%) except QRS duration was <130 ms, and met one of the following two echocardiographic measurements of dyssynchrony: (a) an opposing-wall delay ≥65 msec on tissue Doppler imaging or (b) ≥130 msec delay in the septal-to-posterior wall on M-mode. A total of 172 patients were enrolled, 87 in the CRT group and 85 in the control group. Doppler echocardiography was used to optimize the atrioventricular and interventricular timing delays at baseline, utilizing maximal aortic velocity-time integral for both (also accepting the iterative and Ritter methods for the optimal atrioventricular delay). The primary end-point involved exercise capacity (peak oxygen consumption during cardiopulmonary exercise testing) and was the proportion of patients with ≥1.0 ml/kg/min improvement after 6 months of CRT. Secondary end-points were QOL and NYHA functional class.

The primary end-point was not significantly different in those receiving CRT, (46% vs. 41% in the control, $p = 0.63$), nor was there a difference in quality of life, 6-minute walk, LV dimensions, and ejection fraction. There was a significant improvement in NYHA functional class, in 54% of CRT patients vs. 29% of controls ($p = 0.006$). Subgroup analysis of patients with QRS between 120 and 130 msec (which was prespecified in the protocol design), revealed a significant improvement in peak oxygen consumption, but confidence intervals were wide.

The echocardiographic criteria for dyssynchrony could partly explain the results of this study; 96% patients met criteria for opposing wall delay >65 msec. However, this is a relatively simple method for dyssynchrony assessment, in terms of image acquisition and time requirements, compared to more comprehensive techniques that are also used to identify dyssynchrony by echocardiography, such as measuring the standard deviation of the time to peak myocardial contraction in 12 LV segments or strain rate imaging.[31] This study also followed patients for 6 months and was a relatively smaller study to assess morbidity.[32] An encouraging finding was the improvement in symptoms with CRT, suggesting the need for more information regarding CRT benefit in this patient population. Regardless, we do not have clear evidence at this time supporting the routine use of CRT in moderate-to-severe heart failure with a narrow QRS, based on dyssynchrony parameters from this trial.

PROSPECT Trial

As previously stated, QRS duration is an indirect marker of ventricular dyssynchrony or conduction delay, but a third of patients implanted with resynchronization devices are considered either clinical or echocardiographic "nonresponders."[13,33] The following question has been raised: Is this related to a lack of baseline dyssynchrony, despite meeting QRS criteria? With emerging echocardiographic parameters of dyssynchrony, focus has turned to a direct measurement of mechanical dyssynchrony as a predictor of CRT response. The Predictors of Response to Cardiac Resynchronization Therapy (PROSPECT) trial assessed whether a range of echocardiographic measures of LV mechanical dyssynchrony would predict clinical and echocardiographic endpoints.[34] Inclusion criteria was a standard CRT indication with QRS ≥130 msec. The study recruited 426 patients, all of whom were followed for 6 months.

Patients were considered responders based on either clinical or echocardiographic outcomes. The primary clinical "response" endpoint was a clinical composite score of both subjective and objective measures, including heart failure hospitalization, mortality, NYHA class, and a patient global assessment score[35]; secondary clinical end-points were quality of life, NYHA class, and 6-minute walk. The primary echocardiographic "response" end-point was at least a 15% reduction in LV end-systolic volume at 6 months.

At 6 months, 69% of patients were responders according to the clinical composite outcomes ($p = 0.01$) and 56% by echocardiographic outcomes ($p = 0.03$).[36] The following three echocardiographic parameters predicted a small but significant improvement in both the primary clinical and echocardiographic outcomes: interventricular mechanical delay by pulsed Doppler (IVMD), percentage change in LV filling time per cardiac cycle length (LVFT/RR) as measured by transmitral Doppler, and LV preejection interval (LPEI). Two other parameters were also associated with echocardiographic response, septal-to-posterior wall motion delay on M-mode (SPWMD), and the time delay between the peak systolic velocities in the basal lateral and septal segments ($T_{s\,sep\text{-}lat}$). However, each parameter had a low sensitivity and specificity, leading to the study conclusion that no dyssynchrony measure from the PROSPECT study could help select patients who would respond to CRT. Three core labs were utilized for echocardiographic assessment in the trial, but interlab variability was still high, ranging up to 72%, suggesting that such techniques still require a degree of enhancement for routine use.

REVERSE Study

Cardiac resynchronization therapy has been well established as beneficial in selected patients with moderate-to-severe heart failure, but has not been as extensively studied in less symptomatic heart failure patients. A potential for clinical improvement was suggested by the MIRACLE-ICD II trial,[22] and when compared to NYHA Class III and IV heart failure, Class II CRT patients in two uncontrolled studies had similar improvements in LV function and reverse remodeling after 6 months and 12 months of follow-up, respectively.[37–38] Landolina et al. also found, not unexpectedly, that Class II patients were less likely to improve in functional class, but a low percentage also progressed to Class III heart failure. Conflicting results revealed no clinical or echocardiographic improvement in mild heart failure patients after 3 months of therapy,[39] but brief follow-up could have contributed to these findings. The Resynchronization Reverses Remodeling in Systolic Left Ventricular Dysfunction Study was a randomized controlled, multicenter, double-blind clinical trial designed to assess whether CRT combined with optimal pharmacologic therapy can prevent or slow disease progression compared to medical therapy alone in mild heart failure.[40] Patients with NYHA Class I and Class II heart failure were enrolled, with QRS ≥120 msec, LVEDD ≥55 mm, and LVEF ≤40%. To receive CRT plus ICD, patients were required to have a Class I or II indication according to current guidelines. Patients were followed for 12 months.

The primary end-point was a clinical composite response end-point designed to assess outcomes from interventions in heart failure patients.[35] It takes into account heart failure hospitalizations, mortality, NYHA class, worsening of symptoms to NYHA Class III or IV, and the patient global assessment. Since the study evaluated disease progression, both "unchanged" and "improved" were considered a positive response to CRT from baseline to 12 months. Secondary end-points included LV end-systolic volume index (LVESV in cm² divided by body surface area in m²) as a marker of reverse remodeling, along with NYHA functional class, 6-minute walk, and quality of life.

The study was completed in September 2006, and 610 patients have been randomized.[41] The overall implantation success rate was 96.9%. At this time, published data reviews baseline characteristics from the REVERSE study, but final outcome data is not yet published. Compared to earlier randomized CRT trials, patients in this study are on better pharmacologic therapy with 95.1% on beta-blockers and 97% on angiotensin-converting enzyme inhibitors. Optimization of ACE inhibitors, beta-blockers, and angiotensin blockers was obtained prior to study enrollment, as these drugs promote reverse remodeling.[42] Patients in this study were also younger, had a narrower QRS, and higher systolic blood pressure, yet they had similar LV dysfunction, emphasizing the importance of this trial's results for CRT in asymptomatic and mild heart failure patients.

CONCLUSION

Guidelines recommend CRT for patients with LV ejection fraction less than or equal to 35%, sinus rhythm, and NYHA functional Class III or ambulatory Class IV symptoms despite optimal medical therapy, who have ventricular dyssynchrony, which is currently based on a QRS duration of at least 120 msec.[43–44] Based on the reviewed clinical trial data in this chapter, CRT has been well established as routine therapy in this patient population. Recent trials have demonstrated a survival benefit in advanced heart failure both with and without a defibrillator, and all landmark CRT trials demonstrated a clinical benefit. A few clinical trials have evaluated the use of combined CRT and ICD devices in chronic heart failure,[1,20,45] which is supported by guidelines,[43–44,46] although no study has been appropriately powered to directly compare CRT alone to CRT plus ICD.

Although guidelines are based on QRS duration, promising echocardiographic techniques have suggested the importance of mechanical delay in ventricular dyssynchrony, rather than electrical delay only. The PROSPECT trial did not find positive echo predictors, but we must still define the most reliable and reproducible echocardiographic parameters to best define ventricular dyssynchrony. Another unknown issue is whether dyssynchrony is dynamic, and if a single measurement accurately estimates mechanical delay in an individual patient. Other nonstandard indications with uncertainty include the role of CRT in mild heart failure and if disease progression is altered. Both the REVERSE study and Multicenter Automatic Defibrillator Implantation—Cardiac Resynchronization Therapy (MADIT-CRT) end-points of mortality and heart failure events have further investigated this topic.[47] Due to long-term adverse effects of chronic RV pacing from the DAVID trial,[9] patients with bradycardia indications for pacing might also benefit from CRT. Enrolling studies will provide further advancement on these topics and better define appropriate candidates for resynchronization, reduce the number of nonresponders, and address issues of CRT benefit in mildly symptomatic patients, narrow QRS, atrial fibrillation, and those with chronic pacemaker indications.

PRACTICAL POINTS

1. CRT alone or in combination with an internal cardiac defibrillator (ICD) has been shown to reduce morbidity and mortality in selected patients.

2. COMPANION further substantiated the clinical benefit and reduced morbidity associated with resynchronization therapy in advanced refractory heart failure; additionally, combined CRT and defibrillator therapy was correlated with a survival advantage.

3. CARE-HF confirmed the clinical benefits of CRT (improved functional status, quality of life, and reverse remodeling) but also a survival and morbidity benefit, advocating the routine use of CRT in the chronic heart failure population with moderate symptoms and appropriate QRS duration (>120 ms).

4. Despite improvement in some clinical symptoms with CRT in narrow QRS chronic heart failure patients with moderate symptoms, at this time we do not have clear evidence supporting the routine use of CRT based on dyssynchrony parameters in this patient population.

REFERENCES

1. Bristow MR, Saxon LA, Boehmer J, et al. Cardiac-Resynchronization Therapy With or Without an Implantable Defibrillator in Advanced Chronic Heart Failure (COMPANION). *New Engl J Med.* 2004; 350: 2140–2150.

2. Cleland J, Daubert JC, Erdmann E, et al. The effect of cardiac resynchronization on morbidity and mortality in heart failure. *N Engl J Med.* 2005; 352:1539–1549.

3. Littmann L, Symanski JD. Hemodynamic implications of left bundle branch block. *J Electrocardiol.* 2000;33(Suppl.):115–121.

4. Kashani A, Barold SS. Significance of QRS complex duration in patients with heart failure. *J Am Coll Cardiol.* 2005;46:2183–2192.

5. Bader H, Garrigue S, Lafitte S, et al. Intra-left ventricular electromechanical asynchrony. A new independent predictor of severe cardiac events in heart failure patients. *J Am Coll Cardiol.* 2004;43:248–256.

6. Hochleitner M, Hortnagl H, Ng CK, et al. Usefulness of physiologic dual-chamber pacing in drug-resistant idiopathic dilated cardiomyopathy. *Am J Cardiol.* 1990;66:198–202.

7. Brecker SJ, Xiao HB, Sparrow J, et al. Effects of dual-chamber pacing with short atrioventricular delay in dilated cardiomyopathy. *Lancet.* 1992;340:1308–1312.

8. Innes D, Leitch JW, Fletcher PJ. VDD pacing at short atrioventricular intervals does not improve cardiac output in patients with dilated heart failure. *PACE.* 1994;17:959–965.

9. Wilkoff BL, Cook JR, Epstein AE, et al. Dual chamber pacing or ventricular backup in patients with implantable defibrillator: the Dual Chamber and VVI Implantable DSefibrillator (DAVID) trial. *JAMA.* 2002;288(24):3115–3123.

10. Auricchio A, Stellbrink C, Sack S, et al. The Pacing Therapies for Congestive Heart Failure (PATH-CHF) study: rationale, design, and end-points of a prospective randomized multicenter study. *Am J Cardiol.* 1999;83:130D–135D.

11. Bax JJ, Abraham T, Barold S, et al. Cardiac resynchronization therapy. *J Am Coll Cardiol.* 2005;46(12):2153–2167.

12. Cazeau S, Leclercq C, Lavergne T, et al. for the Multisite Stimulation in Cardiomyopathies (MUSTIC) study investigators. Effects of multisite biventricular pacing in patients with heart failure and intraventricular conduction delay. *N Engl J Med.* 2001;344:873–880.

13. Abraham WT, Fisher WG, Smith AL, et al. for the Multisite Insync Randomized Clinical Evaluation (MIRACLE) investigators and coordinators. Double-blind, randomized controlled trial of cardiac resynchronization in chronic heart failure. *N Engl J Med.* 2002;346: 1845–1853.

14. Yu CM, Chau E, Sanderson JE, et al. Tissue Doppler echocardiographic evidence of reverse remodeling and improved synchronicity by simultaneously delaying regional contraction after biventricular pacing therapy in heart failure. *Circulation.* 2002;105:438–445.

15. The MERIT-HF investigators. Effect of metoprolol CR/XL in chronic heart failure: metoprolol CR/XL randomized intervention trial in congestive heart failure (MERIT-HF). *Lancet.* 1999;353:2001–2007.

16. Auricchio A, Stellbrink C, Block M, et al. Effect of pacing chamber and atrioventricular delay on acute systolic function of paced patients with congestive heart failure. *Circulation.* 1999;99:2993–3001.

17. Linde C, Leclercq C, Rex S, et al. on behalf of the Multisite Stimulation in Cardiomyopathies (MUSTIC) study group. Long-term benefits of biventricular pacing in congestive heart failure: results from the Multisite Stimulation in Cardiomyopathy (MUSTIC) study. *J Am Coll Cardiol.* 2002; 40:111–118.

18. Leclercq C, Walker S, Linde C, et al. Comparative effects of permanent biventricular and right-ventricular pacing in heart failure patients with chronic atrial fibrillation. *Eur Heart J.* 2002; 23:1780–1787.

19. Abraham WT, on behalf of the Multisite Insync Randomized Clinical Evaluation (MIRACLE) investigators and coordinators. Rationale and design of a randomized clinical trial to assess the safety and efficacy of cardiac resynchronization therapy in patients with advanced heart failure: the Multicenter Insync Randomized Clinical Evaluation (MIRACLE). *J Card Fail.* 2000;6:369–380.

20. Young JB, Abraham WT, Smith AL, et al. Safety and efficacy of combined cardiac resynchronization therapy and implantable cardioversion defibrillation in patients with advanced chronic heart failure. The Multicenter Insync ICD Randomized Clinical Evaluation (MIRACLE-ICD) trial. *JAMA.* 2003;289:2685–2694.

21. Moss AJ, Zareba W, Hall JW, et al. Prophylactic implantation of a defibrillator in patients with myocardial infarction and reduced ejection fraction. *N Engl J Med.* 2002;346:877–883.

22. Abraham WT, Young JB, Leon AR, et al. Effects of cardiac resynchronization on disease progression in patients with left ventricular systolic dysfunction, an indication for an implantable cardioverter defibrillator, and mildly symptomatic chronic heart failure. *Circulation.* 2004;110:2864–2868.

23. Bristow MR, Feldman AM, Saxon LA, for the COMPANION steering committee and COMPANION clinical investigators. Heart failure management using implantable devices for ventricular resynchronization: Comparison of Medical Therapy, Pacing, and Defibrillation in Chronic Heart Failure (COMPANION) trial. *J Card Fail.* 2000;6: 276–285.

24. Bardy GH, Lee KL, Mark DB, et al. Amiodarone or an Implantable Cardioverter-Defibrillator for Congestive Heart Failure (SCD-HeFT). *New Engl J Med.* 2005; 352:225–237.

25. Cleland JGF, Daubert JC, Erdmann E, et al. The CARE-HF study (Cardiac Resynchronisation in Heart Failure study): rationale, design, and end-points. *Eur J Heart Fail.* 2001;3:481–489.

26. Cho GY, Song JK, Park WJ, et al. Mechanical dyssynchrony assessed by tissue Doppler imaging is a powerful predictor of mortality in congestive heart failure with normal QRS duration. *J Am Coll Cardiol.* 2005; 46:2237–2243.

27. Beshai JF, Grimm RA. The resynchronization therapy in narrow QRS study (RethinQ study): methods and protocol design. *J Interv Card Electrophysiol.* 2007;19:149–155.

28. Beshai JF, Grimm RA, Nagueh SF, et al. Cardiac-resynchronization therapy in heart failure with narrow QRS complexes. *New Engl J Med.* 2007;357:2461–2471.

29. Yu CM, Chan YS, Zhang Q, et al. Benefits of cardiac resynchronization therapy for heart failure patients with narrow QRS complexes and coexisting systolic asynchrony by echocardiography. *J Am Coll Cardiol.* 2006;48:2251–2257.

30. Bleeker GB, Holman ER, Steendijk P, et al. Cardiac resynchronization therapy in patients with a narrow QRS complex. *J Am Coll Cardiol.* 2006;48:2243–2250.

with an increase in HF hospitalizations, progressive HF deaths, sudden cardiac deaths, and overall mortality.[6–8] We therefore recommend that the lowest dose of diuretic be used before and after CRT therapy as determined by best clinical judgment. Importantly, pharmacologic efforts should be focused on achieving target doses of angiotensin inhibitors (ACEi), beta blockers (BB), angiotensin receptor blockers (ARB), and aldosterone antagonist, aspirin, and statins as it is appropriate to a specific patient's clinical profile.

Once a biventricular pacemaker is implanted, it typically allows for a significant attenuation of diuretic dose. Immediately post-CRT implantation, hemodynamic changes occur including an increase in stroke work, cardiac output, and systolic blood pressure along with a decrease in end-systolic volumes and pulmonary capillary wedge pressure.[9–10] In addition to the long-term biochemical and electromechanical cardiac restructuring frequently seen post-CRT, these short-term hemodynamic shifts quickly result in an environment capable of supporting a new medical regimen.

One consequence of these changes is that the diuretic need is decreased with improved intracardiac filling pressures. These changes require a recalibration to match the decreased demand for diuresis and to avoid excessive intravascular volume loss. After CRT implantation, the previously "optimal" diuretic therapy dosage becomes, in effect, suboptimal and even potentially harmful. If the dose is not decreased, patients frequently will develop intravascular volume depletion, symptomatic hypotension, electrolyte disturbances, and prerenal azotemia.[11] Hence, post-CRT weaning of diuretic therapy is recommended. In some patients, this may allow implementation of higher doses of medications known to chronically improve mortality in HF patients.

For most patients with HF, BB use is an integral component of effective treatment. Bisoprolol, carvedilol, and metoprolol succinate have specifically been shown to improve outcomes in HF patients and are endorsed by the American Heart Association Guidelines for chronic HF. With BB, an improvement in functional class and ejection fraction has also been observed over an expected time-frame of months to years. Notably, with increasing doses of BB subsequent to CRT, patients on beta-blockade have demonstrably fewer hospitalizations and a lower mortality rate.

While the specific mechanisms of action responsible for these improved HF outcomes have yet to be completely elucidated, there are numerous cardiac structural, neurohormonal, and molecular changes associated with beta-blockade. The sympathetic nervous system is activated, in part, as a result of the failing heart's increased adrenergic tone. This tone occurs initially as an intrinsic mechanism intended to improve cardiac function, but over time, this adaptive system degenerates and becomes maladaptive in part, leading to pathological remodeling. BB therapy in conjunction with CRT partially interrupts this maladaptive system and contributes to ventricular reverse remodeling. Structurally, this is seen with an increase in regional contractile functionality, a decrease in chamber size, and potentially with a long-term reduction in mechanical dyssynchrony and an improvement in ejection fraction. On a molecular level, there is mounting evidence of an antiapoptotic effect, a reduction in inflammatory cytokines, a decrease in the level of oxygen free radicals, an improved high-energy phosphate production, and a restoration of intracellular calcium management.[11–12] These alterations ultimately yield improvements in signal transduction. The final product of these molecular changes is a more capable, less dysfunctional myocyte milieu and ventricle.

Conversely, if BB therapy is not carefully uptitrated and individualized to each patient, these drugs can potentially lead to a multitude of well-known adverse effects. After the initiation or recent uptitration of a BB, the optimal fluid balance of a given patient may be tipped askew as a result of increased fluid retention and a temporary decrease in contractile function. Fatigue, hypotension, lightheadedness, and dizziness may also occur. Lastly, bradycardia and heart block can develop. Many times, bradycardia is asymptomatic; however with increasing doses of BB, symptoms as well as insufficient heart rates or blood pressure can limit ideal doses of BB in HF patients. Prior to CRT placement, decreasing or even stopping therapy has sometimes been necessary, although the latter should occur only with persistent, severe symptoms, and after a close review and discontinuation of any other contributing drugs.

Overall, a need currently exists to improve the utilization of BB therapy in HF clinical practice, and CRT may help to improve reaching target doses as well as patient and physician compliance. In the large clinical trials demonstrating improved outcomes with CRT, the rates of BB use ranged from only approximately 30% to 60%.[13] In an analysis of one of the landmark BB mortality trials, the top three given reasons for failure or hesitancy to uptitrate beta-blockade therapy were symptoms of worsening HF, bradycardia, and hypotension.[13] CRT permits beta-blockade in many patients who previously were either unable to initiate therapy or to reach maximum goal dosage secondary to intolerance.[14] Post-CRT, the precipitating conditions of intolerance are in part obviated. The hemodynamic profile is more conducive to the maintenance of an optimal intravascular volume status. Therefore, fluid retention associated with beta-blockade is less of an issue. The increase in systolic blood pressure commonly seen with CRT also decreases the chance of symptomatic drug-induced hypotension and allows for either initiation or uptitration of BB therapy. Lastly, CRT's pacing activity eliminates the concerns of symptomatic bradycardia and heart block. Maximizing beta-blockade may also have its own prognostic incentive as evidence suggests synergistic effects of device and medical therapies including enhanced autonomic effects, improved reverse remodeling, and decreased hospitalization and mortality rates.[15–16]

ACE inhibitor (ACEi) therapy is a cornerstone of HF management. Long-term use may stabilize or potentially improve myocardial function. HF patients on ACEI have reduced hospitalizations and mortality. The majority of patients tolerate this class of drugs with careful titration. For those intolerant, angiotensin receptor blockers (ARB) are a reasonable alternative. In HF patients, valsartan and candesartan specifically have established noninferior outcomes relative to ACEi.[62] Without ACEi or ARB therapy, the renin-angiotensin-aldosterone system (RAAS) operates unopposed, thereby substantially contributing to the progression of HF. RAAS activation is associated with atrial remodeling, ventricular dilatation, hypertrophy, deleterious extracellular matrix changes, systolic dysfunction, and increasing arrhythmogenesis.[17]

CRT permits an increased cohort of HF patients to achieve optimal ACEi or ARB therapy. Intolerance has been a key barrier to this objective. Angiotensin suppression can predispose to hypotension, renal dysfunction, and potentially hyperkalemia. These adverse effects are noted limitations of therapy. In severe HF, high diuretic doses and unfavorable hemodynamics frequently contribute to suboptimal intravascular volume despite total body-volume overload. This further creates an environment conducive to limited, suboptimal medical management. Clinicians frequently find that hypotension occurs less frequently post-CRT. Significant dose-limiting azotemia appears lessened in clinical practice as well. These changes subsequent to CRT frequently lead to successful titration of drug therapy in many post-CRT HF patients. The medical optimization of pharmacologic therapy may also lead to improved patient outcomes in combination with the CRT.

CRT: TROUBLESHOOTING AND IMPLANTATION

Unfortunately, CRT utilization still has a 20% to 30% "nonresponders" rate. The meaning of the term itself is currently debatable. There is not yet an established definition of a nonresponder. Both echocardiographic measures (ejection fraction, mitral regurgitation, ventricular dimensions and volumes), as well as clinical measures (NYHA class, quality of life score, 6-minute walking distance, functional capacity) have been utilized to assess response. A lack of improvement in the chosen parameter has led to the term "nonresponder" in prior CRT studies. Yet, a firm correlation between clinical and echocardiographic improvement does not always exist because an HF patient may clinically improve with no significant change in their echocardiogram or vice-versa. It is also important to note that clinical and imaging improvements do not necessarily occur simultaneously. Current efforts are ongoing to standardize the nonresponder designation.

Nonresponse evaluation should occur if worsening HF and ongoing pathologic ventricular remodeling continue within the first few months post-CRT, or if there is no abatement in symptoms in the first 6 months after implantation. Delineating a potentially correctable cause of nonresponse is an important component of post-CRT management. Volume abnormalities, ongoing coronary ischemia, device placement issues, and suboptimal device programming can

all contribute to lack of response. Lastly, once all identifiable causes are excluded, a selected nonresponder population will inevitably remain with progressive disease. This "true nonresponder" group will require further intervention.

Volume abnormalities may inhibit CRT's beneficial effects. Congestion or intravascular volume depletion can result in maladaptive filling pressures. Clinical decompensation and detrimental remodeling may follow. Avoidance of suboptimal hemodynamics is necessary to maximize CRT response. An evaluation for prerenal azotemia is warranted in nonresponders as well. Post-CRT, over-diuresis can occur without diuretic dose titration. Measures to minimize congestion including fluid and salt restriction, daily weight assessment, and medication compliance should be continued. A limitation of clinical practice is the occasional lack of correlation between current volume assessment measures and true volume status. Ongoing studies are investigating whether implantable continuous hemodynamic monitoring devices will lead to improved patient outcomes. This may be a useful adjunctive tool for the HF caregiver in the future.

Other reasons for poor CRT responses may include ongoing ischemia and lead placement. A CRT nonresponder should be evaluated for ischemia amenable to revascularization. Interventions should be performed on target coronary lesions. While this typically is done at an earlier point in HF management, CRT nonresponse should prompt reassessment in suitable patients. In addition, impaired global perfusion reserve is also thought to trigger intermittent ischemia. SPECT and MR imaging have associated significant nonviability with diminished CRT response.[18–23] CRT can improve metabolism and perfusion, although these effects may augment function as well in nonischemic cardiomyopathy patients.[24] As a separate concern, LV lead placement in scarred myocardium may prevent resynchronization.[25]

COMPLICATIONS OF CRT IMPLANTATION

CRT implantation is associated with early and late complications. Ramifications can prohibit placement, impede response, or prompt corrective interventions. Greater than 90% of CRT devices are successfully implanted (initially) at experienced centers. Placement failure is most commonly caused by technical difficulties implanting the LV lead. Anatomical factors are typically responsible with tortuous venous anatomy precluding access being one of the primary causes. Retrograde venography and noninvasive venous imaging usually allows suitable selection. Additional technical difficulties are frequently encountered as enlarged right atrium distorts the coronary sinus ostium. A resultant inability to either cannulate or support the guiding catheter may occur in up to 4% of cases.[26] Prior studies have reported a 0.4% to 4% incidence of coronary sinus dissection. As the venous system is a low-pressure system, this usually does not have significant long term sequela, as perforation is very uncommon. Suboptimal lead placement can also lead to nonresponse or worsening dyssynchrony. Implant in anterior location or nondyssynchronous region heightens the probability of this complication.[27]

Other problems may arise post-implantation. These may include: 1) CRT nonresponse, with proper lead placement and suitable pacing capture thresholds, 2) lead dislodgement as has been reported in 4% to 12% of patients, 3) phrenic nerve stimulation secondary to lead proximity and inappropriate pacing output. This complication may be seen in 1.6% to 12% of patients and may develop as a consequence of postural changes.[28] Attempts to correct the pacing output should be done if this is encountered. Some refractory cases may require lead repositioning.

OPTIMIZATION OF THE CRT DEVICE

The primary aim of CRT is to favorably alter myocardial pathophysiology by manipulating electrical impulse coordination and reestablishing "synchrony." Dyssynchrony results from progressive HF and further contributes to a refractory condition. The consequences of mechanical dyssynchrony are increased LV volumes, decreased diastolic filling time, increased mitral regurgitation (MR) duration, diastolic MR, and a reduction in systolic function. Suboptimal device programming may result in nonresponse or even deterioration of cardiac function.

A short AV interval reduces cardiac output.[29–30] Since early ventricular contraction results in premature mitral valve closure, the entire atrial volume cannot be utilized. As a result, LV filling is suboptimal and stroke volume is diminished. An AV interval that is too prolonged contributes to progressively severe mitral valvular disease and systolic dysfunction. With delayed ventricular contraction, the mitral valve has incomplete closure. This allows diastolic mitral regurgitation (MR). This then may lead to more severe LV volume overload and worsened systolic function. One of the goals of CRT post-programming is to optimize the AV interval timing to appropriately allow for ventricular contraction with a concordant improvement in hemodynamics.

Since the optimal AV delay varies by individual, CRT calibration to a prespecified interval is not done. Instead, there are numerous techniques currently available using various imaging modalities to assess each individual's optimal AV interval. Echocardiographic techniques are those most commonly utilized.[31–32]

The goal of AV interval optimization is to allow for maximal ventricular filling time. This is accomplished by employing both diastolic and systolic methodologies. From a hemodynamic perspective, improved filling should result in increased stroke volume and cardiac output.[33] Diastolic methods are based upon parameters measured at the mitral inflow. Pulsed-wave Doppler allows visual comparison of the timing and duration of the E wave (passive LV filling) and A wave (active atrial volume contribution). The iterative method aims for mitral valve closure at the end of the A wave. The E

and A wave become temporally separated allowing maximum duration and benefit of each. Difficulty evaluating the A wave for truncation may be a limiting issue in optimization. This limitation also applies to the diastolic filling time technique. The achievement of maximal E/A duration is hampered by difficulty determining when mitral valve closure begins (shortening the A wave). A third diastolic method is measuring the maximal E/A velocity time integral (VTI). While accurate when compared to invasive LV dP/dt, time constraints and reproducibility remain disadvantages. A simplified transmital inflow method exists and employs a technique that avoids A wave truncation.[34] In this technique, the maximal AV delay with preserved ventricular capture is established, this delay is shortened by 5 to 10 msec, and substracted from this new delay is the time difference between the end of the A wave and the onset of systolic mitral regurgitation. This final value has been shown to correlate with optimal AV delay, as determined by invasive monitoring. Finally, a systolic method employs an aortic VTI calculation. This can be done using continuous-wave Doppler with the transducer positioned at the aortic outflow tract. Stroke volume and cardiac output are correlated with aortic VTI, and optimizing AV delay utilizing this methodology results in improved clinical outcomes compared to a standard setting of 120 ms.[35] No method has yet been proven as the most reliable. Selection involves the consideration of each lab's technical experience, reproducibility of results, and procedural time constraints. A current typical approach to AV optimization is to employ the simplified approach both to avoid A wave truncation as well as to take advantage of its rapidity. While AV optimization may improve hemodynamics, ventricular dyssynchrony may still be present. This can be due to persistent delayed LV or RV contraction resulting in interventricular delay. Similarly, intraventricular delay secondary to dyssynchronous LV segmental contractions may be present.

V-V optimization is a more recent technology. Current echocardiographic methods for V-V optimization begin with ventricular delay assessment. Interventricular delay is measured from the initiation of a QRS complex to the beginning of systolic ejection through the aortic and pulmonic outflow tracts. Intraventricular delay is determined by assessment of variability in the onset of LV segmental contractions. Whether changes in interventricular or intraventricular delay leads to better functional or clinical improvement remains uncertain. Evidence is mounting that a reduction in intraventricular dyssynchrony may correlate most consistently with reverse-remodeling.

Once delay is determined, CRT can be programmed to either simultaneous or sequential pacing. The most common current method for evaluating response to delay optimization is aortic VTI (albeit, some controversy still exists). Some studies have demonstrated functional improvement with pre-activation of one ventricle.[36–38] Certain individuals have been shown to respond more favorably to LV pre-activation while others respond best to RV pre-activation. Other studies have concluded that there is either no significant benefit of sequential over simultaneous pacing or that simultaneous pacing has the most significant effect.[39-41]

Forthcoming advances will address the many unanswered questions that include what is the correct order to optimize a device (AV vs. V-V), and what parameters should be used to define improvement. Prior studies have utilized hemodynamics, ejection fraction, as well as reduction in dyssynchrony. As reverse-remodeling ensues in responders, optimization delays may need to be changed further to improve outcomes. Some CRT devices are beginning to include optimization algorithms done automatically in real-time. Other future issues to be addressed include: 1) Will real-time device algorithms prove superior to echocardiogram-based optimization? 2) Will addressing interatrial conduction delay with potentially different atrial lead placement improve AV resynchrony? 3) Does current optimization (done at rest) ever impair exercise tolerance as filling pressures change with tachycardia? Irrespective of the methodology used, the ideal optimization scheme is theoretically accomplished when the clinician has maximized filling, valve timing, cardiac output, and synchrony.

MANAGEMENT OF THE PERSISTENT NONRESPONDER SUBSEQUENT TO CRT

After a complete evaluation for identifiable causes of nonresponse, there will be a population of post-CRT HF patients who continue to have lack of improvement. These patients have further management options dependent on their individual situations. Continued optimal medical therapy, symptom control, and close follow-up with attempted prevention of hospitalizations are indicated for all patients. For those who qualify, an evaluation for cardiac transplantation should be considered. For patients with significant ongoing hemodynamic compromise, consideration should be given to a ventricular assist device (VAD). In some patients, the implementation of a VAD may serve as a "bridge" to transplantation. In others, a VAD may be used as "destination" therapy and has been shown to improve symptoms and survival in the properly selected population. Some patients may require continuous intravenous inotropic support as an outpatient palliative option. Palliative measures in the refractory HF patients should be performed with close communication between the cardiovascular and hospice teams to ensure the achievement of optimal individual comfort and minimization of risk.[19-23]

ATRIAL FIBRILLATION AND CRT

A complicated relationship exists between atrial fibrillation (AF) and HF. The ongoing pathologic remodeling that occurs with HF includes atrial enlargement, "stretch," and interstitial fibrosis. Electrical conditions of increased automaticity, heterogeneous refractoriness, and loss of synchronous conduction result. These structural and functional changes increasingly predispose to the development of atrial fibrillation as HF progress.[42-43] Notably, AF is well known as a contributor to HF and is prevalent in 30% to 50% of Class III/IV HF patients. Hemodynamically, atrial dyssynchrony and variable R-R intervals are associated with decreased cardiac output and increased PCWP. In addition prolonged rapid ventricular response may further exacerbate a patient's cardiomyopathy.

A cohort of patients meet all other criteria for CRT implantation, except that these patients have AF rather than sinus rhythm (SR). In clinical practice, this group of patients has on numerous occasions received a CRT device. Yet only one major clinical trial, MUSTIC-AF, has addressed AF patients. While this initial study demonstrated improved quality of life, functional class, and exercise capacity in this cohort, it was not designed to address mortality. These benefits were subsequently found to be maintained through 12 months. All subsequent landmark CRT trials have utilized patients in SR. While a few small AF trials have suggested mortality benefit with CRT, no major large trial has demonstrated this to date.

Evidence from multiple small studies has suggested comparable benefits in AF and SR patients.[44-46] In many of these studies, part if not all of the AF patients had undergone AVJ ablation to allow 100% paced time. This is in contrast to MUSTIC-AF, in which biventricular pacing greater than 85% of the time correlated with improved outcomes. What is currently unclear is whether AV junctional (AVJ) ablation enables more overall responders or a more optimal response in those demonstrating benefit. In theory, the structural and functional consequences of AF could impede or prohibit CRT response even if present a minority of the time. In a study comparing a population of AF patients >85% paced with another post-AVJ ablation, only those AF patients post-AVJ ablation demonstrated reverse remodeling and improved exercise capacity.[47] Similarly, more responders have been noted in post-AVJ ablation patients in those studies whose AF cohort included both ablated and nonablated patients.[48-50] The Atrio-Ventricular Junction Ablation Followed by Resynchronization Therapy (AVERT) trial is an ongoing randomized, controlled large trial designed to compare AVJ-ablation with CRT versus CRT and pharmacologic therapy alone in those with LV dysfunction and AF.[51]

Current clinical practice is variable in those with severe HF and AF. One common approach is to initially implant a CRT device, subsequently evaluate for clinical improvement, and perform AVJ-ablation in nonresponders. In some cases, CRT response may then develop subsequent to ablation. Further confirmatory studies are certainly still needed.

MITRAL REGURGITATION AND CRT

Mitral regurgitation (MR) is frequently found in conjunction with progressive HF. In many of these patients with progressive cardiomyopathies, the mitral leaflets are morphologically normal. This functional MR may, in part, be reconciled with

CRT. In one of the landmark CRT trials, moderate or severe MR was present in 50% of patients.[52] Notably MR as an independent variable is associated with decreased survival. As such, CRT nonresponders strategies should have some focus on minimizing MR as part of the plan to optimize each patient's HF management.

Pathologic ventricular remodeling is associated with multiple structural alterations that predispose to the development of MR. Progressive ventricular enlargement leads to mitral annular dilation, leaflet tethering, and papillary muscle displacement.[53-54] Impaired contractile ability results in a decreased closing force. If dyssynchrony is present, a suboptimal AV interval can cause incomplete mitral valve closure.

CRT has demonstrated efficacy in improving MR.[55-57] Acutely, resynchronization appears to improve closing force secondary to proper timing of papillary muscle contractions. Over time, reverse-remodeling further allows improved coaptation of the mitral leaflets secondary to correction of the underlying structural abnormalities. Thirty to fifty percent of post-CRT patients may develop these improvements.[55,57]

As previously noted, MR may be a significant contributor to progressive HF and a barrier to effective resynchronization therapy. There is a lack of randomized clinical trials on surgical correction of functional MR. Multiple recent observational and prospective studies have been done on cohorts with severe LV dysfunction and MR evaluating outcomes for mitral valve repair.[58-60] There have been promising results with low reported perioperative mortality, symptomatic improvement, and resultant reverse-remodeling. While there is a lack of data on mortality benefit, one- and two-year survival rates of 70% to 80% have been reported. The most encouraging results have utilized undersized rigid annuloplasty rings, although multiple procedural developments are ongoing.[61] Consultation with an experienced cardiothoracic surgeon is recommended in these cases.

PERI-OPERATIVE MANAGEMENT OF CRT PATIENTS

The peri-operative period for post-CRT HF patients requires close coordination between the cardiac and surgical teams. Guidelines for peri-operative care have been set forth by the ACC/AHA.[63] Prior to surgery, the CRT device should be optimized for maximum cardiac benefit. In clinical practice there is some heterogeneity regarding the continuation of HF medications in the peri-operative period; however, it is imperative to continue all (or almost all) medications initiated prior to surgery, as these medications are in large part responsible for maintenance of a homeostatic cardiac environment. In the absence of an extenuating circumstance, HF medications should not be held.

Immediately prior to surgery, the ICD component of a CRT device should be programmed off, and postoperatively should be turned back on immediately. Consideration must be given to the polarity of device leads as well as electro-

cautery instrument, operative distance to the device, and an individual's pacemaker-dependence. Peri-operatively, patients with severe pulmonary hypertension should have a pulmonary artery catheter placed for hemodynamic monitoring. Lastly, during the postoperative state, serial EKGs as well as cardiac biomarkers should be checked for two to three days for peri-operative MI surveillance.

THE FUTURE OF CRT

The currently indicated criteria for CRT implantation were developed in an attempt to select those patients with the best chance of response. Yet questions remain in regard to each criterion's limitation.[64] Two ongoing clinical trials are investigating whether CRT is beneficial in Class II or asymptomatic Class I HF patients.[65-67] The utility of CRT in those patients with atrial fibrillation occurs in clinical practice with mixed results, although multiple small studies as well as clinical experience suggest benefit. Adjunctive AV nodal ablation may provide greater benefit in this cohort. Whether or not such ablation should be routinely performed is further being evaluated in a prospective, randomized clinical trial. In addition, approximately 30% of HF patients with evidence of mechanical dyssynchrony have a narrow QRS complex. An area of additional controversy is whether these patients would also benefit from CRT. Early studies suggested benefit, but a recent large randomized controlled trial failed to replicate these results.[68] Lastly, whether CRT should remain a limited option for those with LV dysfunction or expanded to include HF patients with a preserved ejection fraction is unknown. Several registry and retrospective studies are underway to address this issue.

CONCLUSION

Management of the post-CRT HF patient entails specific interventions for continued optimal medical care. Secondary to hemodynamic and electromechanical changes, "optimal" medical therapy requires that it be re-adjusted subsequent to device implementation. If required, diuretics typically should be prescribed at decreased dosages. Beta-blockers, ACEi, and ARBs can frequently be titrated to target doses. Monitoring for nonresponse will identify patients with potential barriers to effective therapy. A consistent, algorithmic approach to exclude correctable causes of nonresponse should be done. Assessment for the presence of volume abnormalities, myocardial ischemia, device placement issues, suboptimal device programming, atrial fibrillation, and persistent severe MR should all be considered. Focused correction of individual obstacles may thereafter lead to CRT response. Multidisciplinary collaboration with electrophysiology, interventional cardiology, cardiothoracic surgery, and hospice providers will ensure extensive and optimal care of this complex patient population.

PRACTICAL POINTS

1. CRT typically allows for a significant attenuation of diuretic dose.
2. CRT permits beta-blockade as well as ACEi or ARB therapy in many patients who previously were either unable to initiate therapy or to reach maximum goal dosage.
3. Nonresponse evaluation should occur if worsening HF continues within the first few months post-CRT, or if there is no abatement in symptoms in the first 6 months after implantation.
4. Delineating a potentially correctable cause of non-response is an important component of post-CRT management.
5. The ideal CRT optimization scheme should maximize filling, valve timing, cardiac output, and synchrony.
6. Persistent nonresponders should be evaluated on an individual basis for cardiac transplantation, ventricular assist device, chronic inotropic support, or further palliative options.

REFERENCES

1. Cleland J, Daubert JC, Erdmann E, et al. The effect of cardiac resynchronization on morbidity and mortality in heart failure. *N Engl J Med.* 2005; 352:1539–1549.
2. Bristow MR, Saxon LA, Boehmer J, et al. Cardiac-resynchronization therapy with or without an implantable defibrillator in advanced chronic heart failure. *N Engl J Med.* 2004; 350:2140–2150.
3. Cazeau S, Leclercq C, Lavergne T, et al. Effects of multisite biventricular pacing in patients with heart failure and intraventricular conduction delay. *N Engl J Med.* 2001; 344:873–880.
4. Abraham WT, Fisher WG, Smith AL, et al. Cardiac resynchronization in chronic heart failure. *N Engl J Med.* 2002; 346:1845–1853.
5. Young JB, Abraham WT, Smith AL, et al. Combined cardiac resynchronization and implantable cardioversion defibrillation in advanced chronic heart failure: the MIRACLE ICD Trial. *JAMA.* 2003; 289:2685–2694.
6. Hunt SA, Abraham WT, Chin MH, et al. ACC/AHA 2005 Guideline Update for the Diagnosis and Management of Chronic Heart Failure in the Adult: a report of the American College of Cardiology/American Heart Association Task Force on Practice Guidelines (Writing Committee to Update the 2001 Guidelines for the Evaluation and Management of Heart Failure): developed in collaboration with the American College of Chest Physicians and the International Society for Heart and Lung Transplantation: endorsed by the Heart Rhythm Society. *Circulation.* 2005; 112: e154–235.
7. Domanski M, Tian X, Haigney M, et al. Diuretic use, progressive heart failure, and death in patients in the DIG study. *J Card Fail.* 2006; 12: 327–332.
8. Domanski M, Norman J, Pitt B, et al. Diuretic use, progressive heart failure, and death in patients in the Studies Of Left Ventricular Dysfunction (SOLVD). *J Am Coll Cardiol.* 2003; 42: 705–708.
9. Kass DA, Chen CH, Curry C, et al. Improved left ventricular mechanics from acute VDD pacing in patients with dilated cardiomyopathy and ventricular conduction delay. *Circulation.* 1999; 99:1567–1573.
10. Leclercq C, Cazeau S, Le Breton H, et al. Acute hemodynamic effects of biventricular DDD pacing in patients with end-stage heart failure. *J Am Coll Cardiol.* 1998; 32:1825–1831.
11. Aranda JM Jr, Woo GW, Schofield RS, et al. Management of heart failure after cardiac resynchronization therapy. *J Am Coll Cardiol.* 2005, 46:2193–2198.
12. Takemoto Y, Hozumi T, Sugioka K, et al. Beta-blocker therapy induces ventricular resynchronization in dilated cardiomyopathy with narrow QRS complex. *J Am Coll Cardiol.* 2007, 49:778–783.
13. Feldman DS, Elton TS, Sun B, et al. Mechanisms of disease: detrimental adrenergic signaling in acute decompensated heart failure. *Nat Clin Pract Cardiovasc Med.* 2008, 5:208–218.
14. Wikstrand J, Hjalmarson A, Waagstein F, et al. Dose of metoprolol CR/XL and clinical outcomes in patients with heart failure: analysis of the experience in metoprolol CR/XL randomized intervention trial in chronic heart failure (MERIT-HF). *J Am Coll Cardiol.* 2002, 40:491–498.
15. Aranda JM Jr, Woo GW, Conti JB, et al. Use of cardiac resynchronization therapy to optimize beta-blocker therapy in patients with heart failure and prolonged QRS duration. *Am J Cardiol.* 2005, 95:889–891.
16. Fung JW, Chan JY, Kum LC, et al. Suboptimal medical therapy in patients with systolic heart failure is associated with less improvement by cardiac resynchronization therapy. *Int J Cardiol.* 2007, 115:214–219.
17. Adamson PB, Kleckner KJ, VanHout WL, et al. Cardiac resynchronization therapy improves heart rate variability in patients with symptomatic heart failure. *Circulation.* 2003, 108: 266–269.
18. Bax JJ, Abraham T, Barold SS, et al. Cardiac resynchronization therapy part 2: issues during and after device implantation and unresolved questions. *J Am Coll Cardiol.* 2005, 46: 2168–2182.
19. Ypenburg C, Schalij MJ, Bleeker GB, et al. Extent of viability to predict response to cardiac resynchronization therapy in ischemic heart failure patients. *J Nucl Med.* 2006; 47:1565–1570.
20. Ypenburg C, Schalij MJ, Bleeker GB, et al. Impact of viability and scar tissue on response to cardiac resynchronization therapy in ischaemic heart failure patients. *Eur Heart J.* 2007; 28:33–41.
21. Ypenburg C, Roes SD, Bleeker GB, et al. Effect of total scar burden on contrast-enhanced magnetic resonance imaging on response to cardiac resynchronization therapy. *Am J Cardiol.* 2007; 99:657–660.
22. White JA, Yee R, Yuan X, et al. Delayed enhancement magnetic resonance imaging predicts response to cardiac resynchronization therapy in patients with intraventricular dyssynchrony. *J Am Coll Cardiol.* 2006; 48:1953–1960.
23. Bleeker GB, Kaandorp TA, Lamb HJ, et al. Effect of posterolateral scar tissue on clinical and echocardiographic improvement after cardiac resynchronization therapy. *Circulation.* 2006; 113:969–976.
24. Knaapen P, van Campen LMC, deCock CC, et al. Effects of cardiac resynchronization therapy on myocardial perfusion reserve. *Circulation.* 2004; 110:646–651.
25. Sanders P, Morton JB, Davidson NC, et al. Electrical remodeling of the atria in congestive heart failure: electrophysiological and electroanatomic mapping in humans. *Circulation.* 2003; 108:1461–1468.
26. Linder O, Vogt O, Kammeier A, et al. Effect of cardiac resynchronization therapy on global and regional oxygen consumption and myocardial blood flow in patients with non-ischaemic and ischaemic cardiomyopathy. *Eur Heart J.* 2005; 26:70–76.
27. Meisel E, Pfeiffer D, Engelmann L, et al. Investigation of coronary 256 venous anatomy by retrograde venography in patients with malignant ventricular tachycardia. *Circulation.* 2001; 104:442–447.
28. Butter C, Auricchio A, Stellbrink C, et al. Effect of resynchronization therapy stimulation site on the systolic function of heart failure patients. *Circulation.* 2001; 104:3026–3029.
29. Higgins SL, Hummel JD, Niazi IK, et al. Cardiac resynchronization therapy for the treatment of heart failure in patients with intraventricular conduction delay and malignant ventricular tachyarrhythmias. *J Am Coll Cardiol.* 2003; 42:1454–1459.
30. Hasan A. Optimizing cardiac resynchronization therapy. *Current Heart Failure Reports.* 2008, 5:38–43.
31. Burri H, Sunthorn H, Shah D, et al. Optimization of device programming for cardiac resynchronization therapy. *Pacing Clin Electrophysiol.* 2006; 29:1416–1425.
32. Jansen AH, Bracke FA, van Dantzig JM, et al. Correlation of echo-Doppler optimization of atrioventricular delay in cardiac resynchronization therapy with invasive hemodynamics in patients with heart failure secondary to ischemic or idiopathic dilated cardiomyopathy. *Am J Cardiol.* 2006; 97:552–527.
33. Kerlan JE, Sawhney NS, Waggoner AD, et al. Prospective comparison of echocardiographic atrioventricular delay optimization methods for cardiac resynchronization therapy. *Heart Rhythm.* 2006; 3:148–154.
34. Auricchio A, Ding J, Spinelli JC, et al. Cardiac resynchronization therapy restores optimal atrioventricular mechanical timing in heart failure patients with ventricular conduction delay. *J Am Coll Cardiol.* 2002; 39:1163–1169.
35. Meluzin J, Novak M, Mullerova J, et al. A fast and simple echocardiographic method of determination of the optimal atrioventricular delay

in patients after biventricular stimulation. *Pacing Clin Electrophysiol.* 2004; 27:58–64.

36. Sawhney NS, Waggoner AD, Garhwal S, et al. Randomized prospective trial of atrioventricular delay programming for cardiac resynchronization therapy. *Heart Rhythm.* 2004; 1:562–567.

37. Phillips KP, Harberts DB, Johnston LP, et al. Left ventricular resynchronization predicted by individual performance of right and left univentricular pacing: a study on the impact of sequential biventricular pacing on ventricular dyssynchrony. *Heart Rhythm.* 2007; 4:147–153.

38. Vanderheyden M, De Backer T, Rivero-Ayerza M, et al. Tailored echocardiographic interventricular delay programming further optimizes left ventricular performance after cardiac resynchronization therapy. *Heart Rhythm.* 2005; 2:1066–1072.

39. Leon AR, Abraham WT, Brozena S, et al. Cardiac resynchronization with sequential biventricular pacing for the treatment of moderate-to-severe heart failure. *J Am Coll Cardiol.* 2005; 46:2298–2304.

40. Mortensen PT, Sogaard P, Mansour H, et al. Sequential biventricular pacing: evaluation of safety and efficacy. *Pacing Clin Electrophysiol.* 2004; 27:339–345.

41. Baker JH, Turk K, Pire LA, et al. Optimization of interventricular delay in biventricular pacing: results from the RHYTHM ICD V-V Optimization Phase study [abstract]. *Heart Rhythm.* 2005; 2:S205–S206.

42. De Lurgio D, Boehmer J, Higgins S, et al. Simultaneous biventricular pacing with optimized atrioventricular delay results in more reverse remodelling versus other resynchronization modalities in DECREASE-HF [abstract]. *J Card Fail.* 2007; 13(Suppl 2):S141.

43. Efremidis M, Pappas L, Sideris A, et al. Management of atrial fibrillation in patients with heart failure. *J Card Fail.* 2008, 14:232–237.

44. Maisel WH, Stevenson LW. Atrial fibrillation in heart failure: epidemiology, pathophysiology, and rationale for therapy. *Am J Cardiol.* 2003; 91:2D–8D.

45. Delnoy PP, Ottervanger JP, Luttikhuis HO, et al. Comparison of usefulness of cardiac resynchronization therapy in patients with atrial fibrillation and heart failure versus patients with sinus rhythm and heart failure. *Am J Cardiol.* 2007, 99:1252–1257.

46. Molhoek SG, Bax JJ, Bleeker GB, et al. Comparison of response to cardiac resynchronization therapy in patients with sinus rhythm versus chronic atrial fibrillation. *Am J Cardiol.* 2004, 94:1506–1509.

47. Leclercq C, Victor F, Alonso C, et al. Comparative effects of permanent biventricular pacing for refractory heart failure in patients with stable sinus rhythm or chronic atrial fibrillation. *Am J Cardiol.* 2000, 85:1154–1156, A9.

48. Gasparini M, Auricchio A, Regoli F, et al. Four-year efficacy of cardiac resynchronization therapy on exercise tolerance and disease progression: the importance of performing atrioventricular junction ablation in patients with atrial fibrillation. *J Am Coll Cardiol.* 2006; 48: 734–743.

49. Leon AR, Greenberg JM, Kanuru N, et al. Cardiac resynchronization in patients with congestive heart failure and chronic atrial fibrillation: effect of upgrading to biventricular pacing after chronic right ventricular pacing. *J Am Coll Cardiol.* 2002; 39:1258–1263.

50. Gasparini M, Auricchio A, Metra M, et al. Long-term survival in patients undergoing cardiac resynchronization therapy: the importance of performing atrio-ventricular junction ablation in patients with permanent atrial fibrillation. *Eur Heart J.* 2008; 29:1644–1452.

51. Kies P, Leclercq C, Bleeker GB, et al. Cardiac resynchronisation therapy in chronic atrial fibrillation: impact on left atrial size and reversal to sinus rhythm. *Heart.* 2006; 92:490–494.

52. Hamdan MH, Freedman RA, Gilbert EM, et al. Atrioventricular junction ablation followed by resynchronization therapy in patients with

congestive heart failure and atrial fibrillation (AVERT-AF) study design. *Pacing Clin Electrophysiol.* 2006; 29:1081–1088.

53. Woo GW, Petersen-Stejskal S, Johnson JW, et al. Ventricular reverse remodeling and 6-month outcomes in patients receiving cardiac resynchronization therapy: analysis of the MIRACLE study. *J Interv Card Electrophysiol.* 2005; 12:107–113.

54. Otsuji Y, Kumanohoso T, Yoshifuku S, et al. Isolated annular dilation does not usually cause important functional mitral regurgitation: comparison between patients with lone atrial fibrillation and those with idiopathic or ischemic cardiomyopathy. *J Am Coll Cardiol.* 2002; 39:1651–1656.

55. Yiu SF, Enriquez-Sarano M, Tribouilloy C, et al. Determinants of the degree of functional mitral regurgitation in patients with systolic left ventricular dysfunction: A quantitative clinical study. *Circulation.* 2000; 102:1400–1406.

56. Lancellotti P, Melon P, Sakalihasan N, et al. Effect of cardiac resynchronization therapy on functional mitral regurgitation in heart failure. *Am J Cardiol.* 2004; 94:1462–1465.

57. Ypenburg C, Lancellotti P, Tops L, et al. Mechanism of improvement in mitral regurgitation after cardiac resynchronization therapy. *Eur Heart J.* 2008; 29:757–765.

58. Vinereanu D, Turner M, Bleasdale R, et al. Mechanisms of reduction in mitral regurgitation by cardiac resynchronization therapy. *Journal of the American Society of Echocardiography.* 2007; 20:54–62.

59. Romano MA, Bolling SF. Update on mitral repair in dilated cardiomyopathy. *J Card Surg.* 2004; 19:396–400.

60. De Bonis M, Lapenna E, La Canna G, et al. Mitral valve repair for functional mitral regurgitation in end-stage dilated cardiomyopathy: role of the "edge-to-edge" technique. *Circulation.* 2005; 112(9 Suppl): I402–1408.

61. Bishay ES, McCarth PM, Cosgrove DM, et al. Mitral valve surgery in patients with severe left ventricular dysfunction. *Eur J Cardiothorac Surg.* 2000; 17:213–221.

62. Maggioni AP, et al. Effects of valsartan on morbidity and mortality in patients with heart failure not receiving angiotensin-converting enzyme inhibitors. *J Am Coll Cardiol.* 2002; 40, 1414–1421.

63. Eagle K, Berger P, Calkins H, et al. ACC/AHA Guideline Update for Perioperative Cardiovascular Evaluation for Noncardiac Surgery—Executive Summary A Report of the American College of Cardiology/ American Heart Association Task Force on Practice Guidelines (Committee to Update the 1996 Guidelines on Perioperative Cardiovascular Evaluation for Noncardiac Surgery). *Circulation.* 2002; 105; 1257–1267.

64. Linde C. Future directions in cardiac resynchronization therapy. *Current Heart Failure Reports.* 2008, 5:51–55.

65. Linde C, Gold M, Abraham WT, et al. Baseline characteristics of patients randomized in The Resynchronization Reverses Remodeling In Systolic Left Ventricular Dysfunction (REVERSE) study. *Congest Heart Fail.* 2008; 14:66–74.

66. Moss AJ, Brown MW, Cannom DS, et al. Multicenter automatic defibrillator implantation trial-cardiac resynchronization therapy (MADIT-CRT): design and clinical protocol. *Ann Noninvasive Electrocardiol.* 2005; 10(4 Suppl):34–43.

67. Hamdan MH, Freedman RA, Gilbert EM, et al. Atrioventricular junction ablation followed by resynchronization therapy in patients with congestive heart failure and atrial fibrillation (AVERT-AF) study design. *Pacing Clin Electrophysiol.* 2006; 29:1081–1088.

68. Beshai JF, Grimm RA, Nagueh SF, et al. Cardiac-resynchronization therapy in heart failure with narrow QRS complexes. *N Engl J Med.* 2007; 357:2461–2471.

CHAPTER

13

The Cost Effectiveness of Cardiac Resynchronization Therapy

Dhruv S. Kazi • Mark A. Hlatky

Heart failure is a significant public health problem in the United States, with roughly 5 million Americans living with it. Despite improved understanding of its pathophysiology, heart failure remains a major cause of morbidity and mortality, and is currently responsible for at least 20% of all hospital admissions among persons older than 65.[1] Cardiac resynchronization therapy (CRT) represents a new therapeutic approach to the management of heart failure, and has been shown in randomized clinical trials to reduce symptoms, heart failure hospitalizations, and heart failure deaths.[1-9] The effect of this novel but expensive therapy on total cost of care is an important consideration as the prevalence of heart failure—and the use of CRT—increases in the general population. We summarize the data on the economic outcomes of CRT and discuss its cost-effectiveness.

CONTEXT

Because health care resources are limited, economic principles can be applied to assess how to use these resources most efficiently. Committing resources to a particular use implies that they are no longer available for other uses. This is the concept of opportunity cost—the true cost of utilizing resources is the cost of not being able to put them to their best alternative use.

A second key economic principle is the law of diminishing marginal returns (Fig. 13.1), which says that the benefit obtained from providing an additional unit of goods or services decreases progressively with the quantity of resources used. As shown in Figure 13.1, the optimal point for the system to operate is when marginal benefit equals marginal cost. In the medical context, care is considered to be cost-effective when the value obtained from additional expenditures remains "reasonable"—at point C rather than point D in Figure 13.1.

While the development of new diagnostic and therapeutic technologies forms the basis of modern medical progress, it is also a major driving force behind the rapid increase in health care costs. Historically, the approval of new medical technology has required only the demonstration of safety and efficacy. However, as governments struggle to rein in health care expenses, the additional benchmark of cost-effectiveness has been added in many countries, either as a requirement for approval (in Australia and Ontario, Canada, for example) or for adoption by the health care system (in England). Demonstration of cost-effectiveness is not, however, required in the United States. Proponents of considering cost-effectiveness argue that, if a new technology is to be adopted, it should demonstrate not only superiority in safety or efficacy compared with available therapeutic options, but also that it adds value for the patient (or the health care system or society) commensurate with its additional cost.

The value of a new technology like CRT can be gauged by comparing it with an existing therapeutic alternative (optimal pharmacologic therapy, OPT), and calculating the incremental cost-effectiveness ratio (ICER). The numerator of the ICER is the total net cost of using the new therapy compared with using the alternative therapy, and the denominator of the ICER is the total net effectiveness of using the new therapy compared with using the alternative therapy:

Incremental Cost Effectiveness Ratio (ICER)

$$= \frac{\text{Cost}_{CRT} - \text{Cost}_{OPT}}{\text{Outcome}_{CRT} - \text{Outcome}_{OPT}}$$

Three key concepts emerge from the above equation.

First, the choice of comparators is paramount when assessing a new technology. For instance, consider two new technologies, cardiac resynchronization without and with defibrillation capability (CRT-P and CRT-D, respectively). The CRT-D device is almost three times as expensive as the CRT-P device, and has a shorter battery life, thereby incurring higher initial as well as long-term costs. While performing a health care economic evaluation, should both these new technologies be compared with optimal pharmacologic therapy, or should the most expensive technology be compared with the second most expensive technology? A prudent purchaser would first compare CRT-P with OPT, and then compare CRT-D with CRT-P to judge whether the significant

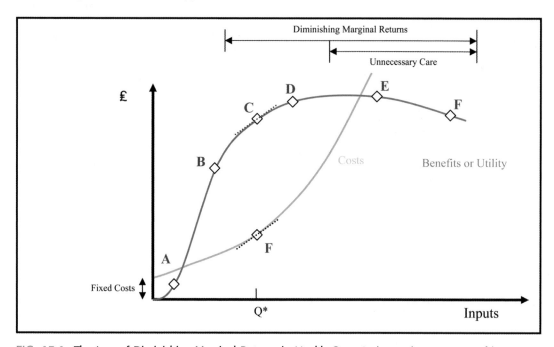

FIG. 13.1. **The Law of Diminishing Marginal Returns in Health Care.** As increasing amounts of inputs are committed to health care, costs (grey curve) rise progressively. The benefits (red curve), on the other hand, do not. Moving from A to B and from B to C requires an equal increase in inputs, but the benefits gained from moving from B to C are substantially lower. Moving from E to F is actually harmful—in health care, as in life, more is not always better. The optimal point for the system to operate is where the cost of producing one additional unit of the goods or services (the marginal cost) is equal to the benefit obtained from producing that additional unit (marginal benefit), at point Q*.

cost of adding the defibrillation capability is justifiable.[10] Cost-effectiveness is a relative measure, not an absolute measure; a therapy can only be "cost-effective" compared with an alternative (Table 13.1).

Second, the ICER is based on assessing the complete costs and the complete benefits of each treatment, not merely

TABLE 13.1   The Choice of Comparator

Therapy	Cost ($)	Effectiveness (QALY)	ICER – Relative to OPT ($/QALY)	ICER – Relative to CRT-P ($/QALY)
OPT	46,000	2.3	-	-
CRT-P	59,900	3.01	19,600	-
CRT-D	82,200	3.15	43,000	160,000

A decision analytic model based on data from the COMPANION trial produced the above costs and effects over a 7-year period. The ICER of CRT-P relative to OPT ($19,600/QALY) shows that it is a cost-effective intervention.[15] If CRT-D were to be compared with OPT, an ICER of $43,000/QALY would also make it appear cost-effective. However, the appropriate comparator for CRT-D is CRT-P—the next-best alternative—and not OPT. When CRT-D is compared to CRT-P, the ICER rises to $160,000/QALY, which is well above the accepted range of $50,000–75,000/QALY. This example highlights the salience of the appropriate comparator in all cost-effectiveness analyses.

their initial costs and short-term outcomes. Cardiac resynchronization has a significant upfront cost (of device implantation), so evaluating its cost-effectiveness over a short time-horizon, say of one or two years, may not provide a complete and balanced picture of its value in patient care. In particular, the high initial costs related to implanting the device may be offset over time by reducing hospitalizations, including costly admissions to the intensive care unit. The need for regular interrogations and periodic battery replacements, and the potential for device-related complications, however, could increase overall costs of device therapy. Thus a long-term perspective is essential to obtain a complete picture of costs and benefits of CRT. While measuring costs and effects over the lifetime of the patient would be ideal, the key is that the follow-up in the analysis be sufficiently long to capture all of the relevant costs and benefits, and thereby provide an unbiased assessment of the cost-effectiveness of the device.

The ICER is usually expressed as dollars per life-year added, which then should be compared to a benchmark in order to interpret the result. Several countries (such as the United Kingdom and the Netherlands) have determined a monetary threshold above which a new technology is no longer considered cost-effective. Although there is no hard and fast threshold for cost-effectiveness in the US, most analysts consider $50,000 to $75,000 per quality-adjusted life year (QALY) to be acceptable, but not cost-effectiveness ratios that exceed $100,000/QALY. These are only rough guides, however, as there is no formal national framework in the United States for systematic health care economic evaluation.

COSTS

The cost of CRT includes the cost of the device and its initial implantation, as well as the costs added by subsequent complications, regular interrogations, and generator replacements, and the costs associated with routine heart failure care, including medications, clinic visits, and hospitalizations. The substantial upfront costs of the device and its implantation may be offset over time by the costs associated with care saved by improved heart failure symptoms. While patients who live longer and have a better quality of life may be able to stay in the labor force and contribute to the economy, these indirect costs associated with changes in productivity are usually omitted from cost-effectiveness studies because they would systematically undervalue treatments for patients who are not working. Home health care is included as a direct medical cost, so a therapy that increases the number of patients who can care for themselves may produce substantial savings. These various costs are borne by different parties but it is best to evaluate the total cost of a new technology from the societal perspective—to consider all medical costs irrespective of who bears them (hospital, patient, or a third-party payer).

EFFECTIVENESS

The clinical effectiveness used in the denominator of the incremental cost-effectiveness ratio is conventionally measured by the extent to which either the quantity or quality of the patient's life is increased. Quality Adjusted Life Years (QALYs) are preferred as a measure of effectiveness in many analyses because they capture both of these dimensions of improved patient outcomes.[11] QALYs are calculated by multiplying the life-expectancy of the patient with a preference weight that reflects the patient's quality of life on a scale from 0 (death) to 1 (perfect health). For instance, if a patient spends 2 extra years in a health condition associated with preference-weight of 0.3, he would have gained $2 \times 0.3 = 0.6$ QALYs. The preference weights used to calculate QALYs can be obtained using formal elicitation techniques (e.g., the standard-gamble) or quality of life questionnaires (e.g., Minnesota Living With Heart Failure questionnaire).[12]

Cardiac resynchronization therapy has been demonstrated in clinical trials to improve functional capacity, symptoms, and quality of life, and to reduce heart failure hospitalizations, and all-cause mortality.[9] Given its impact on both quality of life and longevity, the effects of CRT are frequently expressed in the combined unit of QALYs.

COST-EFFECTIVENESS OF CARDIAC RESYNCHRONIZATION THERAPY

The cost and outcomes data used to calculate the ICER may be collected alongside the clinical data while conducting a randomized clinical trial (RCT), which makes individual-level data available for the analysis. As with the clinical data obtained from an RCT, the cost data thus collected may provide an objective measure of the expenses associated with the intervention. However, trial-based assessments of cost-effectiveness have several important limitations. The costs incurred in an RCT may be driven by the study protocol, and are dependent on the characteristics of the patients recruited to the study as well as the clinical centers where the trial is being conducted (which are usually academic centers, and have higher costs). More importantly, RCTs tend to have relatively short durations of follow-up (the longest RCT data available for cardiac resynchronization is less than 3 years of follow-up). These issues may be circumvented by developing a model of the natural history of the disease and the impact of the intervention being studied—which can then incorporate average costs and outcomes from published RCTs or meta-analyses thereof. Moreover, by varying the input parameter, either individually or simultaneously as a group, one can test the robustness of the results provided by the model.

While these arguments make decision-analytic models an attractive approach to health care economic evaluations, these models too have limitations. The most important limitation is that the results of these models are often highly dependent on the assumptions made while developing the model and the choice of input parameters. Thus the underlying assumptions of decision analytic models must always be critically examined, and close attention must be paid to the results of sensitivity analyses.

The cost-effectiveness of CRT has been evaluated by randomized clinical trials as well as by decision analytic modeling.

Randomized Clinical Trial

The Cardiac Resynchronization in Heart Failure (CARE-HF) trial was a randomized clinical trial conducted at 82 clinical centers in 12 European countries.[1] A total of 813 patients with New York Heart Association Class III or IV heart failure due to left ventricular systolic dysfunction (LVEF <0.35) and cardiac dyssynchrony were randomized to CRT-P plus medical therapy (n = 409) versus medical therapy alone (n = 404). The cost-effectiveness analysis was specified a priori as a secondary outcome in the protocol and included data from all patients enrolled in the trial.[13] Cost of medical care was estimated from the utilization of major medical resources, with costs based on the United Kingdom's National Health Service reference costs. The cost of the device was assumed to be the mean list price across the devices and countries involved in the trial, and was spread over the potential lifetime of the device accounting for patient survival so that only those costs incurred during the study period were included in the cost-effectiveness analysis. Quality of life data was collected prospectively using validated questionnaires (the EQ-5D and Minnesota Living With Heart Failure questionnaires). Patient survival was extrapolated using an exponential model for survival; linear regression was used to extrapolate the quality of life data. Future costs and benefits were discounted at 3.5%. During a mean follow-up of 29.4 months, patients assigned to CRT had significantly increased costs (€4,300, 95% CI: 1,300–7,500), as well as longer survival (0.10 years, 95% CI: −0.01–0.21), and improved quality of life and QALYs (0.22, 95% CI: 0.13–0.32). The incremental cost-effectiveness ratio was calculated as €19,300 per QALY gained (95% CI: 5,500–45,400) and €43,600 per life-year gained (95% CI: −146,200–223,900). These results were sensitive to the cost of the device, implantation procedure, and hospitalization. For instance, the ICER for CRT improved to €18,000/QALY when the CRT device cost was assumed to be €5,000 and deteriorated to €65,000/QALY when the device cost was assumed to be €25,000, assuming all other parameters were held constant.

Decision Analytic Models

One of the first decision-analytic models to evaluate the cost-effectiveness of CRT-P compared with medical therapy produced an incremental cost-effectiveness of $107,800/QALY (interquartile range: $79,800 to $156,500).[14] However, this model was limited in several ways, most importantly in that it did not account for the improved quality of life associated with CRT, and data from the CARE-HF trial were not available when the model was published.

Three subsequent decision-analytic models have incorporated results from large randomized clinical trials.[15–17] As expected, these models have produced disparate results, based on the model assumptions (See Table 13.2 for a summary of available data).

A model based on the results of the COMPANION trial and with an analytic horizon of 7 years produced an incremental cost-effectiveness of $19,600 per QALY for CRT-P relative to OPT, and $160,000 per QALY for CRT-D relative to CRT-P,[3, 10, 15] suggesting that while CRT-P is cost-effective, the addition of the defibrillator component increases the initial and long-term costs substantially, with only a modest improvement in outcomes.

Yao et al. designed a model that combined the data from the COMPANION and CARE-HF trials (recall that CARE-HF did not have a CRT-D arm).[16] In their model, from a lifetime perspective in a 65-year-old patient, the incremental cost-effectiveness of CRT-P compared to OPT was €7,500 (95% CI: €5,300–€11,800) per QALY gained, while the incremental cost-effectiveness of CRT-D compared with CRT-P was €47,900 (95% CI : €35,700–€79,400) per QALY gained. In this model, the cost-effectiveness of device implantation varied inversely with age. This is particularly true for CRT-D devices—the ICER relative to CRT-P at age 75 was €73,300—because older patients have a higher mortality even if sudden cardiac death is averted by the defibrillator.

A recently published complex model that incorporated data from randomized clinical trials used a UK healthcare perspective to evaluate the cost-effectiveness of CRT-P and CRT-D in a mixed age cohort over a lifetime.[17] Compared with OPT, CRT-P conferred an additional 0.70 QALYs for an additional £11,600 per person, producing an estimated ICER of £16,700 per QALY (range £14,600–20,300). CRT-D versus CRT-P conferred an additional 0.29 QALYs for an additional £11,700 per person, giving an ICER of £40,200 per QALY (range £26,600–59,400). When the cost and effectiveness of all three treatment strategies are compared with each other, the estimated net benefit from CRT-D was less than with the other two strategies, until the willingness-to-pay threshold exceeds £40,200/QALY (which is considerably higher than the 15-20,000 pounds sterling per QALY traditionally used in the UK).

UNCERTAINTY IN HEALTH CARE ECONOMIC EVALUATIONS

An economic evaluation can only be as good as the data used, so uncertainties about clinical efficacy of CRT imply uncertainty in the assessment of its cost-effectiveness. Although the input parameters in a decision-model are drawn from randomized clinical trials, data for some important parameters are scanty. For instance, one key issue is whether CRT-P reduces sudden cardiac death in patients with heart failure as well as reducing deaths from progressive heart failure. The incremental benefit obtained from using CRT-D instead of CRT-P will be smaller to the extent that CRT-P prevents sudden death. The impact of uncertainty in these parameters on cost-effectiveness can be tested using sensitivity analyses, where the results of the model are recalculated after systematically varying values of input parameters, thereby identifying the variables with the greatest impact on the ICER. When the results of the model are highly sensitive to the exact value of a parameter, it indicates that better data are needed. In the models described above, the incremental cost-effectiveness ratio was sensitive to the cost of device implantation and its complications, and the efficacy of the therapy (e.g., relative risk of heart failure hospitalization with CRT).

A second source of uncertainty are the core assumptions embedded in the model.[18] For instance, does the model consider the possibility that a patient may undergo cardiac transplantation? If so, does it incorporate the cost of the transplantation and posttransplant care? Such assumptions produce what is called structural uncertainty, which cannot be tested by sensitivity analyses. Structural uncertainty can be extremely difficult to overcome—and requires that the structure of the model be carefully examined prior to accepting its results at face value.

FUTURE DIRECTIONS

Between one third and one half of patients who receive CRT do not respond with improved symptoms or cardiac

TABLE 13.2 Cost-Effectiveness of CRT in Published Randomized Clinical Trials and Decision Analytic Models

Model	Reference	Strategy	Cost (range if available)	Effect (Life-Years)	Effect (QALYs)	ICER (per Life Year Gained)	ICER (per QALY)	Comment
Randomized Clinical Trial:								
Analysis based on CARE-HF	[2],[14]	OPT	€15,795 (3,684–18,185)	1.92 (1.51–2.52)	1.19 (0.65–1.73)	-	-	Time horizon for analysis was 29.4 months, the mean duration of follow-up in CARE-HF.
		CRT-P	€20,110 (9,443–22,540)	2.02 (1.62–2.53)	1.42 (1.01–1.92)	€43,596 (–146,236–223,849)	€19,319 (5,482–45,402)	
Decision Analytic Models:								
Based on Early RCTs	[15]	OPT	$34,400 (31,100–37,700)	-	2.64 (2.47–2.82)	-	-	Considered lifetime costs and benefits, but did not consider improvements in quality of life with CRT.
		CRT-P	$64,400 (59,000–70,200)	-	2.92 (2.72–3.14)	-	$107,800 (79,800–156,500)	
Based on COMPANION	[4],[11],[16]	OPT	$46,000	3.37	2.30			Time horizon for analysis was 7 years.
		CRT-P	$59,900	3.87	3.01	$27,800*	$19,600*	
		CRT-D	$82,200	4.15	3.15	$79,600*	$159,200*	
Based on data from CARE-HF and COMPANION	[17]	OPT	€39,060	6.1	4.08			Considered lifetime costs and benefits.
		CRT-P	€53,996	8.23	6.06	€7011 (5,346–10,003)	€7,538 (5,325–11,784)	
		CRT-D	€87,350	9.16	6.75	€35,874 (27,709–56,353)	€47,909 (35,703–79,438)	
Based on a meta-analysis of all available RCTs	[18]	OPT	£9,367	4.9	3.10			Considered lifetime costs and benefits.
		CRT-P	£20,997	5.8	3.80	£12,922*	£16,735*	
		CRT-D	£32,687	6.2	4.09	£40,310*	£40,310*	

*Calculated from published data.

€, Euros; $, Dollars (US); £, Pounds Sterling (UK). As of April 2008, $1 = €0.64 = £0.5.

Table 13.2 summarizes the major cost-effectiveness analyses of cardiac resynchronization in the peer-reviewed literature. Note the variability in estimates of cost-effectiveness among the studies. The incremental cost-effectiveness ratios for CRT-P are as compared with OPT, whereas the ICERs for CRT-D are as compared with CRT-P. OPT, optimal pharmacologic therapy for heart failure; CRT-P, cardiac resynchronization therapy without defibrillation capability; CRT-D, cardiac resynchronization therapy with defibrillation capability; QALY, quality-adjusted life year.

function. Clearly, if one could predict beforehand which patients would respond to CRT, the nonresponders could be spared an expensive procedure and the associated risk of adverse events, thus improving the effectiveness and cost-effectiveness of CRT. Likewise, if one could accurately quantify patients' risk of sudden cardiac death, one could limit the implantation of CRT-D to patients with a risk high enough to justify the additional cost. No tests are presently universally accepted as being accurately predictive of these factors.

The randomized clinical trials that form the basis of the economic evaluations have had relatively short durations of follow-up, so the long-term cost and effects of cardiac resynchronization remain uncertain. For instance, it is unknown whether the 44% reduction in deaths from progressive heart failure continues beyond the first few years or whether the underlying disease eventually progresses to a point where CRT is no longer effective. The long-term cost-effectiveness of CRT will be much more favorable to the extent that the device continues to be effective indefinitely. Only long-term clinical data can establish this point, including newer clinical trials with longer follow-up periods.

A lingering question is whether the efficacy of cardiac resynchronization demonstrated in randomized clinical trials—where carefully selected patients were treated by experts in specialized centers—can be achieved in widespread practice in the general population. For instance, the typical heart failure patient in clinical practice is almost a decade older and has many more co-morbidities than patients enrolled in randomized clinical trials. Whether these more typical patients can achieve the same degree of benefit as seen in clinical trials is an unknown, especially because they may be at a greater risk of procedural complications due to their overall state of health. Furthermore, in clinical trials, the physicians who implanted CRT devices were highly experienced experts from high-volume centers, and may well have better outcomes than average. It is therefore important to document outcomes of CRT implantation in general community practice. Currently, the Center for Medicare and Medicaid Services requires that its insurees who receive an implantable cardioverter defibrillator (ICD) for primary prevention be included in the National Cardiovascular Data ICD Registry, which is maintained by the American College of Cardiology in partnership with the Heart Rhythm Society. The registry would be even more useful if it included more devices (CRT-P and CRT-D), broader indications for device therapy (not just those for primary prevention), and more patients (not just Medicare beneficiaries). The collection of long-term follow-up data, not just data at implantation, is key to judge the effectiveness of device therapy. The importance of such a registry, with information on the effectiveness as well as safety of these devices in the community, is highlighted by the recent ICD recalls and advisories.[19-20]

Clinical trials thus far have focused largely on patients with NYHA Class III and Class IV failure,[9] with the majority of recruited patients belonging to NYHA Class III. The role of CRT, and by extension of CRT-D, in patients who were either underrepresented in the clinical trials or excluded all together—such as patients with NYHA Class I and Class II heart failure, those with atrial fibrillation or bradyarrhythmias, narrow QRS complexes, right bundle branch block, or chronic kidney disease—continues to evolve. A registry would also help in this regard. While retrospective analyses are never as robust as randomized clinical trials, regression analyses on a large, complete dataset may suggest variables that need to be most closely examined in future prospective clinical trials.

CONCLUSIONS

We live in times of burgeoning health care costs, and it seems inevitable that every new intervention will be the object of rigorous economic scrutiny. Insurance companies (and increasingly, consumers as well) want to maximize the returns on every dollar, pound, or euro invested in health care. While the merits of this focus on economic efficiency—and in particular its implications for equity—continue to be debated,[21-23] the reality is that the need for objective economic analysis of new technology is here to stay.

Approximately 1% to 3% of all patients discharged alive after their index hospitalization for HF and 15% to 20% of patients seen in specialized heart failure clinics meet CRT trial eligibility criteria.[24-27] Of these patients, approximately one half also meet trial eligibility criteria for an ICD.[28] The magnitude of the public health burden of heart failure and the substantial upfront as well as ongoing costs associated with cardiac resynchronization underline the need to carefully consider the economic implications of widespread adoption of this therapy.

CRT-P improves both quality of life and survival (primarily by reduction in pump-failure deaths) in patients with symptomatic systolic heart failure despite optimal medical management (New York Heart Association functional Class III and IV, and left ventricular ejection fraction <0.35), with a prolonged QRS complex (> 120ms), and in doing so, has been shown in multiple models and in different settings to be cost-effective relative to optimal pharmacologic therapy.

CRT-D, which additionally incorporates an implantable defibrillator, reduces the risk of sudden cardiac death. However, CRT-D is substantially more expensive than CRT-P, and it is unclear whether there is an improvement in outcomes sufficient to justify the near-doubling of costs. Ongoing trials will compare CRT-D with an ICD, but there are no ongoing studies that will compare CRT-D with CRT-P. Given the uncertainty about the clinical and economic impact of CRT-D relative to CRT-P, a comparative randomized clinical trial would be ideal. From a practical point of view, however, it is unlikely that many physicians would feel comfortable randomizing patients with heart failure to CRT-P now that trials have shown that ICDs are effective in this population.

In conclusion, the weight of the available evidence suggests that CRT-P is safe, effective, and cost-effective in patients with advanced symptomatic systolic heart failure with a wide QRS complex. CRT-D improves outcomes compared with optimal medical therapy, but it is uncertain whether the small incremental benefit of CRT-D over CRT-P justifies the substantial increase in costs.

PRACTICAL POINTS

1. The cost of a new treatment can only be assessed in the context of its effect on clinical outcomes.
2. Clinical effectiveness can be measured using "quality adjusted life-years," which give weight to both increases in life-expectancy as well as increases in quality of life.
3. Net cost of CRT includes the cost of inserting the device and the cost of any subsequent device complications and follow-up, as well as the cost savings (if any) from reducing clinical complications.
4. Cost-effectiveness analysis compares CRT therapy with the next-best alternative.
5. The cost-effectiveness of CRT is evaluated by comparing the net costs with net clinical effectiveness.
6. The cost-effectiveness of CRT-P relative to medical therapy appears attractive, but the cost-effectiveness of CRT-D relative to CRT-P is uncertain.

REFERENCES

1. Cleland JG, Daubert JC, Erdmann E, et al. The effect of cardiac resynchronization on morbidity and mortality in heart failure. *N Engl J Med.* 2005;352:1539–1549.
2. Cazeau S, Leclercq C, Lavergne T, et al. Effects of multisite biventricular pacing in patients with heart failure and intraventricular conduction delay. *N Engl J Med.* 2001;344:873–880.
3. Bristow MR, Saxon LA, Boehmer J, et al. Cardiac-resynchronization therapy with or without an implantable defibrillator in advanced chronic heart failure. *N Engl J Med.* 2004;350:2140–2150.
4. Auricchio A, Stellbrink C, Sack S, et al. Long-term clinical effect of hemodynamically optimized cardiac resynchronization therapy in patients with heart failure and ventricular conduction delay. *J Am Coll Cardiol.* 2002;39:2026–2033.
5. Abraham WT, Young JB, Leon AR, et al. Effects of cardiac resynchronization on disease progression in patients with left ventricular systolic dysfunction, an indication for an implantable cardioverter-defibrillator, and mildly symptomatic chronic heart failure. *Circulation.* 2004;110:2864–2868.
6. Abraham WT, Fisher WG, Smith AL, et al. Cardiac resynchronization in chronic heart failure. *N Engl J Med.* 2002;346:1845–1853.
7. Young JB, Abraham WT, Smith AL, et al. Combined cardiac resynchronization and implantable cardioversion defibrillation in advanced chronic heart failure: the MIRACLE ICD Trial. *JAMA.* 2003;289:2685–2694.
8. Higgins SL, Hummel JD, Niazi IK, et al. Cardiac resynchronization therapy for the treatment of heart failure in patients with intraventricular conduction delay and malignant ventricular tachyarrhythmias. *J Am Coll Cardiol.* 2003;42:1454–1459.
9. McAlister FA, Ezekowitz J, Hooton N, et al. Cardiac resynchronization therapy for patients with left ventricular systolic dysfunction: a systematic review. *JAMA.* 2007;297:2502–2514.

10. Hlatky MA. Cost effectiveness of cardiac resynchronization therapy. *J Am Coll Cardiol.* 2005;46:2322–2324.
11. Basic Types of Economic Evaluation. In: Drummond MF, Torrance GW, O'Brien BJ, et al. *Methods for Economic Evaluation of Health Care Programmes.* 3rd. ed. New York, NY: Oxford University Press; 2005:7–26.
12. Oliver A. At The End Of The Beginning: Eliciting Cardinal Values For Health States. In: LSE Health and Social Care Discussion Paper Number 2 London, UK. : London School of Economics and Political Science; 2002. http://www.lse.ac.uk/collections/LSE Health And Social Care/pdf/DiscussionPaperSeries/DP2_2002.pdf. Last updated February 1, 2002. Accessed March 5, 2007.
13. Calvert MJ, Freemantle N, Yao G, et al. Cost-effectiveness of cardiac resynchronization therapy: results from the CARE-HF trial. *Eur Heart J.* 2005;26:2681–2688.
14. Nichol G, Kaul P, Huszti E, et al. Cost-effectiveness of cardiac resynchronization therapy in patients with symptomatic heart failure. *Ann Intern Med.* 2004;141:343–351.
15. Feldman AM, de Lissovoy G, Bristow MR, et al. Cost effectiveness of cardiac resynchronization therapy in the Comparison of Medical Therapy, Pacing, and Defibrillation in Heart Failure (COMPANION) trial. *J Am Coll Cardiol.* 2005;46:2311–2321.
16. Yao G, Freemantle N, Calvert MJ, et al. The long-term cost-effectiveness of cardiac resynchronization therapy with or without an implantable cardioverter-defibrillator. *Eur Heart J.* 2007;28:42–51.
17. Fox M, Anderson R, Dean J, et al. The clinical effectiveness and cost-effectiveness of cardiac resynchronisation (biventricular pacing) for heart failure: systematic review and economic model. In: Health Technology Assesment; 2007. http://www.ncchta.org/fullmono/mon1147.pdf. Accessed January 1, 2008.
18. Critical Assessment of Economic Evaluation. In: Drummond MF, SMJ, Torrance GW, O'Brien BJ, Stoddard GI, ed. *Methods for the Economic Evaluation of Health Care Programmes.* New York, NY: Oxford University press; 2005:27–54.
19. Recommendations from the Heart Rhythm Society Task Force on Device Performance Policies and Guidelines. Endorsed by the American College of Cardiology Foundation (ACCF) and the American Heart Association (AHA) and the International Coalition of Pacing and Electrophysiology Organizations (COPE). Heart Rhythm Society 2007. (http://www.hrsonline.org/uploadDocs/HRSTaskForceRecsFull.pdf. Accessed August 30, 2007.)
20. Steinbrook R. The controversy over Guidant's implantable defibrillators. *N Engl J Med.* 2005;353:221–224.
21. Harris J. "QALYfying the value of life." *J Med Ethics.* 1987;13:117–123.
22. Williams A. The 'fair innings argument' deserves a fairer hearing! Comments by Alan Williams on Nord and Johannesson. *Health Econ.* 2001;10:583–585.
23. Nord E. Concerns for the worse off: fair innings versus severity. *SocSciMed.* 2005;60:257–263.
24. Pedone C, Grigioni F, Boriani G, et al. Implications of cardiac resynchronization therapy and prophylactic defibrillator implantation among patients eligible for heart transplantation. *Am J Cardiol.* 2004;93:371–373.
25. Cardiac Resynchronization Therapy and Implantable Cardiac Defibrillators in Left Ventricular Systolic Dysfunction. Evidence Report/Technology Assessment No. 152 (Prepared by the University of Alberta Evidence-based Practice Center under Contract No. 290-02-0023). Agency for Healthcare Research and Quality. AHRQ Publication No. 07-E009. Rockville, MD, 2007. http://www.ahrq.gov/clinic/tp/defibtp.htm. Accessed August 27, 2007.
26. McAlister FA, Tu JV, Newman A, et al. How many patients with heart failure are eligible for cardiac resynchronization? Insights from two prospective cohorts. *Eur Heart J.* 2006;27:323–239.
27. Grimm W, Sharkova J, Funck R, et al. How many patients with dilated cardiomyopathy may potentially benefit from cardiac resynchronization therapy? *Pacing Clin Electrophysiol.* 2003;26:155–157.
28. Toma M, McAlister FA, Ezekowitz J, et al. Proportion of patients followed in a specialized heart failure clinic needing an implantable cardioverter defibrillator as determined by applying different trial eligibility criteria. *Am J Cardiol.* 2006;97:882–885.

Cardiac Resynchronization Therapy: A Regulatory Perspective

William H. Maisel

Despite remarkable advances in the pharmacologic treatment of patients with severe heart failure (HF), persistently high rates of mortality and repeat hospitalization stimulated the need for additional therapies. Cardiac resynchronization therapy (CRT) has undergone extensive evaluation and is of proven clinical benefit for selected patients.[1–7] The devices used to deliver the therapy are technologically sophisticated and were developed through collaboration among physicians, patients, industry, and regulators. Health care providers play a role not only in the clinical use of a device but also at times in device design, production, use, and safety by expressing their need for certain products, by providing practical input and feedback into product design, by participating in device-related research, and by reporting device-related adverse events.[8] Physicians and other health care providers should understand the rules that govern the device premarket evaluation and approval processes, investigational research, and device postmarket surveillance.

PREMARKET EVALUATION

The U.S. Food and Drug Administration (FDA) is charged with ensuring the safety and effectiveness of medical devices in the United States and regulates more than 1,700 types of devices, 500,000 medical device models, and 23,000 manufacturers.[8] The goal is to get good, safe, effective devices to patients as quickly as possible.

Congress enacted the Medical Device Amendments of 1976 to better allow the FDA to establish the safety and effectiveness of medical devices.[8] The legislation was based on the idea that the degree of device regulation should correlate with the degree of risk posed by the device. Therefore, FDA premarket evaluation and approval, conducted by the Center for Devices and Radiologic Health (CDRH), depends on the complexity of the device and the perceived risk to the patient. Three regulatory classes (I, II, and III) were defined by the legislation.[8] All devices are subject to "general controls" including proper labeling and adherence to predefined Good Manufacturing Practices, such as a demonstration of adequate packaging and storage. Class I devices are low-risk de-

vices with minimal potential for harm and include such items as stethoscopes and tongue blades. Class II devices are moderate-risk devices and include a broad range of products, such as computed tomography scanners and gastroenterology endoscopes, that must meet or exceed certain predefined product performance standards. Products categorized as Class III are perceived to be higher-risk devices, and include pacemakers and ICDs including CRT devices. Their safety and efficacy can be ensured only by a thorough premarket evaluation and approval process.

Before receiving FDA approval to market a new medical device in the United States, manufacturers must demonstrate that the device is safe (its benefits outweigh the risks) and effective (it reliably does what it is intended to do). Data to support safety and effectiveness may include device design verification and validation studies, observational studies, randomized clinical trials, epidemiology studies, animal studies, bench research, engineering or manufacturing tests, and statistical risk analyses. The FDA is required by Congress to use the "least burdensome" approach, meaning that manufacturers are required to provide only data that are necessary to demonstrate safety and effectiveness.

When a device is ready for clinical testing, the FDA issues an Investigational Device Exemption (IDE). This exemption grants permission to use the device in humans in an experimental situation to assess its safety. An Investigational Device Exemption can be used only at a specific institution after approval by the institution's Institutional Review Board (IRB). Violations of federal regulations during use of an investigational device under an Investigational Device Exemption could result in disqualification of investigators, Institutional Review Boards, and institutions from current or future research.

Important differences exist between the drug and device regulatory approval processes. Typically, premarket evaluation of drugs includes clinical trials involving thousands of patients. Once approved, a drug may remain on the market, essentially unaltered, for decades. In contrast, the medical device product life cycle—from conception to obsolescence—is short. For example, since ICDs were first FDA approved in 1985, the generators have decreased in size eightfold and increased in computer memory capacity by a factor of 500. It is therefore critical that new devices reach the market (and the patients they benefit) quickly but safely.

The FDA bases its approval decision on "valid scientific evidence," weighing evidence on clinical effectiveness and safety. The development and clinical acceptance of CRT was characterized by a number of challenges relating to both the design and interpretation of clinical trials performed to evaluate the efficacy and safety of CRT. Because FDA approval of expanded CRT clinical indications into new clinical populations may be equally challenging, it is instructive to understand and review the regulatory approval process of the initial CRT devices.

Early CRT trials were designed to establish evidence of functional improvements (improved New York Heart Association [NYHA] Class, improved 6-minute walk test, etc.) and improvements in quality of life (QOL). Trials were conducted on a background of optimal pharmacologic therapy (OPT). Selected published CRT clinical trial experience is summarized in Table 14.1. The results of these pivotal studies underscore the importance of trial design in endpoint interpretation and clinical (and regulatory) acceptance. Subjective end-points are susceptible to patient and observer bias, highlighting the importance of blinding and appropriate control groups. Indeed, in many studies, the control arms that did not receive CRT also experienced an initial clinical improvement. The relatively short-term end-points (3 to 6 months) for the initial trials demonstrated proof-of-concept but failed to provide meaningful insight into long-term efficacy. Crossover trial designs (all patients get LV lead and are then randomized to therapy ON then OFF or vice versa), as used in many early CRT trials, have the advantage of requiring smaller sample sizes to demonstrate an effect. However, the patient groups must be well-matched at baseline in order to determine whether there is a true treatment effect.

Because subjective end-points are more susceptible to bias, "hard" end-points, such as mortality or heart failure hospitalization, are favored because they are both more objective and clinically relevant. In addition to evidence of a statistically significant beneficial treatment effect, the magnitude of the treatment effect must be clinically relevant. The evidence of acute physiologic improvements in stroke volume, cardiac output, narrowing of the QRS complex, and reduction in dyssynchrony must translate into meaningful long-term clinical improvement. Both the COMPANION[5] and CARE-HF[6] trials, for example, designated all-cause mortality as a secondary endpoint. In the COMPANION trial, no significant difference was observed in all-cause mortality between CRT and OPT (hazard ratio, 0.76; 95% confidence interval, 0.58-1.01; p = 0.06) whereas the CARE-HF trial demonstrated a statistically significant improvement in mortality with CRT over OPT (hazard ratio, 0.64; 95% confidence interval, 0.48-0.85; p<0.002). Differences in trial duration, patient populations, and absolute event numbers may partially explain the apparent discrepancy.

While efficacy is a requisite component of any new therapy, a reasonable assurance of safety is equally (if not more) important and often more difficult to measure. Clinical trials involving thousands of patients can often demonstrate efficacy but are substantially underpowered and/or poorly controlled in order to adequately quantify important, albeit infrequent, safety issues. CRT trials are no different. Although prespecified safety end-points were met in the early pivotal clinical CRT trials, assessments of safety and estimates of rates of rare or infrequent events (such as coronary sinus injury or cardiac perforation) are difficult to acquire during premarket evaluation, prompting the need for postmarket registries to collect

TABLE 14.1 **Selected Cardiac Resynchronization Therapy Trials for the Assessment of Functional Improvement and Quality of Life**

Study/Year	Patient Population (n)	Trial Design	Primary Efficacy End-points(s)	Outcomes Treatment	Control
MUSTIC-SR/ 2001	NYHA Class III; LVEF <0.35; QRS>150ms	Randomized (0-14d after implant); single-blind; crossover design		6-minute walk (m) @ 3 mos.	
			Active-inactive group (n=29)	384±79	336±128[a]
			Inactive-active group (n=29)	413±117	316±142[a]
			Combined groups	399±100	326±134[b]
MIRACLE/ 2002	NYHA Class III/IV; LVEF ≤0.35; QRS≥130ms	Randomized (1-14d after implant); double-blind; parallel control design		Change @ 6 mo. in: NHYA class	
			% Improved ≥2grades	16%	6%[b]
			% Improved 1 grade	52%	32%
			% No change	30%	59%
			Median QOL score	−18	−9[c]
			6-minute walk (m)	+39	+10[d]
MIRACLE-ICD/ 2003	NYHA Class III/IV;LVEF ≤0.35; QRS≥130ms and candidate for ICD	Randomized (1-14d); double-blind; parallel control design		Change @ 6 mo.	
			Median NHYA class	−1	0[e]
			Median QOL score	−17.5	−11[f]
			6-minute walk (m)	55	53[a]

[a] P = ns (treatment vs. control); [b] P <0.001 (treatment vs. control); [c] P = 0.001; [d] P = 0.005; [e] P = 0.007; [f] P = 0.02

devices used in electrophysiology labs. It was created to detect and communicate problems rapidly and may help identify not only device malfunctions, but also human factors that contribute to adverse patient outcomes. Reported problems and observations are shared throughout the network. The potential advantage for the FDA is that it increases the malfunction reporting rate and more directly connects them with device users to facilitate quicker and more thorough understanding of performance issues.

Remote monitoring systems offer great promise for improved postmarket data collection. Remote monitoring may serve to 1) reduce the need for clinic visits, 2) enable remote data transfer, 3) provide automated or semi-automatic patient alerts, and 4) permit early identification of generator and lead performance issues. Some patients may be reassured by the availability of remote monitoring. The quality of remote monitoring data is generally excellent and particularly useful for evaluating trends. Data interpretation may be challenging and additional clinical information may be required for accurate interpretation. False positives (for example, a set screw issue or the failure to plug the SVC port that is inappropriately classified as a lead performance issue) and false negatives (lead change between remote monitoring check) may occur.

Because of the potential for a number of different registries to collect data, efforts to standardize definitions will increase the potential to aggregate data from disparate sources including the NCDR ICD Registry, CMS databases, FDA, industry, and independent registries. This may provide an opportunity to amplify signals or confirm findings when performance issues arise. It may also facilitate efforts to link the NCDR ICD Registry to longitudinal databases such as administrative claims databases or remote monitoring systems. Barriers to success include not only technical data management challenges, but also issues related to patient confidentiality and the current lack of clinical follow-up in national registries.

ASSESSING DEVICE PERFORMANCE

ICD generators and leads must survive for years in a hostile environment and effectively pace and defibrillate when needed. However, because they serve a life-sustaining function, physicians and patients have appropriately high expectations for reliable device performance. Measuring device performance is important for clinical decision making, to set realistic expectations for patients and physicians, for transparency, and to monitor and improve performance. Importantly, many factors affect ICD generator and lead performance, including not only device design and manufacturing, but also physician and patient factors. In some cases, such as those involving lead dislodgements or perforations, differentiating device performance from a procedural or iatrogenic complication may be difficult. Frequently used terms in discussions of device performance are defined in Table 14.3. The definitions are more applicable to arrhythmia device generators than to leads.

TABLE 14.3 Definitions of Terms Frequently Used to Describe Device Performance

Term	Definition
Device performance	A measure of how well a device meets the user expectations that not only include specific device failures but also perceived quality, usability, robustness, and conformance to applicable labeling.
Device malfunction	Failure of a device to meet its performance specifications or otherwise perform as intended. Performance specifications include all claims made in the labeling of the device.
Device reliability	A measure of a device to be free of specific hardware and software failures, typically expressed at a given point in time or a failure rate per unit of time (e.g., failure rate per month).
Device failure	A device that does not perform its intended function as a result of a specific hardware and/or software failure.

Postmarket monitoring of ICD generator and lead performance has received much attention. In general, monitoring of generator performance—because they may be explanted and returned to the manufacturer for analysis—is easier than it is for leads. Postmarket monitoring of lead performance is more difficult because malfunctioning leads are often abandoned, and if they are removed, they may be damaged during explantation. This makes assessment of lead malfunction rates difficult and makes analysis of lead failure mechanisms more challenging.

Studies of ICD generator performance have been performed, although specific studies of CRT-D devices are lacking. According to FDA manufacturer annual reports from the years 1990–2002, 8,489 of 415,780 implanted ICDs were removed in the United States due to malfunction.[11] Battery/capacitor abnormalities and electrical issues are the most common types of malfunction. The average annual ICD malfunction replacement rate of 20.7 replacements per 1,000 implants is significantly higher than the pacemaker malfunction replacement rate of 4.6 replacements per 1,000 implants,[11] not surprising given the increased complexity of defibrillators. A meta-analysis of device registries yielded similar findings, demonstrating a 20-fold higher ICD malfunction rate compared to the pacemaker malfunction rate (26.5 versus 1.3 malfunctions per 1,000 person years).[12]

It is more difficult to describe ICD lead performance because study results have varied widely. Reported ICD lead "survival" varies from 91% to 99% at 2 years, 85% to 98% at 5 years, and 60% to 72% at 8 years.[13] Overall, typical ICD leads implanted in the 1990s are expected to have an ~1%/year failure rate (5% at 5 years, 10% at 10 years, etc.), although some have reported ICD lead survival of <90% at

5 years.[9,14] Certain patient populations, such as pediatrics, are expected to have higher failure rates due to the small stature, fast growth rates, and high activity levels of the patients. Specific prospective studies of LV lead performance are limited, although most manufacturers report LV lead survival (excluding dislodgements, infection, etc.) exceeding 98% at 3 years.

REGULATORY ACTION

When the FDA identifies a problem or potential problem with a medical device, it may conduct a more in-depth investigation, often with the assistance of the manufacturer, to help determine the root cause of the problem. Problems may be due to manufacturing defects, poor product design, misleading labeling, confusing instructions, patient sensitivity, or other causes. In many cases, the manufacturer first identifies the problem and notifies the FDA.

Depending on the nature and scope of the problem, the FDA may choose to issue a public health advisory or a safety alert.[8] A public health advisory is issued when a device with the potential for risk is identified. A safety alert, on the other hand, is issued when a device has actually caused serious injury or death. The FDA may also use several enforcement methods to obtain manufacturer compliance. Warning letters may be issued for regulatory violations. When violations are recurrent or pose a serious health threat, medical product may be seized (when products are not in compliance with regulations) or injunctions (when manufacturers or personnel are not in compliance with regulations) may be issued. Mandatory recalls and premarket approval suspension or withdrawal may be invoked when a reasonable probability of serious harm exists.

Recalls and safety alerts (collectively referred to as "advisories") affecting pacemakers and ICDs are common, although importantly, most advisories are issued when the risk of actual device failure is < 1%. Since 1990, more than 1 million pacemakers and ICDs have been affected by an advisory.[15] ICDs are recalled more frequently than pacemakers (16.4 versus 6.7 advisories per 100 person-years).[16] Hardware malfunctions and computer errors account for 95% of device recalls.[16]

CLINICAL MANAGEMENT AND COMMUNICATION OF ICD PERFORMANCE ISSUES

A past survey of physicians regarding the clinical management of pacemaker and ICD generator recalls demonstrated great variation; some physicians replaced all devices, while others replaced none or very few.[17] While the rate of death from generator failure is exceedingly low, the clinical consequences of device replacement vary by procedure, operator, and patient characteristics. Similarly, ICD lead failure can result in failure to pace, failure to defibrillate, and inappropriate shocks. LV

TABLE 14.4 Factors to Consider in the Risk-Benefit Analysis of Advisory Device Removal

Factors
Underlying rhythm/Pacemaker dependence
Prior history of arrhythmia
Risk of future arrhythmia
Risk of replacement procedure
Risk of malfunction in advisory device
Malfunction associated with sudden or gradual loss of function
Malfunction mechanism known/understood
Can reprogramming device mitigate the risk?
Risk of malfunction in replacement device
Patient anxiety

lead failure can result in an exacerbation of heart failure. Death from ICD lead failure is thought to be very rare.

The clinical results of ICD generator and lead abnormalities can be potentially catastrophic, but so can prophylactic device replacement. Generator replacement alone for advisory devices is associated with a measurable major complication rate of up to 5.8%.[18] The risk of infection is higher for generator replacements than for initial implants. The risks of lead extraction include the potential for catastrophic events such as cardiac tamponade, severe vascular injury, and death. In fact, extraction of the Telectronics Accufix™ atrial J lead resulted in more deaths than the lead malfunction itself. Mortality associated with extraction of larger leads in experienced hands approaches 1%.

A number of factors contribute to the calculus of whether an advisory ICD generator or lead should be replaced or followed conservatively (Table 14.4). In addition, because of the risks of extraction and the potential complications from adding additional leads, the decision of when to prophylactically replace an otherwise normally functioning advisory ICD or LV lead is a difficult one.

The 2006 HRS Task Force on Device Performance Policies and Guidelines underscore the importance of timely and thorough communication by industry with patients, physicians, and regulators which is critical to maintaining trust and eliminating as much uncertainty as possible.[19] It is also recommended that physicians know not only general risks associated with device replacement, but the specific risks at their own institution, as these may vary from center to center depending not only on physician skill but patient population.

A number of factors affect the decision and timing about whether or not to issue advisory notices regarding specific performance issues. Industry, in collaboration with Heart Rhythm Society and regulators, has developed specific policies and procedures related to advisory notices and consults with standing committees of "independent" experts for advice regarding the need and timing of communication. In most cases, the root cause of a device performance issue needs to be understood in order to answer the key questions that affect clinical notification and management.

CONGRESSIONAL OVERSIGHT OF FDA

When concern arose among the public, manufacturers, and Congress about prolonged delays accompanying the FDA device approval process, Congress enacted the FDA Modernization Act of 1997.[8] This Act expedited review times by setting time limits on the FDA at various steps in the approval process; by requiring expedited review of devices representing breakthrough technologies or devices for which no alternative exists; by allowing a manufacturer to request in writing, before application for device approval, the specific data that will be required for approval; and by allowing the FDA to use third-party reviewers to evaluate lower-risk devices. This provides an instructive example as to how Congress can set priorities for the FDA.

Congressional oversight of the FDA occurs by enactment of legislation, by control of the FDA budget, and by confirmation of the FDA commissioner. Each of these processes often but not always occurs in partisan fashion. The ease or difficulty of the FDA device approval process affects the speed and cost at which new devices can be brought to market and, therefore, has broader economic implications for manufacturers and the U.S. economy.

The challenge to the FDA has been and remains striking a balance between "rushing a product to market" to allow patients to benefit from medical advances and simultaneously ensuring patient safety. Congressionally legislated time limits for review and approval decisions on new devices, therefore, can "tip the balance" toward speed or safety.

CONCLUSIONS

Cardiac resynchronization therapy has improved and extended the lives of numerous patients. The clinical demands placed on CRT devices are substantial. Careful premarket evaluation and close postmarket monitoring of device performance are critical to set realistic expectations for patients and physicians, for clinical decision making, for transparency, and to monitor and improve performance. Nevertheless, because of the complexity of the devices, occasional software "glitches" and performance issues will inevitably arise. In addition, the FDA will be challenged to expedite important product advances to market so that patients may benefit. The FDA, Congress, manufacturers, the public, and health care providers each play a vital role in the process of bringing new and innovative therapies to the patient's bedside.

PRACTICAL POINTS

1. The U.S. Food and Drug Administration (FDA) is charged with ensuring the safety and effectiveness of medical devices in the United States including cardiac resynchronization therapy.

2. Premarket evaluation is based on the idea that the degree of device regulation should correlate with the degree of risk posed by the device and is intended to bring new and modified devices to market safely.

3. Small, short-term premarket clinical studies may be useful for assessing acute or subacute device performance (such as acute pacing thresholds), but they are inadequate for assessing long-term device performance because they are of insufficient size and are not designed to account for all implant, patient, and physician variables that can affect outcome.

4. The goal of postmarket surveillance is to enhance public health by reducing the incidence of medical device adverse experiences.

5. The current postmarket surveillance system relies not only on the FDA and manufacturers but also on hospitals, long-term and ambulatory medical care facilities, health care providers, and patients to report adverse events from medical devices.

6. Postmarket surveillance is designed to identify uncommon but potentially serious device-related adverse events.

7. Careful premarket evaluation and close postmarket monitoring of device performance are critical for setting realistic expectations for patients and physicians, for clinical decision making, for transparency, and for monitoring and improving performance.

REFERENCES

1. Linde C, Braunschweig F, Gadler F, et al. Long term improvements in quality of life by biventricular pacing in patients with chronic heart failure: results from the Multi-site Stimulation in Cardiomyopathy study (MUSTIC). *Am J Cardiol.* 2003; 91: 1090–1099.
2. Nelson GS, Berger RD, Fetics BJ, et al. Left ventricular or biventricular pacing improves cardiac function at diminished energy cost in patients with dilated cardiomyopathy and left bundle branch block. *Circulation.* 2000; 102: 3053–2059.
3. Linde C, Leclercq C, Rex S, et al. Long-term benefits of biventricular pacing in congestive heart failure: results from the Multisite Stimulation In Cardiomyopathy (MUSTIC) study. *J Am Coll Cardiol.* 2002; 40:111–118.
4. St. John Sutton MG, Plapper T, Abraham WT, et al. Effect of cardiac resynchronization therapy on left ventricular size and function in chronic heart failure. *Circulation.* 2003; 107: 1985–1990.
5. Bristow MR, Saxon LA, Boehmer J, et al. Cardiac-resynchronization therapy with or without an implantable defibrillator in advanced chronic heart failure. *N Engl J Med.* 2004; 350: 2140–2150.
6. Cleland JGF, Daubert JC, Erdmann E, et al. The effect of cardiac resynchronization on morbidity and mortality in heart failure. *N Engl J Med.* 2005; 352: 1539–1549.
7. Abraham WT, Young JB, Leon AR, et al. Effects of cardiac resynchronization on disease progression in patients with left ventricular systolic dysfunction, an indication for an implantable cardioverter-defibrillator and mildly symptomatic chronic heart failure. *Circulation.* 2004; 110:2864–2868.
8. Maisel WH. Medical Device Regulation: An introduction for the practicing physician. *Ann Int Med.* 2004; 140: 296–302.
9. Maisel WH, Hauser R. Proceedings of the ICD Lead Performance Conference. *Heart Rhythm.* 2008; 5: 1331–1338.
10. Hammill SC, Kremers MS, Stevenson LW, et al. Review of the Registry's Second Year, Data Collected, and Plans to Add Lead and Pediatric ICD Procedures. *Heart Rhythm.* 2008; 5: 1359–1363.

11. Maisel WH, Moynahan M, Zuckerman BD. Pacemaker and ICD generator malfunctions. Analysis of Food and Drug Administration annual reports. *JAMA*. 2006; 295: 1901–1906.

12. Maisel WH. Pacemaker and ICD generator reliability: Meta-analysis of device registries. *JAMA*. 2006; 295: 1929–1934.

13. Maisel WH, Kramer DB. ICD lead performance. *Circulation*. 2008; 117: 2721–2723.

14. Kleemann T, Becker T, Doenges K, et al. Annual rate of transvenous defibrillation lead defects in implantable cardioverter-defibrillators over a period of >10 years. *Circulation*. 2007; 115: 2474–2480.

15. Maisel WH. Safety issues involving medical devices: Implications of recent implantable cardioverter-defibrillator malfunctions. *JAMA*. 2005; 294: 955–958.

16. Maisel WH, Sweeney MO, Stevenson WG, et al. Recalls and safety alerts involving pacemakers and implantable cardioverter-defibrllator generators. *JAMA*. 2001; 286: 793–799.

17. Maisel WH. Physician management of pacemaker and implantable cardioverter-defibrillator advisories. *Pacing and Clinical Electrophysiology*. 2004; 27: 437–442.

18. Gould PA, Krahn AD. for the Canadian Heart Rhythm Society Working Group on Device Advisories. Complications associated with implantable cardioverter-defibrillator replacement in response to device advisories. *JAMA*. 2006;295:1907–1911.

19. Carlson MD, Wilkoff BL, Maisel WH, et al. Recommendations from the Heart Rhythm Society Task Force on Device Performance Policies and Guidelines. *Heart Rhythm*. 2006; 3: 1250–1273.

The Role of Cardiac Resynchronization Devices in Monitoring Patients with Chronic Heart Failure

Philip B. Adamson • Emilio Vanoli

Management of patients with chronic heart failure initially focuses on determining an etiology for left ventricular dysfunction followed by establishing life-saving medication and device therapies intended to reduce the chances of progressive pump dysfunction and sudden cardiac death.[1] Beta-blockers, angiotensin, antagonism with ACE-inhibitors, or angiotensin receptor blockers, and aldosterone blockade form the basis for neurohormonal intervention for selected heart failure patients, and many times result in significant improvement in quality of life and pump function, along with reduced mortality.[1] Coupled with neurohormonal inhibition, device therapies further reduce mortality[1-5] and, in the case of cardiac resynchronization therapy (CRT),[4-6] improve morbidities of this chronic disease syndrome.

Patients with persistent left ventricular systolic dysfunction and symptomatic heart failure, after adequate neurohormonal intervention, complicated with interventricular conduction delays, have a consensus recommendation for correction of ventricular electromechanical dyssynchrony (QRS > 120 msec) using cardiac resynchronization therapy (CRT) achieved with atrioventricular sequential biventricular pacing.[1,4-6] It is clear that CRT, with or without implantable cardioverter defibrillator (ICD) therapy, reduces symptoms and hospitalizations due to worsening of heart failure. It also improves ventricular function in over 70% of patients and significantly reduces risk of death.[1,4-6] Despite significant advances in heart failure disease management from optimal medical and device therapies, frequent hospitalizations remain a significant problem with very important clinical, economic, and social consequences. The most common reason for patients to require hospitalization is worsening congestion resulting from excessive volume accumulation.[7] In this context, the next and most involved step in long-term heart failure management is monitoring patients to avoid volume congestion in hopes of reducing the need for hospitalization. To prevent volume congestion, follow-up of patients with heart failure still relies mostly on traditional methods, such as frequent physical examination, daily weight monitoring, and reporting of symptoms. These tools have marginal predictive value when estimating volume or hospitalization

risks,[8-11] providing the rationale for incorporating new data in long-term heart failure disease management.

The focus of this chapter is to review diagnostic information available from implanted CRT devices with consideration for how these parameters may help assess ambulatory patients with heart failure. A suggested means to coordinate information processing is provided to achieve optimal outcomes with an emphasis on developing a strategy for triaging follow-up in hopes of reducing the need for hospitalization to achieve normal volume status. Several important lessons can be learned about monitoring heart failure patients by reviewing studies examining heart failure disease management strategies.

HEART FAILURE DISEASE MANAGEMENT: MONITORING STRATEGY TRIALS

Several approaches to heart failure disease management have been evaluated in clinical studies and include a variety of frequent encounter strategies designed to reduce the need for hospitalization, as summarized in Table 15.1.[12-18] Among several excellent studies, one very interesting trial was the Specialized Primary and Networked Care in Heart Failure (SPAN-CHF) trial, which prospectively randomized heart failure patients from a mix of academic and community practice sites to usual care or an intervention arm.[14] Patients were enrolled during an index heart failure hospitalization and were randomly assigned to groups that received follow-up care that normally occurred at the site or to a second group that had a nurse case manager, who visited the patient's home with education materials and home situation assessment. In the intervention arm, nurses telephoned patients once or twice a week to reinforce the home visit information and to make sure that patients were taking their medications, adhering to dietary restrictions, and weighing in daily. With the intervention outlined in SPAN-CHF, there was a significant 52% reduction in heart failure hospitalizations during the 90-day intervention, but the effect on this end-point was lost once the nurse calls stopped, even though patients had telephone numbers to call any time for help.[14] Interestingly, total hospitalizations for any cause were no different between the

TABLE 15.3 Implanted Device Compon
Which Direct Physiologic I
Is Sensed or Derived Infor
Computed

Device Component	Information Provided or
Atrial Lead	Heart Rate, Atrial Pacing, A tion/tachycardia
Right Ventricular Lead	Heart Rate, Ventricular pa(lar arrhythmias, Ventricu to Atrial Fibrillation
Left Ventricular Lead	Ventricular pacing and LV
Pulse Generator	Heart Rate Variability, Acti racic Impedance

Direct Physiologic Information from Implanted Devices

Heart Rate

Resting heart rates may have prognostic valı
with chronic heart failure.[20–21] Traditional sim
measurements are influenced by both clinical
mental factors, which may limit understanding
rate may be associated with clinical interventio
sis. In contrast, device-based heart rate calcula

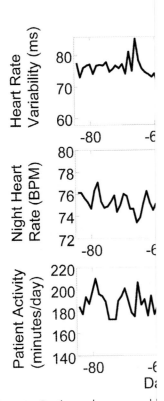

FIG. 15.1. Continuously measured l
(SDAAM), night heart rate and patie
leading to hospitalization. Used with
autonomic assessment in patients
measured by an implanted cardiac r

TABLE 15.1 Summary of Key Disease Management Studies and Their Basic Results

Trial/Study	Intervention	n	Population	Result
SPAN-CHF[1]	Nurse visit, then weekly calls	200	Immediately post-hospitalization	52% reduction in HF hospitalizations, no change in all-cause hospitalization
WHARF[2]	Telemonitoring	280	NYHA Class III-IV post-hospitalization	No change in hospitalizations, 56.2% reduction in mortality
TEN-HMS[3]	Usual care vs. weekly nurse calls vs. telemonitoring	426	Immediately post-hospitalization	No change in HF hospitalizations, 16%-18% absolute reduction in mortality favoring weekly nurse calls and telemonitoring
Rich et al.[4]	Intensive education with home nursing visits and frequent follow-up	282	Elderly hospitalized patients	13.2% absolute reduction in readmission rate
Fonarow et al.[5]	In-patient management and organized follow-up	214	Hospitalized NYHA Class IV with referral for transplant	85% reduction in hospitalizations (historic control)

Note inconsistent reductions in heart failure (HF) hospitalizations and mortality.
[1]Kimmelstiel C, Levine D, Perry K, et al. Randomized, controlled evaluation of short and long-term benefits of heart failure disease management within a diverse provider network: The SPAN-CHF trial. *Circulation*. 2004;110:1450–1455.
[2]Goldberg LR, Piette JD, Walsh MN, et al. Randomized trial of a daily electronic home monitoring system in patients with advanced heart failure: The Weight Monitoring in Heart Failure (WHARF) trial. *Am Heart J*. 2003;146:705–712.
[3]Cleland JG, Louis AA, Swedberg K, et al. Noninvasive home telemonitoring for patients with heart failure at high risk of recurrent admission and death: The Trans European Network-Home-Care Management (TEN-HMS) study. *J Am Coll Cardiol*. 2005;45:1654–1664.
[4]Rich MW, Beckham V, Wittenberg C, et al. A multidisciplinary intervention to prevent the readmission of elderly patients with congestive heart failure. *N Engl J Med*. 1995;333:1190–1195.
[5]Fonarow GC, Stevenson LW, Alden JA, et al. Impact of a comprehensive heart failure management program on hospital readmissions and functional status of patients with advanced heart failure. *J Am Coll Cardiol*. 1997;30:725–732.

intervention and control group. Neurohormonal intervention in SPAN-CHF was similar between the control and intervention groups throughout the trial. Therefore, the reduction in heart failure hospitalizations was likely due to better volume management in the intervention group, rather than from maximizing life-saving medications.[14]

SPAN-CHF demonstrated that nurse calls are very effective in reducing heart failure hospitalizations, but, in most health care systems, this intervention is not reimbursable and requires funding from sources other than pay-for-service billing, which seriously limits widespread application. However, the SPAN-CHF and other trials clearly demonstrate that intensive focus on volume management in patients with heart failure reduces episodes of heart failure decompensation.

Another similarly designed trial, the Trans-European Network-Home-Care Management System (TEN-HMS), was conducted in three countries characterized by nationalized health care systems (Germany, the Netherlands, and the United Kingdom).[15] Patients with a recent heart failure hospitalization were randomly assigned to one of three groups intended to implement long-term heart failure management strategies, including institution and uptitration of life-saving medical therapies to appropriate dosing. The first of the three groups consisted of a transtelephonic information management system in which the patient's blood pressure, pulse, cardiac rhythm, and weight were transmitted twice daily to a centralized data management server via Internet access and then transmitted to the patient's responsible study site.[15]

Automated monitoring of the physiologic information allowed preset parameters of weight change, blood pressure values, or rhythm changes to alert nurses at each study center of a change in patient status. Then providers contacted patients for assessment with final medical decision-making determined by combining information gained from monitored physiologic parameters and from direct patient contact.

The second randomized group consisted of telephone calls monthly from a specially trained heart failure nurse provider, who assessed the patient's symptoms and current medication dosing and adherence. The nurse contacts were intended to ensure that the long-term plan for the patient's heart failure management initially instituted during the index hospitalization was successfully implemented during the follow-up period. Additionally, it was thought that nurse contact might provide opportunities to identify volume changes earlier in hopes to avoid congestion leading to acute care hospitalization. The automated monitoring group and nurse contact group were initially hypothesized for comparison, and the third group was added as a control.[15]

The third randomization group was considered "usual care," in which the patient's long-term heart failure management plan, again established in the index hospitalization, became the responsibility of the patient's primary care provider. Interestingly, the primary end-point of the trial, which was days lost because of death or hospitalization in acute care hospitalizations for any reason during 450 days of follow-up, was not significantly different in any of the groups, but mortality

(which was a component of the prima
markedly higher in the usual care group cc
telephone management or automated inf
ing.[15] As a matter of fact, those patients ra
ing care or automated telephone care wei
likely to survive the 12-month follow-up
who received their post-hospitalization
primary care providers.[15] No significant
tality or the primary end-point was founc
care group and the automatic telemonito

To further understand the effect in TEN
analysis found that monitoring daily wei
using two rule of thumb approaches includ
weight gain in one day or 5 pounds in thre
average convergence divergence algorithi
quate sensitivity nor specificity to be clinic
monitoring of patients with heart failure, a
heart failure decompensation leading to h

A more recent trial, The Home or Hosp
(HHH), was a European Community-fur
randomized, controlled clinical trial, coi
Poland, and Italy, to assess the feasibility
home telemonitoring of clinical and phy
ters, which was compared to usual care
events in 461 patients with chronic syst
Home telemonitoring was administered
three randomized strategies: (1) monthly
(2) phone contact plus weekly transmii
and (3) phone contact, weekly transmii
and monthly 24-hour recording of cardic
Patients completed 81% of vital signs tra
as 92% of cardiorespiratory recordings, b
there was no significant effect of home
reducing bed-days occupancy for hear
death plus heart failure hospitalization
reduction of cardiac events was, howev
Italian cohort.[18]

SUMMARY

Several important lessons can be learne
strategy trials. Primarily frequent (more
contact with patients with chronic he
studies results in a significant reduction
pitalization to manage volume exacerbati
quent nurse calls to this population ma
mortality. Patient contact has several go;
sesses patient volume (congestion symj
perfusion (blood pressure, symptoms), a
ommended medical and lifestyle recoi
medications, activity, etc.) Although dail
was a component of most managemen
performance of this measurement in pro
tion is consistently poor.[10–11, 19]

crease risks of major complications, such as cerebrovascular accident, or contribute to acute decompensation. In clinical studies, using implanted device data for the diagnosis of sustained atrial high rate events is superior to symptom-based monitoring,[23] but results from ongoing trials will eventually clarify how medical management will impact complications such as stroke or heart failure decompensation. For example, ventricular response to atrial fibrillation is an important marker of successful therapy,[24–25] and device-based monitoring allows continuous assessment of ventricular rate during activities of daily living. Routine Internet-based surveillance can discover unexpected arrhythmias and prompt therapies focusing on rate and rhythm control with possible impact on embolic event rates.

Recent clinical trials demonstrated that, for many patients, rate control of atrial fibrillation is an equal or superior treatment strategy compared to persistent attempts to maintain normal sinus rhythm.[24–25] This seems true for patients with and without heart failure who experience chronic persistent atrial fibrillation. Successful ventricular rate control was carefully defined in prospective trials by using heart rates obtained at rest and during 6-minute hall walk testing.[24–25] In contrast to these approaches, implanted device information continuously monitors ventricular response to atrial fibrillation during patient's daily activities, thus increasing the probability of successful management of chronic persistent atrial fibrillation.

Heart rhythm monitoring has also other very important applications. For instance, the incidence of ventricular arrhythmias is very important information for electrophysiologists and heart failure practitioners, including the incidence of appropriate or inappropriate therapy delivery. Prognosis after appropriate ICD therapy for potentially lethal ventricular arrhythmias is significantly worse, but the higher mortality in treated patients is mostly due to worsening heart failure, rather than sudden death.[26] Therefore, this higher risk group may be a population in whom frequent assessment is appropriate.

Amount of Ventricular Pacing

Particularly important in ensuring the benefit of CRT devices is the amount of biventricular pacing, which is another critical factor to monitor. Patients with persistent rapid ventricular response to atrial fibrillation or those with frequent ventricular premature contraction may inhibit the ability to deliver biventricular pacing. In this context, recent data demonstrate that high percentage ($> 92\%$) of biventricular pacing in patients with a CRT device is associated with improved prognosis.[27] Therefore, monitoring the amount of biventricular pacing can directly influence medical therapies designed to slow conduction of atrial fibrillation or maximization of other medications designed to decrease ventricular ectopy. Device-based monitoring of the amount of ventricular pacing provides a novel means to maximize the effect of this therapy.

In contrast, right ventricular apical pacing may be detrimental to patients with structural heart disease.[28] Efforts to minimize right ventricular apical pacing in devices such as single or dual chamber ICD's can also be monitored using device-based diagnostics.

DERIVED DATA FROM IMPLANTED DEVICES

Intrathoracic Impedance

Theoretical Background

Intrathoracic impedance is a computed device-based parameter that may help assess the amount of lung water and attendant clinical stability in heart failure patients receiving CRT. Intrathoracic impedance is essentially the resistance of electrical flow through the thorax and is determined by lung conductivity and tissue resistance.[29] Intrathoracic impedance is calculated as the impedance of a subthreshold electrical impulse generated by the right ventricular lead as that impulse travels from the lead toward the implanted pulse generator. Device-based intrathoracic impedance is theoretically superior to transthoracic measurements since the vector and distance between the lead and the pulse generator are constant. This improves reproducibility of the parameter measurements, thus making daily comparison a more meaningful and reliable marker of "lung water." Limiting this technology is the fact that computations are affected by pocket edema, which precludes the use of this marker for several weeks following CRT implantation.

Intrathoracic impedance measurements as a device-based diagnostic may serve as a marker of "lung water" based on the hypothesis that pulmonary circulatory engorgement and pulmonary edema progressively increase as patients decompensate.[29–30] Increased lung water leads to decreased intrathoracic impedance reflecting persistent pulmonary congestion. Animal studies demonstrated that changes in intrathoracic impedance directly correlated to changes in left ventricular filling pressure.[29] These findings were confirmed in only very limited human studies in which pulmonary capillary wedge pressure and volume of diuresis required to restore optivolemic status correlated well to changes in intrathoracic impedance in patients hospitalized for decompensated heart failure.[30] Continuous monitoring of intrathoracic impedance found changes apparent an average of 18 days before patients presented with symptoms severe enough for hospitalization.[30]

One commercially available method to frequently monitor intrathoracic impedance, called "The Optivol Fluid Index," (Medtronic, Inc) uses a cumulative sum method, which measures daily intrathoracic impedance and compares the daily measurement with a 30-day running average, thought to reflect the patient's own "baseline" values. Differences in daily impedance values that are persistently below the running average accumulate until an arbitrary threshold is crossed suggesting significant increases in lung volume.[30] Clinically, threshold crossings are accessible remotely by Internet-based information systems using data that is uploaded from the patient's home or by face-to-face encounters using a programmer to directly interrogate the device, but this represents a significant limitation in that finding a threshold crossing requires either frequent monitoring (monthly) or the fortunate random discovery of significant changes. Outside the United States, a patient notification system is available, which causes the device to sound an audible alert when the threshold is crossed.

Evidence Base for Intrathoracic Impedance in Patients with Heart Failure

No prospective trials are planned to determine if using intrathoracic impedance to guide medical intervention prevents the need to hospitalize patients with heart failure. Therefore, recommendations for clinical use can only be based on nonrandomized and unblinded feasibility studies that are also limited in scope by the small populations studied. For example the first such study performed in 34 heart failure patients by Yu et al. found a consistent correlation between filling pressures and degree of volume overload with intrathoracic impedance measurements.[30] In this study there were 24 hospitalizations in 9 patients, and changes in intrathoracic impedance were apparent an average of 18 days before hospitalization, while worsening dyspnea was reported on average 3 days before severe decompensation.[30] An accurate assessment of intrathoracic impedance's predictive value was not possible. It was unclear from this trial how often intrathoracic thresholds are crossed in the presence of other diseases or not related to ongoing pathologies at all.

In a prospective observational trial called The European Observational InSync Sentry Study, the audible device alert system was used to determine if the threshold crossing of the Optivol Fluid Index to monitor intrathoracic impedance predicted worsening heart failure.[31] Patients in this trial were instructed to contact study personnel if the device alert sounded alarm and the patients were evaluated for worsening heart failure signs or symptoms. The study found that threshold crossings using the Optivol Fluid Index feature in patients indicated for CRT therapy was 60% sensitive with 60% positive predictive value for predicting worsening heart failure. The false-positive rate was 38% during the follow-up period.[31]

These results must be tempered by the fact that individual investigators were allowed to alter the alert threshold or turn off the alarm system depending on the specific patient's experience. The trial did discover that important non-heart failure-related clinical events may cause changes in intrathoracic impedance. These important events included pneumonia, left ventricular lead dislodgement, and new onset atrial fibrillation.[31] Other studies also determined that pulse generator pocket edema, pocket inflammation, or trauma could also cause false-positive changes in intrathoracic impedance.

Another small trial designed to evaluate the performance of intrathoracic impedance in predicting heart failure events included 115 patients followed for 9 months using the patient alert system.[32] Worsening heart failure status requiring modifications in medical therapy was used as the endpoint to calculate predictive statistics. In the follow-up period, 49 device alerts occurred and only 15 of those were associated with clinically determined worsening heart failure.[32] Interpretation of the results from this study were limited by the following two main factors: 1) the period of time elapsing between the device alert and the time when patients were examined to determine worsening heart failure and 2) the use of traditional tools to determine volume status, which are known to poorly predict actual cardiac filling pressures.[8–9] Investigators immediately assessed patients to find presence or absence of physical examination findings consistent with volume overload. Patients at this time would likely appear normal since threshold crossings may occur an average of 18 days before heart failure status decompensates to the point of producing physical signs or symptoms of congestion.[30] Clinical signs and symptoms of heart failure may be a very late phenomenon that is only apparent when patients are well advanced in a congestive decompensation.

In this light, derived device diagnostics, such as intrathoracic impedance or heart rate variability, seem to sense changes in status long before patients have symptoms or physical signs develop. As a result, remote changes in medial therapies based solely on changes in derived diagnostics may be limited, such that these data may only be useful for initiation of unscheduled clinical assessment or may increase the frequency of clinical encounters. Data from clinical trials are not sufficient to support the possibility that alterations in potentially toxic medications, such as diuretics, to maintain normal volume over time can be made based solely on derived diagnostic data.

Finally, the first small case-control series of patients studied to determine if intrathoracic impedance predicted the need for heart failure hospitalization enrolled 27 patients followed for one year.[33] Impedance changes were associated with a 61% true-positive rate when predicting hospitalization for heart failure. Hospitalizations were 9 times less likely in those patients with device-based audible alert system activated. This is encouraging information, but not sufficient to support use of derived data to guide remote management of specific medical interventions.

Clinical Application and Limitations of Intrathoracic Impedance

Intrathoracic impedance measurements are currently available in one manufacturer's devices and can serve as a "trigger" to notify providers of a change in stability that requires more frequent follow-up. Problems other than heart failure decompensation can also influence intrathoracic impedance measurements, such as pneumonia, lead dislodgement, and pulse generator pocket edema. Furthermore, no data exists demonstrating that remote response to changing impedance, by changing diuretics for example, is a safe or effective approach. Therefore, the clinical utility of intrathoracic impedance is as a marker of ongoing stability and should be used to alter follow-up plans or initiate contact by nurse providers (Fig. 15.2).

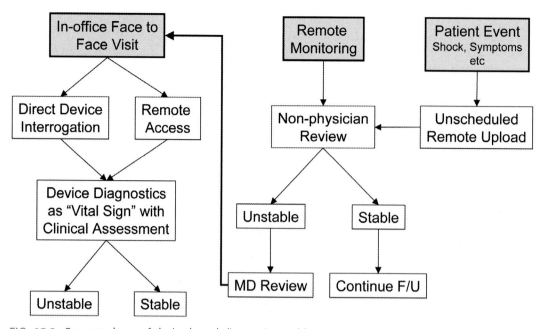

FIG. 15.2. Suggested use of device-based diagnostics and how remote monitoring may influence clinical follow-up.

Heart Rate Variability

Atrial-to-atrial depolarization intervals can be measured from the atrial lead of a CRT device and can be used to compute heart rate variability (HRV), which is an indirect marker of cardiac autonomic control.[34–35] Higher variability suggests stronger vagal control, while reduced variability suggests vagal withdrawal and an autonomic imbalance favoring the sympathetic nervous system. Heart rate variability is known to predict cardiovascular mortality in patients after myocardial infarction or with heart failure.[22, 34–35] (Fig. 15.3), but until continuous measurements were possible, any association between changes in heart rate variability and worsening heart failure status was not known.

The first clinical study to examine device-based heart rate variability computed the standard deviation of the atrial-to-atrial median (SDAAM) intervals using the medians of 5-minute device recordings.[36] The study involved patients who were randomly assigned CRT therapy or not after the device was implanted as part of the MIRACLE trial.[6] Continuously measured SDAAM was significantly higher after 3 months in those receiving CRT suggesting that improvement in overall cardiovascular status also resulted significant change in autonomic control of the heart.[36] Subsequent studies using slightly different methods of quantifying heart rate variability[37] confirmed this "shift" in autonomic control towards vagal control, which implies a more stable, less sympathetic dependent system.

Because HRV responded to CRT delivery, it was hypothesized that other changes in clinical status may influence continuous assessment of cardiac autonomic control. In this context, further evaluation of continuously measured device-based HRV included prediction of both mortality (Fig. 15.3)

and impending decompensation requiring hospitalization.[22] (Fig. 15.1). Continuous HRV assessment suggested that adaptive reflexes can be tracked as patients progress in the early stages of decompensated heart failure. It is probable that these reflex autonomic responses to the initial decline in cardiac performance are key adaptive elements that prevent symptoms of congestion early in the decompensation process. Sympathetic activation and vagal withdrawal may serve to temporarily improve cardiac performance as volume accumulates and can be overwhelmed if conditions persist. Autonomic adaptations, as shown by changes in HRV measurements, were identified as early as 21 days prior to the development of worsening symptoms requiring hospitalization.[22]

Along with decline in previously stable HRV measurements, patients with persistently low HRV (SDAAM <50 msec) are at much higher risk for hospitalization in the subsequent 12 months as demonstrated in Figure 15.4.[22] This suggests that both changes in HRV and basal values powerfully stratify mortality risk, assess baseline clinical stability predicting longer-term risk for hospitalization and can be used to remotely discover impending decline in clinical stability (Fig. 15.5).

Suggested Clinical Application of Device-Based Heart Rate Variability

Device based heart rate variability can serve, clinically, as a means to assess long-term patient stability and need for follow-up as demonstrated in Figure 15.5.[38] Data can be obtained either from direct device interrogation in an office setting or using Internet-based information systems for remote assessment. Both the absolute value of SDAAM

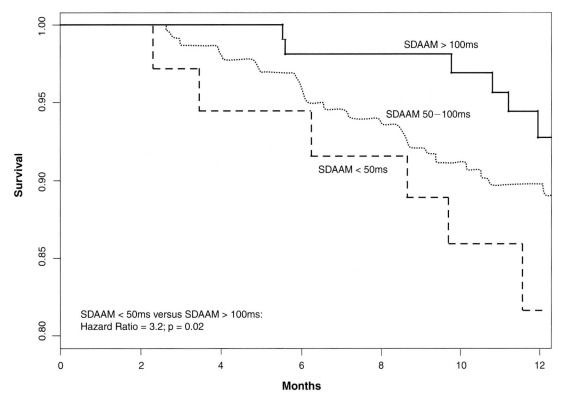

FIG. 15.3. Association of baseline heart rate variability measurements in predicting 12-month mortality. Patients with SDAAM greater than 100 ms were 3.2 times more likely to survive compared to those with SDAAM less than 50 ms. Used with permission from Adamson PB, Smith AL, Abraham WT, et al. Continuous autonomic assessment in patients with symptomatic heart failure: prognostic value of heart rate variability measured by an implanted cardiac resynchronization device. *Circulation.* 2004;110:2389-2394.

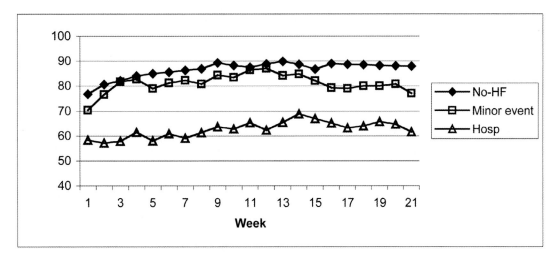

FIG. 15.4. Continuous measurement of heart rate variability stratifies risk for heart failure event in ambulatory patients. These data from 262 patients suggested that individuals with persistently low heart rate variability were more likely to require hospitalization in the 21-week follow-up period. Used with permission from Adamson PB, Smith AL, Abraham WT, et al. Continuous autonomic assessment in patients with symptomatic heart failure: prognostic value of heart rate variability measured by an implanted cardiac resynchronization device. *Circulation.* 2004;110:2389–2394.

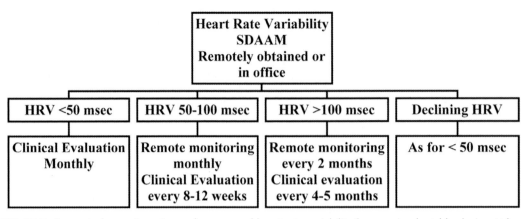

FIG. 15.5. Suggested use of continuously measured heart rate variability from an implantable device. Values refer to the SDAAM.

and its change over time are important markers of clinical stability.

Clinical Limitations

Measurement of HRV by an implanted device requires a predominance of sinus rhythm. Therefore, HRV cannot be measured if an individual experiences atrial rhythm disorders (atrial fibrillation) or if atrial pacing is required for greater than 80% of the 24 hours. Studies generally used automatic detection algorithm that compared daily heart rate variability with a patient reference line and accumulated differences in an algorithm to detect subtle but persistent changes in the parameter.[22] Change detection algorithms are not always available, which forces the user to visually identify variability changes that persist over time, undoubtedly decreasing the sensitivity of the test in common clinical use.

CONCLUSIONS

Heart rate variability, then, may be useful to either remotely or in direct patient contact, stratify risk for clinical decompensation. Persistent decline or chronically low SDAAM values call for more frequent follow-up to ensure appropriate clinical intervention when needed. Patients with changing or low heart rate variability should be considered to be at high risk for volume overload exacerbation and hospitalization. Continuously measured heart rate variability can be a very useful tool to determine longer-term risk for decompensated heart failure and can be integrated into clinical practice by remote review or direct device interrogation.

INTEGRATION OF DEVICE DATA INTO CLINICAL PRACTICE

Successful utilization of device-based diagnostic data requires a system that efficiently provides information to practitioners responsible for patient care and action on physiologic data. This system requires cooperation between electrophysiologists

and heart failure providers.[39] Many times electrophysiologists or pacemaker clinics are responsible for obtaining and monitoring remotely uploaded device information. Internet information systems, however, allow heart failure providers to gain access to Internet-based device uploads by obtaining website access privileges from manufacturers. This allows the provider with primary responsibility for heart failure management to make clinical decisions based on device-based information at the same level as a "vital sign." This information can be remotely reviewed or obtained during an office visit by direct interrogation of the device. For example if atrial rhythm is a concern in a clinical encounter but cannot be determined by usual testing or examination, the device can be directly interrogated to determine the underlying rhythm. Programmer availability is an issue, but usually can be overcome by planning between pacemaker and heart failure clinics.

Using Device Information in Daily Practice

Details of how device diagnostics can be implemented into a practice system that can serve heart failure providers depends on several factors specific to the local environment, such as solo versus group practice, availability and training of nonphysician providers to review data, electronic versus paper medical records systems, etc. Additionally, communication and cooperation between heart failure providers and implanting physicians determines the extent to which device data can be clinically used. Finally, the comfort level of non-implanting physicians in interrogating and following implanted devices is certain to increase as physicians are trained to acquire and interpret signals from devices.[40]

A practice model should consider several important points when being tailored to fit a specific environment. The heart failure provider should consider how device-based diagnostics may triage the time interval between face-to-face visits. This requires a thoughtful consideration of how frequently the patient should upload device information from home. Traditionally, implanted devices are monitored remotely to check specific electrophysiologic parameters, such as battery life and lead impedance. For a heart failure monitor to impact clinical practice, the device-based information should be made available in a frequency that will safely allow less frequent face-to-face encounters by identifying patients with changing physiology who need to be seen before scheduled follow-up appointments or to predict risk for heart failure events. For example, patients with continuously measured heart rate variability measurements (SDAAM) greater than 100 msec are at very low risk for heart failure hospitalization in the next 12 months. Office visits for these patients can be much less frequent than those with low heart rate variability (less than 50 msec) who may require very frequent evaluation either by telephone or in-office evaluation.

Unfortunately, there is no consensus about frequency of follow-up for patients with heart failure even without remotely acquired device diagnostics. It is clear from several studies, as noted previously, that organized disease management systems utilizing physician and nonphysician providers to frequently see and contact patients with heart failure effectively prevents decompensation and the need for hospitalization. Furthermore, there are no clinical trial data to guide frequency of remote evaluation of device diagnostics. Therefore, recommendations can only be based on data that is currently available about when a specific parameter changes during the process of decompensation and how well a specific device diagnostic predicts risk of subsequent events. To create an algorithmic approach to heart failure follow-up it is convenient to categorize patients with heart failure managed as outpatients into the following two potential groups based on their predicted event rates: 1) clinically unstable and 2) clinically stable patients. Patients, of course, can change status depending on the success of the management strategy (Fig. 15.2).

Unstable patients are at high risk for heart failure decompensation and are characterized by low heart rate variability (SDAAM < 50 msec) or intermediate values (between 50 and 100 msec), high resting heart rate, low daily activity levels and recent frequent changes in medications, particularly diuretics, to effectively manage volume. Most patients in the unstable group are those in whom active attempts to restore optimal volume require close monitoring of the effects of diuretic dose changes. Many disease management systems provide weekly or more frequent encounters for these patients to monitor the effectiveness of medical changes and avoid side-effects such as dehydration or potassium depletion. Current device-based information systems may reduce the need for face-to-face office encounters if patients transmit weekly with special attention to heart rate variability, intrathoracic impedance, activity and night heart rate. The interval between in-office visits can be safely extended by relying on remote diagnostics (Figs. 15.2 and 15.5). This strategy for unstable patients can be coupled with telephone contact and patient involvement using daily weights and home-measured systemic pressure. Home health care, when available, also augments the safety of this approach.

Unstable individuals may benefit from several monitoring inputs in order to avoid hospitalization. In this elevated risk population, device diagnostics is only one piece of information that forms the basis of successful out-patient management of volume exacerbation. Intrathoracic impedance measurements may have maximal application in the unstable group of patients as clinical study evidence suggests changes in this parameter are apparent up to 18 days before symptoms lead to hospitalization. Future device applications to support heart failure disease management will likely be based on implantable hemodynamic monitoring systems, which promise to reduce the probability for heart failure patients to become unstable by providing information useful to prevent exacerbation, as well as guide therapeutic intervention intended to restore optimal volume.[41–49]

Without device information, unstable patients may benefit from office visits every 4 weeks with volume assessment as the focus of the visit and nurse telephone contact at 2-week intervals. With device-based information systems an adequate assessment of volume can be accomplished by review of transmitted data at 4 weeks and the scheduled office visit can be extended to 8-12 weeks. If changes in volume status are detected remotely, then nurse managers can contact patients to determine if nonheart failure co-morbidities, such as pneumonia or chronic lung disease exacerbations are responsible for changes in device-based information. In response to changes in device diagnostics, alterations in medical management to control volume can be accomplished remotely or in an office visit arranged sooner than scheduled, depending on the clarity of the situation.

It is important to recall that many times physiologic and derived device information can change before patients develop symptoms associated with volume overload. This early warning system provides the basis for a preventive strategy that may allow less intense changes in volume management compared to changes required when patients are in the throes of acute exacerbation. The benefits of device-based information review for the unstable patient is to extend the time for in-office follow-up, to direct nurse manager contact to those patients with changing status thus effectively preventing progression of congestion to acutely decompensated heart failure.

The general group of heart failure patients are those who are stable and at low risk for decompensation. This group is characterized by high heart rate variability (SDAAM >100 msec), no recent changes in medical management, stable nighttime heart rates, and normal intrathoracic impedance. Daily activity counts from the implanted device may not be specifically helpful to determine low risk individuals. The in-office follow-up of this group without device data is often every 12 weeks coupled with patient involvement of measuring daily weights. Device diagnostics may be helpful to extend office visit intervals to 4 or 5 months with remote review of data at 2-month intervals between visits (Fig. 15.5).

Health care providers, either public, like in many European countries, or private patients, may financially benefit from remote monitoring with a reduction in office visit costs and travel expenses. This is especially true for patients living in rural areas at significant distances from provider offices. In terms of the social benefit of an integrated disease management, patients will benefit from preventing heart failure decompensation by decrease in disease progression and, theoretically, by decreased exposure to situations in which mortality risk is elevated, such as acute care hospitalization.[50]

Disease management of heart failure will continue to improve as sensor sophistication improves, especially in light of hemodynamic monitoring systems that may represent the most important device-based advancement in the near future.[41–49] Ultimately, disease management paradigms will undoubtedly include providing the patient with understandable device based information to daily manage their disease without need for continuous provider review or involvement.[46] This approach, similar to patient self-management of other chronic diseases such as diabetes mellitus, is based on physician driven algorithms for therapy, especially diuretic dosing, and is most promising for efficient cost-effective prevention of decompensation events.

Data Flow and Infrastructure

Patients initiate the data exchange sequence by manually or automatically uploading information from their device using a home interrogation system (Fig. 15.6). Area telemetry systems allow the provider to schedule interrogation and uploading of information without the need for the patient to interact with their home monitoring system. That data is stored, then, on a secured Internet website sponsored by the device's manufacturer. There are no industry standards for information exchange in Web-based device information, so there is no cooperation between manufacturers and no ability to interface information into electronic medical records. Therefore, Internet information is usually printed from the Website and scanned into the electronic medical record or placed in a paper record file. Scanned information in an electronic medical record system can be routed to the individual responsible for review. This person, who can be a specially trained nurse, advanced practice provider or physician, then reviews the diagnostic information to influence medical decision making (Figs. 15.2 and 15.6). In most situations, a specially trained nurse can review device diagnostics and forward only information from patients with unclear status to the responsible provider. The heart failure nurse provider can initiate a telephone call to the patient if changes in device diagnostics are noted and use predetermined algorithms to alter medical management.

The value of remote review of heart failure diagnostics is now recognized and is a billable activity, which helps support the infrastructure required to manage large populations of heart failure patients. Using remotely obtained device diagnostics can substantially reduce the need for frequent face-to-face encounters and, hopefully, reduce the overflow of patients typically found in the emergency rooms of high-level disease management centers. Furthermore, device diagnostics may provide a superior means to "stage" severity and stability of heart failure status serving to triage follow-up needs. Providers in general cardiology or even internal medicine practices can have access to such data and may benefit by increasing the frequency of surveillance in a practice system that cannot accommodate the intense follow-up needs required to successfully manage heart failure patients in outpatient settings. Device information management allows a unique opportunity for collaboration between the multiple caregivers for patients with complex heart failure syndromes.

CONCLUSIONS

The clinical value of implanted devices intended to deliver therapies, such as cardiac resynchronization or sudden death prophylaxis, is significantly improved by integrating

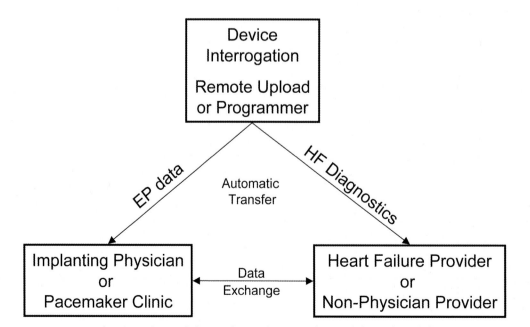

FIG. 15.6. Suggested cooperation and data exchange for optimal use of device-based diagnostics in clinical settings.

CHAPTE[R]

16

Niraj Varma • [

[I]n patients wit[
the presence
branch bloc[
conduction or provo[
In contrast, overall s[
with pre-excitation o[
cardiac resynchroniz[
cal activation sequen[
prognostic effects. H[
activation normally [
during pacing, are r[
may be necessary to [
electrical activation o[
responses observed i[
pacing may increase [
LBBB despite similar [
up to one third of pa[
face ECG recordings [
address these issues.][
mapping of ventricul[
noninvasively, called [
has been recently des[

ECGI provides r[
mapping of cardiac e[
ECGI images epicard[
(activation sequences[
surface electrocardio[
been validated exter[
humans by comparis[
open-heart surgery[18][
struction accuracy [
obtained in human s[
a noninvasive imagi[
ventricle cardiac acti[
methodology has be[
acquires more than 2[
diograms using a mi[
and body-surface ele[
neously by a thoraci[
data and the geome[
developed to compu[

monitoring features into heart failure disease management. For example, an implantable cardioverter defibrillator will never provide therapy for tachyarrhythmias in more than 80% of the implanted patients, but now it can provide continuous monitoring of heart rate, heart rate variability, activity, intrathoracic impedance, incidence of atrial arrhythmias, rate response to chronic persistent atrial fibrillation in addition to the incidence of ventricular tachyarrhythmias. Enhancement of heart failure disease management includes proper staging of current disease stability and assistance in follow-up without the requirement for face-to-face evaluation or indiscriminate telephone calls to large populations of patients. With the current and worsening epidemic of heart failure and widespread indications for device therapies for these patients, utilizing device monitoring features will be a component of a strategy to manage heart failure as an outpatient disease with emphasis on preventing decompensation, rather than reacting to advanced volume exacerbation.

PRACTICAL POINTS

1. Frequent monitoring of heart failure patients reduces hospitalization and, possibly, overall mortality.
2. Monitoring of patients receiving stable standard-of-care medical and device therapies generally focuses on volume management to avoid abnormal volume overload, which requires hospitalization.
3. Current monitoring strategies require contact with large populations of patients, many of whom are very stable, in order to identify those with changing stability or volume accumulation.
4. Implanted therapeutic devices sense a large amount of physiologic information, which can be exploited to remotely provide important diagnostic feedback to providers.
5. Device-based diagnostic information can generally be classified as *direct* physiologic information (such as heart rate, arrhythmias, pacing) or *derived* data calculated from the physiologic signal (heart rate variability, activity, intrathoracic impedance).
6. Direct physiologic data may lead to immediate clinical action, such as rate control of atrial fibrillation, while derived data provides a marker of clinical stability, which can used to identify patients with more frequent follow-up needs.
7. Appropriate use of device-based diagnostics requires data sharing between implanting physicians and those primarily responsible for heart failure management.
8. Future systems will likely involve a larger number of sensors, including hemodynamic monitoring systems, to provide a comprehensive disease management program that can be obtained remotely.

REFERENCES

1. Hunt SA, Abraham WT, Chin MH, et al. 2009 focused update incorporated into the ACC/AHA 2005 Guidelines for the Diagnosis and Management of Chronic Heart Failure in the Adult: A report of the American College of Cardiology/American Heart Association Task Force on Practice Guidelines developed in collaboration with the international society for heart and lung transplantation. *J Am Coll Cardiol.* 2009;53:e1–e90.
2. Moss AJ, Zareba W, Hall WJ, et al. Prophylactic implantation of a defibrillator in patients with myocardial infarction and reduced ejection fraction. *N Engl J Med.* 2002;346:877–883.
3. Bardy GH, Lee KL, Mark DB, et al. Amiodarone or an implantable cardioverter-defibrillator for congestive heart failure. *N Engl J Med.* 2005; 352:225–237.
4. Bristow MR, Saxon LA, Boehmer J, et al. Cardiac-resynchronization therapy with or without an implantable defibrillator in advanced chronic heart failure. *N Engl J Med.* 2004;350:2140–2150.
5. Cleland JG, Daubert JC, Erdmann E, et al. The effect of cardiac resynchronization on morbidity and mortality in heart failure. *N Engl J Med.* 2005;352:1539–1549.
6. Abraham WT, Fisher WG, Smith AL, et al. Cardiac resynchronization in chronic heart failure. *N Engl J Med,* 2002;346:1845–1853.
7. Fonarow GC, Abraham WT, Albert NM, et al. Factors identified as precipitating hospital admissions for heart failure and clinical outcomes: Findings from OPTIMIZE-HF. *Arch Intern Med.* 2008;168: 847–854.
8. Capomolla S, Ceresa M, Finna G, et al. Echo-Doppler and clinical evaluations to define hemodynamic profile in patients with chronic heart failure: accuracy and influence on therapeutic management. *Eur J Heart Fail.* 2005;7:624–630.
9. Stephenson LW, Perloff JK. The limited reliability of physical signs for estimating hemodynamics in chronic heart failure. *JAMA.* 1989;261:884–888.
10. Lewin J, Ledwidge M, O'Loughlin C, et al. Clinical deterioration in established heart failure. What is the value of BNP and weight gain in aiding diagnosis? *Eur J Heart Fail.* 2005;7:953–957.
11. Chaudhry SI, Wang Y, Concato J, et al. Patterns of weight change preceding hospitalization for heart failure. *Circulation.* 2007;116:1549–1554.
12. Rich MW, Beckham V, Wittenberg C, et al. A multidisciplinary intervention to prevent the readmission of elderly patients with congestive heart failure. *N Engl J Med.* 1995;333:1190–1195.
13. Fonarow GC, Stevenson LW, Alden JA, et al. Impact of a comprehensive heart failure management program on hospital readmissions and functional status of patients with advanced heart failure. *J Am Coll Cardiol.* 1997;30:725–732.
14. Kimmelstiel C, Levine D, Perry K, et al. Randomized, controlled evaluation of short and long-term benefits of heart failure disease management within a diverse provider network: The SPAN-CHF trial. *Circulation.* 2004;110:1450–1455.
15. Cleland JG, Louis AA, Swedberg K, et al. Noninvasive home telemonitoring for patients with heart failure at high risk of recurrent admission and death: The Trans European Network-Home-Care Management (TEN-HMS) study. *J Am Coll Cardiol.* 2005;45:1654–1664.
16. Goldberg LR, Piette JD, Walsh MN, et al. Randomized trial of a daily electronic home monitoring system in patients with advanced heart failure: The Weight Monitoring in Heart Failure (WHARF) trial. *Am Heart J.* 2003;146:705–712.
17. Hauptman PJ, Rich MW, Heidenreich PA, et al. The heart failure clinic: A consensus statement of the Heart Failure Society of America. *J Card Fail.* 2008;14:801–815.
18. Mortara A, Pinna GD, Johnson P, et al. Home telemonitoring in heart failure patients: the HHH study (Home or Hospital in Heart Failure). *Eur J Heart Fail.* 2009;11:312–318.
19. Zhang J, Goode KM, Cuddihy PE, et al. Predicting hospitalization due to worsening heart failure using daily weight measurements: analysis of the Trans-European Network-Home-Care Management System (TEN-HMS) study. *Eur J Heart Fail.* 2009;11:420–427.
20. Fox K, Borer JS, Camm AJ, et al. Resting heart rate in cardiovascular disease. *J Am Coll Cardiol.* 2007;50:823–830.
21. Metra M, Torp-Pederson C, Swedberg K, et al. Influence of heart rate, blood pressure and beta-blocker dose on outcome and the differences in outcome between carvedilol and metoprolol tartrate in patients with chronic heart failure: results from the COMET trial. *Eur Heart J.* 2005; 26:2259–2268.

22. Adamson PB, Sm
sessment in patie
heart rate variab
tion device. Circ

23. Ziegler PD, Koeh
termittent moni
1445–1452.

24. Roy D, Talajic N
atrial fibrillation

25. Wyse DG, Waldo
rhythm control
347:1825–1833.

26. Poole JE, Johnsc
defibrillator sho
359:1009–1017.

27. Koplan BA, Kapl
all cause mortali
with heart failur
Coll Cardiol. 200

28. Wilkoff BL, Coc
tricular backup
Dual Chamber a
2002;288:3115–

29. Wang L, Lahtin
system to measu
failure canine m

30. Yu CM, Wang I
in patients wit
feasibility of e
2005;112:841–8

31. Vollmann D, Na
racic impedance
of deteriorating

32. Ypenburg C, Ba
monitoring to p
99:554–557.

33. Maines, M Cata
ids accumulatio
rillator in redu
case-control stu

34. Katona PG, Jih I
parasympatheti

35. Heart rate varia
pretation and cl
ology and the N
Circulation. 199

36. Adamson PB, Kl
therapy improve
failure. Circulat

TABLE 16.1 Patient Characteristics

Patient	1	2	3	4	5	6	7	8
Disease	CAD	CAD	CAD	DCM	CAD	CAD	CAD	DCM
LVEF %	20	10	25	15	25	30	15	15
Response	R	NR	R	NR	R	NR	NR	NR
Native Rhythm: Intrinsic Conduction (ms)								
QRS	160		180	140	180		140	130
RV Activation	40		51	30	29		38	32
LV Activation	90		144	101	141		111	88
RV Pacing (ms)								
QRS	200		150	190	190	160	170	
RV Activation	70		36	90	88	63	64	
LV Activation	130		124	133	149	139	135	
CRT (ms)								
QRS	120	160	120	200	150	160	120	140
RV Activation	68	75	42	69	88	61	60	52
LV Activation	79	148	87	130	68	134	59	78

CAD, coronary artery disease; DCM, dilated cardiomyopathy; LVEF, left ventricular (LV) ejection fraction; R, responder to CRT (cardiac resynchronization therapy); NR, nonresponder; RV, right ventricular; Activation, mean ventricular activation time from the beginning of QRS (for intrinsic beats) or pacing artifact (for paced beats). (Compiled with permission from Oster HS, Taccardi B, Lux RL, Ershler PR, Rudy Y. Electrocardiographic imaging: Noninvasive characterization of intramural myocardial activation from inverse-reconstructed epicardial potentials and electrograms. Circulation. 1998;97:1496–1507.)

could not spread directly to the inferior LV but slowly propagated transseptally from the RV to reach the LV lateral and posterior walls by spreading inferoposteriorly from anterior LV. In three patients (4, 7, and 8) (not illustrated here; see reference 21) LV epicardial activation started from the septoapical region, spreading laterally and ending at the lateral or posterolateral base. In patient #5, the activation wavefront spread superiorly from inferior LV rather than from the apical region, ending at the midanterolateral wall.

Propagation of wavefronts was determined sometimes by line(s)/region(s) of conduction block or slowed conduction. These were visualized by ECGI. In patients 4, 5, 7, and 8, activation that crossed the septum from RV was prevented from spreading directly to the LV by an anterior line(s)/region(s) of block. It reached the lateral wall by way of either apical or inferior LV. Latest activation was at the inferoposterior base. This "U-shaped" activation was also reported based on endocardial mapping.[5] Some lines remained unchanged with change of pacing mode, suggesting fixed boundaries of anatomical origin. On other occasions, line(s)/region(s) of block shifted to other locations, disappeared, or emerged later during pacing (see next page). This phenomenon pointed to a functional mechanism. Lines of block were sometimes multiple, generating complex conduction barriers. For example, in patient #6 (Fig. 16.2), two lateral lines of block forced electrical activation to propagate in a counterclockwise

direction regardless of the pacing mode. Previous reports with endocardial mapping using invasive techniques also revealed heterogenous LV activation patterns with differing location and extents of specific ventricular delays.[5, 7, 25] These phenomena may be due to lesions of the specialized conduction tissue, presence of scar regions, and slow cell-to-cell conduction[26] resulting from LV disease. In conclusion, LV activation was conspicuously heterogenous despite surface ECG indicating similar QRS patterns of LBBB.

Right Ventricular (RV) Pacing

RV pacing (RVP) has been postulated to simulate LBBB though few direct comparisons have been made. In this study, RVP did not change QRS duration (177 ± 20 ms versus LBBB: 155 ± 22 ms, p = NS) and LV activation (135 ± 9 ms versus LBBB: 113 ± 25 ms, p = NS) significantly compared to intrinsic conduction during LBBB. However, areas of LV (functional) conduction delays changed with RV pacing compared to corresponding intrinsic rhythm. In patient #5, pacing dissolved the anterior line of blockage present during intrinsic conduction. In contrast, a similar line was induced by RV pacing in patient #1, when it had not been present before (Fig. 16.1). In one case, RV pacing reduced LV activation time. The RV was also affected by RV pacing, because RV activation times increased significantly to 69 ± 20 ms (p <0.02). These results indicate that RV pacing exerts significant and unpredictable effects on ventricular excitation and should not be regarded as simply equivalent to LBBB.[27] This may help explain the increase in mortality observed with RV pacing in patients with LBBB and LV dysfunction.[2, 8]

Resynchronization with Biventricular Pacing

LV activation patterns with biventricular pacing were different among patients. However, QRS width did not change significantly in response to CRT (intrinsic conduction 155 ± 22 versus CRT 146 ± 28 ms, p = NS). The widely used measure of QRS duration is only a reflection on the body surface of the total duration of ventricular activation and not a reliable marker of LV activation. This may underlie the weakness of QRS in predicting response to CRT.[28]

Variations in LV activation with CRT are illustrated in Figure 16.1. For example, patient #5 was a responder to CRT. Activation spread from the lateral wall LV pacing site and ended locally at the basal LV after 110 ms. On the anterior LV, latest activation occurred at 138 ms, immediately adjacent to a line of block (which was also present during LBBB). In this case, this line of block did not preclude response to CRT because posterolateral LV activation occurred rapidly, indicating successful paced pre-excitation of the lateral/posterolateral LV, which is the desired effect of LV pacing. LVEF increased from 25% to 40%, and LV internal dimension decreased by 10%, indicating successful clinical effect.

A lack of response to CRT poses a significant management problem.[29] This may have diverse etiologies. An electrical evaluation of paced response as a potential cause for CRT failure has been rarely investigated. The current series identifies potential electrical causes for lack of response to LV pacing despite "optimal" LV lead placement (defined in conventional practice as obtaining good pacing thresholds in the target area). In patient #4, LV pacing from an anterior position slowed LV lateral wall activation relative to native rhythm. Activation time to the basal LV doubled. The region of slow conduction only appeared during pacing, indicating dependence of propagation of the paced wavefront on the electrical substrate adjacent to the pacing lead. Thus, pacing exerted changes in conduction in the target posterolateral LV wall, which was not present during intrinsic activation, indicating a functional mechanism for conduction slowing. In patient #6 (Fig. 16.2), ECGs recorded during CRT and RV pacing were similar. This would initially seem to suggest that the LV lead was nonfunctional. However, isolated LV pacing indicated excellent paced capture thresholds. ECGI provided an explanation for these findings. Propagation of LV paced wavefronts was severely limited. Thus, during simultaneous biventricular pacing (Fig. 16.2C), RV paced wavefronts had already reached the LV, as LV pacing breakthrough was just initiating. The LV paced wavefront was delayed and had a negligible effect on overall activation. However, sequential pacing with LV preactivation (Fig. 16.2D) permitted LV pacing contribution to

biventricular activation. Hence, despite a conventionally "optimal" LV pacing site, the region of capture was surrounded by an encircling area of slow conduction, which severely limited propagation of the paced activation wavefront. Patient #2 with a history of anterior and anterolateral wall LV infarction (LV ejection fraction 10%, end-diastolic internal diameter 8.2 cm) improved two functional classes (NYHA IV to II) within 4 weeks of CRT. However, ECGI results of ventricular electrical activation did not reconcile with this clinical effect (Fig. 16.3). Excitation generated by the anteriorly located LV lead activated the RV but not the LV because of fixed anterior anatomic blockage. These lines of conduction slowing and blockage, acting as boundaries, severely limited paced wavefront propagation to a viable target area. Thus, LV pacing had a negligible pre-excitatory effect on the posterolateral LV. Postimplant echocardiography in subsequent follow-up provided the explanation. Progressive deterioration occurred with LV dilatation and diminishing ejection fraction. The patient deceased from heart failure 9 months later. This apparent paradox illustrates a placebo clinical response (well recognized in device trials[9]) with subjective benefit occurring despite lack of electrical or echocardiographic evidence.

Lead position has been reported to affect resynchronization therapy in some series.[30] In the current study, preexcitation of the posterolateral LV in patients with anteriorly located LV leads (patients 2, 3, 4, and 6), was less effective than in patients with lateral leads (patients 1, 5, 7, and 8). This may have resulted from the high likelihood of encountering regions of conduction block and slow conduction (anatomic and functional) in the anterolateral aspects that interfered with propagation from the anterior to the lateral wall. Under these conditions, RV activation was more influenced than LV activation, which did not differ substantially from intrinsic conduction in LBBB. This ECGI finding may explain the higher probability of clinical benefit with lateral compared to anterior lead placement.[30]

Cardiac Resynchronization with Left Ventricular (LV) Pacing

Ventricular activation was assessed in response to LV pacing in three patients with intact atrioventricular conduction, in whom the device was programmed for LV pacing alone with optimized AV delay. This permitted fusion between intrinsic excitation and the LV paced beat. The degree of fusion varied depending on the balance between the length of the PR interval versus programmed atrial-ventricular delay (Fig. 16.4). An important effect was that this pacing mode, which eliminated RV pacing, avoided paced activation delays in the RV itself.

IMPLICATIONS

This study, using ECGI's unique ability to provide 3-D reconstruction and high-resolution mapping of ventricular

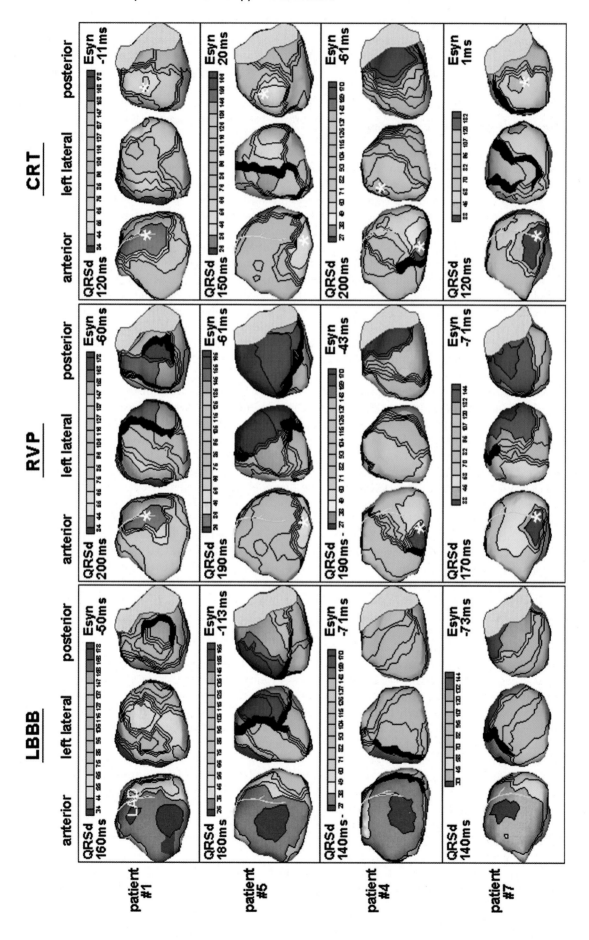

excitation, revealed complexities of electrical substrate in patients with heart failure. Wide and unpredictable variations were observed in ventricular activation both during intrinsic conduction and in response to pacing. These factors may have prognostic and therapeutic implications and may contribute to the varied responses to CRT.

Patients have been selected for CRT on the basis of QRS width and/or depiction of mechanical dyssynchrony. However, both of these measures have significant limitations as selection criteria,[28, 31–32] Once selected, LV leads at implantation are conventionally deployed to the posterolateral LV although this may be limited by epicardial vessel anatomy and local pacing capture thresholds. Propagation of wavefronts to and from these sites is a potentially critical element but this has not been well characterized. The current study illustrates that target areas may vary in location and response to LV pacing may be heterogenous. These factors constitute further potential limitations to effective LV pacing and may affect clinical responses.

Target Areas

The optimal LV pacing lead site is theoretically the latest site of activation. This has been assumed to be the inferolateral LV in patients with LBBB[4–6, 33] and to be responsible for mechanical dyssynchrony.[34] ECGI exposed limitations to this conventional line of thinking. Similar LBBB patterns appearing on the surface ECG during intrinsic conduction (or RV pacing) concealed very different LV activation sequences. This is consistent with results from endocardial mapping.[35] Hence, empiric LV lead placement directed to the inferolateral LV may not always target the region of latest activation. This may be a mechanism contributing to the observation that epicardial stimulation of this area (without electrical mapping) did not always yield maximum contractility improvement,[36] In contrast, LV lead placement directed to endocardial sites of latest conduction delay yielded greater increases in contractility, especially when this late activated area was large[35] and was associated with superior clinical outcome.[30, 37]

FIG. 16.1. Epicardial isochrone maps for four representative patients. Patients 1 and 5 were CRT responders, and patients 4 and 7 nonresponders. Intrinsic conduction with LBBB (left panels), right ventricular pacing (RVP, middle panels) and biventricular pacing during cardiac resynchronization therapy (CRT, right panels) are depicted. Epicardial surfaces of both ventricles are displayed in three views: anterior, left lateral, and posterior. There is overlap between adjacent views. Left anterior descending (LAD) coronary artery is shown. Thick black markings indicate line/region of conduction block. Pacing sites are marked by asterisks. **QRSd,** QRS duration. **Esyn,** Electrical synchrony index. Esyn corresponds to the mean activation time difference between lateral RV and LV free walls, i.e., indexes interventricular resynchronization directly from measurements on the heart. Interventricular synchrony is indicated when Esyn equals zero, RV pre-excitation by a negative Esyn and LV pre-excitation by positive Esyn value.

Left Panels Intrinsic Conduction During LBBB Ventricular activation of right ventricle (RV) was followed by a much delayed left ventricular (LV) activation, indicating left bundle branch block (LBBB). Several different LV activation patterns are depicted. Patient 1 had LV breakthrough at 49 ms (left lateral view). Combined wavefronts advancing from apical, inferior, and superior LV all contributed to overall LV activation, which ended at the posterolateral wall. In patient #5, the LV activation wavefront spread superiorly from the inferior LV to end anterolaterally. Patients 4 and 7 demonstrated apical-to-basal epicardial conduction. Wavefronts emerged from a septoapical origin, spread laterally to end at the lateral or posterolateral base.

Middle Panels Response to Right Ventricular Pacing (RVP) Note RVP changed areas of slow conduction/lines of block compared to intrinsic activation, indicating that this pacing mode is not simply equivalent to LBBB. For example, in patient #1, a line of block appears anteriorly, but in patient # 5 a preexisting line of block is shortened. These data point to the functional nature of conduction block in these regions.

Right Panels Responses to Biventricular Pacing (CRT) Patients 1 and 5 were responders with lateral LV lead positions. In patient #1, CRT dissolved the anterior line of block evident during RVP, activating the anterior and anterolateral LV relatively evenly compared to intrinsic conduction. Interventricular synchrony improved (Esyn less negative). In patient #5, Esyn became positive (from −113 to 20 ms) indicating LV pre-excitation, though an anterior line of blockage persisted. In contrast, patients 4 and 7 were nonresponders. In patient #4, LV pacing resulted in marked slowing of the paced wavefront in the lateral LV wall, in contrast to intrinsic conduction when conduction was relatively rapid in the same area. Esyn changed marginally from −71 to −61 ms, indicating ineffective resynchronization in this nonresponder. QRS duration prolonged. In patient #7, CRT induced a line of functional blockage in the anterolateral LV (not apparent with RVP). Despite this, Esyn improved because the LV lead was sited laterally. (Compiled with permission from Oster HS, Taccardi B, Lux RL, Ershler PR, Rudy Y. Electrocardiographic imaging: Noninvasive characterization of intramural myocardial activation from inverse-reconstructed epicardial potentials and electrograms. *Circulation.* 1998;97:1496–507.)

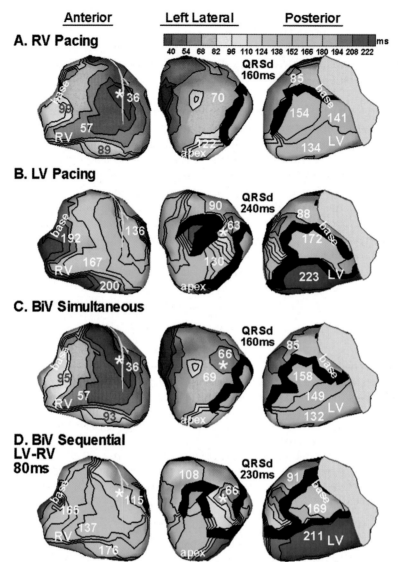

FIG. 16.2. Imaging (anterior, left lateral, and posterior views) in patient #6, during different pacing modes. **A.** Right ventricular (RV) pacing, **B.** Left ventricular (LV) pacing, **C.** Cardiac resynchronization therapy with simultaneous biventricular (BiV) pacing, **D.** Cardiac resynchronization therapy with LV pacing preset of 80 ms relative to RV pacing (sequential pacing mode). Activation times (in ms) of selected regions are indicated on the map. In this patient, 12-lead ECGs recorded after implant were similar during simultaneous biventricular pacing and during RV pacing. Imaging revealed the underlying mechanism. During simultaneous biventricular pacing (**C**), RV pacing breakthrough occurred 30 ms earlier than LV breakthrough. The RV paced wavefront had arrived at the LV lead location just when LV pacing breakthrough was commencing. Consequently, LV pacing did not influence overall ventricular activation. Thus ventricular activation was similar in RV pacing and simultaneous biventricular pacing (**A** and **C**). In contrast, when LV pacing occurred 80 ms prior to RV pacing, LV activation resembled that during LV pacing alone (**D** and **B**, respectively), except that RV activation advanced slightly (30 ms) due to RV electrode effect. The modulating effect of complex conduction barriers on paced wavefront propagation was illustrated. A line of blockage across the LV lateral free wall was present consistently over all pacing modes. It prevented any anterior activation from propagating inferiorly to the midlateral region. This area was activated by a wavefront propagating from the inferior LV (for RV or biventricular simultaneous pacing, **A** and **C**), or possibly by an intramural wavefront (for LV or biventricular sequential pacing, **B** and **D**). In addition, during LV or biventricular sequential pacing, a line of blockage between lateral and inferior LV prevented lateral activation from propagating inferiorly. This was a functionally determined line of unidirectional blockage, because wavefront propagation in the reverse direction was permitted in the other two pacing modes. Because of these complex barriers, global activation could propagate around the heart only in a counterclockwise fashion. Inferior LV could be activated only by wavefront spreading from the RV. In terms of electrical synchrony, biventricular sequential pacing was better than biventricular simultaneous pacing in this patient. (Compiled with permission from Oster HS, Taccardi B, Lux RL, Ershler PR, Rudy Y. Electrocardiographic imaging: Noninvasive characterization of intramural myocardial activation from inverse-reconstructed epicardial potentials and electrograms. *Circulation.* 1998;97:1496–507.)

Isochrones during Biventricular Pacing

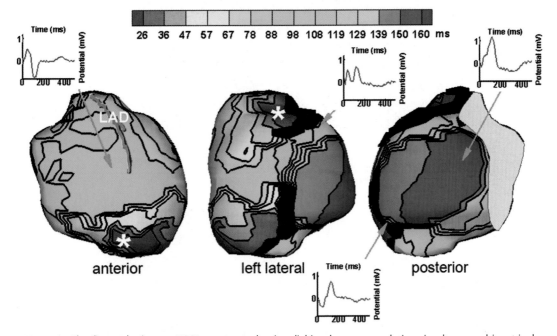

FIG. 16.3. The figure depicts an ECGI-constructed epicardial isochrone map during simultaneous biventricular pacing (CRT). Epicardial surfaces of both ventricles are displayed in three views: anterior, left lateral, and posterior. There is overlap between adjacent views. The left anterior descending (LAD) coronary artery is marked. Selected ECGI-reconstructed epicardial electrograms are indicated by arrows. Pacing sites (RV and LV, asterisks), as expected, are the earliest ventricular sites to be activated (red). Thereafter, LV activation is irregular with development of regions of conduction block (thick black markings) and slowing (crowded isochrones) displaying fractionated local electrograms. These delay activation of a large territory of the lateral/posterolateral LV. In fact, this region is activated terminally (blue) despite pacing from an immediately adjacent site. Electrograms are preserved in this area indicating epicardial viability. Hence, LV pacing failed to achieve target area pre-excitation. (Reproduced with permission from Varma N, Jia P, Rudy Y. Placebo CRT. *J Cardiovasc Electrophysiol.* 2008;19:878.

Paced Responses

LV lead placement at a site with good paced capture thresholds is regarded as effective lead placement. This approach assumes that LV pacing causes homogenous global LV activation. However, the presence of LV disease may modulate propagation. Thus, posterolateral transmural scar was reported to negate CRT effect, presumably due to inexcitability of this target area, although electrical activation was not investigated.[38] Interestingly, ECGI has demonstrated that disordered electrical activation may not consistently match scar distribution.[21] For example, variations in propagation may occur in nonscar areas. An important finding in the current study was that LV paced wavefronts differed considerably among patients, likely determined by altered electrical substrate in the presence of LV pathology, and these characteristics may have significant clinical sequelae. Thus, in some patients, LV pacing encountered complex conduction barriers. Lines of blockage varied in extent, number, and location. Anteriorly directed LV lead positions more frequently encountered anterior LV lines of block, rendering them less effective in posterolateral LV pre-excitation. However, lines of blockage did not always preclude response (for example, patient #5) possibly indicating that location and extent of lines of blockage and/or slow conduction zones were critical modulating elements. Importantly, some of these zones of slow conduction developed in response to pacing (functional mechanism) and were not predictable from maps in intrinsic conduction. Prolonged propagation of depolarization was reported to correlate with poorer hemodynamic response to pacing compared to when global activation was rapid.[39] Hemodynamics improved when these "slow conduction" areas were avoided and paced wavefronts were permitted to emerge and recruit adequate tissue mass. These data underscore the importance of recognizing differing patterns of ventricular activation in response to pacing.

This study demonstrated significant RV (as well as LV) activation delays with RV pacing, either alone or in conjunction with simultaneous biventricular pacing. This may be avoided by LV pacing alone with critically timed atrioventricular (AV) delays resulting in fusion of the propagated paced wavefront with intrinsic conduction via an intact right bundle (Fig.16.4). This CRT mode may avoid RV hemodynamic deficit associated with simultaneous biventricular pacing.[40]

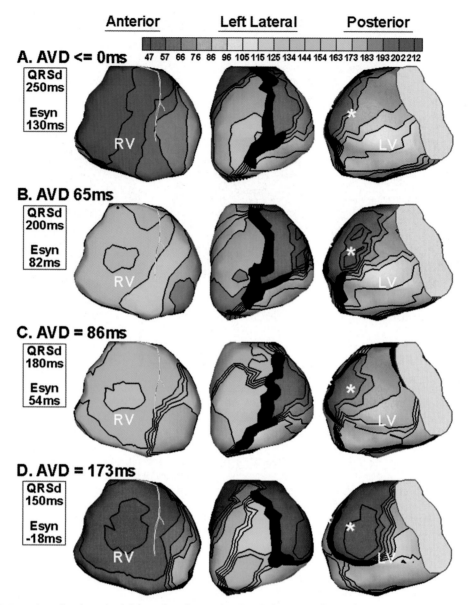

FIG. 16.4. Imaging (anterior, left lateral, and posterior views) during atrially synchronized LV pacing in patient #5, who had underlying LBBB. This series of LV paced beats with progressively increased atrioventricular (AV) delays demonstrates increasing degree of fusion of LV paced activation with RV activation via intrinsic right bundle branch conduction. Thus, **A** shows pure LV paced activation without fusion, and **B** through **D** demonstrate progressively greater fusion. Esyn improved as fusion increased (**D**). **A:** LV paced activation sequence without fusion. **B–D:** Fusion beats with progressively earlier intrinsic right ventricular (RV) activation (time of RV breakthrough) relative to LV pacing, resulting in progressively greater degree of fusion. **B:** Right ventricular breakthrough at 153 ms after LV pacing. **C:** RV breakthrough at 132 ms after LV pacing. **D:** RV breakthrough at 45 ms after LV pacing. **QRSd**, QRS duration. **Esyn**, Electrical synchrony index. Esyn corresponds to the mean activation time difference between lateral RV and LV free walls, i.e., indexes interventricular resynchronization directly from measurements on the heart. Interventricular synchrony is indicated when Esyn equals zero, RV pre-excitation by a negative Esyn, and LV pre-excitation by positive Esyn value. (Compiled with permission from Oster HS, Taccardi B, Lux RL, Ershler PR, Rudy Y. Electrocardiographic imaging: Noninvasive characterization of intramural myocardial activation from inverse-reconstructed epicardial potentials and electrograms. *Circulation.* 1998;97:1496–1507.)

FUTURE

CRT is an electrical therapy toward a hemodynamic goal. Thus, its effects will be modulated by altered electrical characteristics of diseased LV tissue. These are depicted in only rudimentary fashion by the ECG, which when used as the basis for selection of candidates for CRT, is at best only a modest predictor of hemodynamic improvement.[41] The current study, using high-resolution noninvasive mapping of ventricular activation, points to a selection method permitting both identification of areas of terminal epicardial LV depolarization (which may be variably located) and assessment of LV activation in response to LV pacing (which may be affected by electrical substrate). These may form key determinants of response to CRT.

Case #2 illustrates that assessment of response to pacing therapies based on clinical criteria may be erroneous, and conventional echocardiographic demonstration of evidence of remodeled mechanical function may take several months to manifest.[42] In contrast, ECGI acutely revealed severely limited paced wavefront propagation to a viable target area and lack of intended electrical effect of LV pacing. This evaluation presaged CRT failure. In the future, noninvasive electrical imaging may have significant utility during implant procedures. Dynamic 3-D mapping may facilitate identification of optimal target regions and LV pacing lead deployment and programming of timing to produce a maximal global region of near-simultaneous activation and LV synchronization. This may improve response rate to CRT.

CONCLUSION

ECGI provided unique insight into ventricular activation during LV dysfunction. During intrinsic conduction, LV activation was variable. Alteration by RV pacing indicated that this pacing mode was not simply equivalent to LBBB. The modulating effect of electrical substrate was demonstrated because both RV pacing and CRT sometimes created regions of slow LV conduction, indicating functional electrical characteristics of local tissue. Complex electrophysiologic barriers, possibly dependent on paced wavefront geometry and its direction of propagation, may determine outcome of pacing therapies.

PRACTICAL POINTS

1. CRT is an electrical therapy and its success will be governed by electrical parameters.
2. Electrical activation of the heart is incompletely described by the QRS complex on the surface ECG. In contrast, noninvasive imaging with ECGI provides detailed ventricular mapping.
3. ECGI demonstrated that variability in LV conduction delays and success of intended LV preexcitation pacing may contribute to inconsistent CRT response in different individuals.
4. Electrical substrate may modulate the transduction of electrical stimulation into hemodynamic effect.

ACKNOWLEDGMENTS

In addition to the authors, Charulatha Ramanathan, Raja N. Ghanem, and Kyungmoo Ryu also participated in the ECGI study on which this chapter is based. The study was supported by NIH-NHLBI Merit Award R37-HL-033343 and Grant RO1- HL-49054 to Y.R.

REFERENCES

1. Baldasseroni S, Opasich C, Gorini M, et al. Left bundle-branch block is associated with increased 1-year sudden and total mortality rate in 5,517 outpatients with congestive heart failure: a report from the Italian network on congestive heart failure. *Am Heart J.* 2002;143: 398–405.
2. Wilkoff BL, Cook JR, Epstein AE, et al. Dual-chamber pacing or ventricular backup pacing in patients with an implantable defibrillator: the Dual Chamber and VVI Implantable Defibrillator (DAVID) Trial. *JAMA.* 2002;288:3115–3123.
3. Cleland JG, Daubert JC, Erdmann E, et al. The effect of cardiac resynchronization on morbidity and mortality in heart failure. *N Engl J Med.* 2005;352:1539–1549.
4. Durrer D, van Dam RT, Freud GE, et al. Total excitation of the isolated human heart. *Circulation.* 1970;41:899–912.
5. Auricchio A, Fantoni C, Regoli F, et al. Characterization of left ventricular activation in patients with heart failure and left bundle-branch block. *Circulation.* 2004;109:1133–1139.
6. Vassallo JA, Cassidy DM, Marchlinski FE, et al. Endocardial activation of left bundle branch block. *Circulation.* 1984;69:914–923.
7. Vassallo JA, Cassidy DM, Miller JM, et al. Left ventricular endocardial activation during right ventricular pacing: effect of underlying heart disease. *J Am Coll Cardiol.* 1986;7:1228–1233.
8. Hayes JJ, Sharma AD, Love JC, et al. Abnormal conduction increases risk of adverse outcomes from right ventricular pacing. *J Am Coll Cardiol.* 2006;48:1628–1633.
9. Abraham WT, Fisher WG, Smith AL, et al. Cardiac resynchronization in chronic heart failure. *N Engl J Med.* 2002;346:1845–1853.
10. Ramanathan C, Ghanem RN, Jia P, et al. Noninvasive electrocardiographic imaging for cardiac electrophysiology and arrhythmia. *Nat Med.* 2004;10:422–428.
11. Ramanathan C, Jia P, Ghanem R, et al. Activation and repolarization of the normal human heart under complete physiological conditions. *Proc Natl Acad Sci UA.* 2006;103:6309–6314.
12. Burnes JE, Taccardi B, Rudy Y. A noninvasive imaging modality for cardiac arrhythmias. *Circulation.* 2000;102:2152-6.
13. Burnes JE, Taccardi B, Ershler PR, et al. Noninvasive electrocardiographic imaging of substrate and intramural ventricular tachycardia in infarcted hearts. *J Am Coll Cardiol.* 2001;38:2071-8.
14. Burnes JE, Taccardi B, MacLeod RS, et al. Noninvasive ECG imaging of electrophysiologically abnormal substrates in infarcted hearts: A model study. *Circulation.* 2000;101:533-40.
15. Ghanem RN, Burnes JE, Waldo AL, et al. Imaging dispersion of myocardial repolarization, II: noninvasive reconstruction of epicardial measures. *Circulation.* 2001;104:1306-12.
16. Oster HS, Taccardi B, Lux RL, et al. Electrocardiographic imaging: Noninvasive characterization of intramural myocardial activation from inverse-reconstructed epicardial potentials and electrograms. *Circulation.* 1998;97:1496-507.
17. Oster HS, Taccardi B, Lux RL, et al. Noninvasive electrocardiographic imaging: reconstruction of epicardial potentials, electrograms, and isochrones and localization of single and multiple electrocardiac events. *Circulation.* 1997;96:1012-24.

18. Ghanem RN, Jia P, Ramanathan C, et al. Noninvasive electrocardiographic imaging (ECGI): comparison to intraoperative mapping in patients. *Heart Rhythm.* 2005;2:339-54.

19. Wang Y, Cuculich PS, Woodard PK, et al. Focal atrial tachycardia after pulmonary vein isolation: Noninvasive mapping with electrocardiographic imaging (ECGI). *Heart Rhythm.* 2007;4:1081-1084.

20. Intini A, Goldstein RN, Jia P, et al. Electrocardiographic imaging (ECGI), a novel diagnostic modality used for mapping of focal left ventricular tachycardia in a young athlete. *Heart Rhythm.* 2005;2:1250-1252.

21. Jia P, Ramanathan C, Ghanem RN, et al. Electrocardiographic imaging of cardiac resynchronization therapy in heart failure: observation of variable electrophysiologic responses. *Heart Rhythm.* 2006;3:296-310.

22. Ritter P, Padeletti L, Gillio-Meina L, et al. Determination of the optimal atrioventricular delay in DDD pacing. Comparison between echo and peak endocardial acceleration measurements. *Europace.* 1999;1:126-130.

23. Nagao K, Toyama J, Kodama I, et al. Role of the conduction system in the endocardial excitation spread in the right ventricle. *Am J Cardiol.* 1981;48:864-170.

24. Myerburg RJNK, Gelband H. Physiology of canine intraventricular conduction and endocardial excitation. *Circulation Research.* 1972;30:217-243.

25. Rodriguez LM, Timmermans C, Nabar A, et al. Variable patterns of septal activation in patients with left bundle branch block and heart failure. *J Cardiovasc Electrophysiol.* 2003;14:135-141.

26. Akar FG, Spragg DD, Tunin RS, et al. Mechanisms underlying conduction slowing and arrhythmogenesis in nonischemic dilated cardiomyopathy. *Circulation Res.* 2004;95:717-725.

27. Varma N. Left ventricular conduction delays in response to right ventricular apical pacing. Influence of LV dysfunction and bundle branch block. *J Cardiovasc Electrophysiol.* 2008;19:114-122.

28. Kass DA. Predicting cardiac resynchronization response by QRS duration: the long and short of it. *J Am Coll Cardiol.* 2003;42:2125-2127.

29. Aranda JM Jr, Woo GW, Schofield RS, et al. Management of heart failure after cardiac resynchronization therapy: integrating advanced heart failure treatment with optimal device function. *J Am Coll Cardiol.* 2005;46:2193-2198.

30. Butter C, Auricchio A, Stellbrink C, et al. Effect of resynchronization therapy stimulation site on the systolic function of heart failure patients. *Circulation.* 2001;104:3026-3029.

31. Beshai JF, Grimm RA, Nagueh SF, et al. Cardiac-resynchronization therapy in heart failure with narrow QRS complexes. *N Engl J Med.* 2007;357:2461-2471.

32. Chung ES, Leon AR, Tavazzi L, et al. Results of the Predictors of Response to Cardiac Resynchronization Therapy (PROSPECT) Trial. *J Cardiac Failure.* 2007;3:793.

33. Wyndham C, Smith T, Meeran M, et al. Epicardial activation in patients with left bundle branch block. *Circulation.* 1980;61:696-703.

34. Leclerq CKD. Retiming the failing heart: principles and current clinical status of cardiac resynchronization. *J Am Coll Cardiol.* 1999;39:194-201.

35. Tse HF, Lee KL, Wan SH, et al. Area of left ventricular regional conduction delay and preserved myocardium predict responses to cardiac resynchronization therapy. *J Cardiovasc Electrophysiol.* 2005;16:690-695.

36. Dekker AL, Phelps B, Dijkman B, et al. Epicardial left ventricular lead placement for cardiac resynchronization therapy: optimal pace site selection with pressure-volume loops. *J Thorac Cardiovasc Surg.* 2004;127:1641-1647.

37. Singh JP, Fan D, Heist EK, et al. Left ventricular lead electrical delay predicts response to cardiac resynchronization therapy. *Heart Rhythm.* 2006;3:1285-1292.

38. Bleeker GB, Kaandorp TA, Lamb HJ, et al. Effect of posterolateral scar tissue on clinical and echocardiographic improvement after cardiac resynchronization therapy. *Circulation.* 2006;113:969-976.

39. Lambiase PD, Rinaldi A, Hauck J, et al. Non-contact left ventricular endocardial mapping in cardiac resynchronisation therapy. *Heart.* 2004;90:44-51.

40. Lee KL, Burnes JE, Mullen TJ, et al. Avoidance of right ventricular pacing in cardiac resynchronization therapy improves right ventricular hemodynamics in heart failure patients. *J Cardiovasc Electrophysiol.* 2007;18:497-504.

41. Nelson GS, Curry CW, Wyman BT, et al. Predictors of systolic augmentation from left ventricular preexcitation in patients with dilated cardiomyopathy and intraventricular conduction delay. *Circulation.* 2000;101:2703-2709.

42. Varma N, Jia P, Rudy Y. Placebo CRT. *J Cardiovasc Electrophysiol.* 2008;19:878.

INDEX